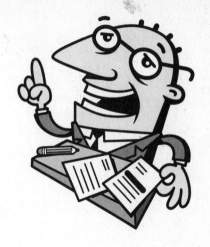

Medical-Surgical Nursing
Demystified

Demystified Series

Accounting Demystified
Advanced Calculus Demystified
Advanced Physics Demystified
Advanced Statistics Demystified
Algebra Demystified
Alternative Energy Demystified
Anatomy Demystified
asp.net 2.0 Demystified
Astronomy Demystified
Audio Demystified
Biology Demystified
Biotechnology Demystified
Business Calculus Demystified
Business Math Demystified
Business Statistics Demystified
C++ Demystified
Calculus Demystified
Chemistry Demystified
Circuit Analysis Demystified
College Algebra Demystified
Corporate Finance Demystified
Databases Demystified
Data Structures Demystified
Differential Equations Demystified
Digital Electronics Demystified
Earth Science Demystified
Electricity Demystified
Electronics Demystified
Engineering Statistics Demystified
Environmental Science Demystified
Everyday Math Demystified
Fertility Demystified
Financial Planning Demystified
Forensics Demystified
French Demystified
Genetics Demystified
Geometry Demystified
German Demystified
Home Networking Demystified
Investing Demystified
Italian Demystified
Java Demystified
JavaScript Demystified
Lean Six Sigma Demystified
Linear Algebra Demystified

Macroeconomics Demystified
Management Accounting Demystified
Math Proofs Demystified
Math Word Problems Demystified
MATLAB® Demystified
Medical Billing and Coding Demystified
Medical Terminology Demystified
Medical-Surgical Nursing Demystified
Meteorology Demystified
Microbiology Demystified
Microeconomics Demystified
Nanotechnology Demystified
Nurse Management Demystified
OOP Demystified
Options Demystified
Organic Chemistry Demystified
Personal Computing Demystified
Pharmacology Demystified
Physics Demystified
Physiology Demystified
Pre-Algebra Demystified
Precalculus Demystified
Probability Demystified
Project Management Demystified
Psychology Demystified
Quality Management Demystified
Quantum Mechanics Demystified
Real Estate Math Demystified
Relativity Demystified
Robotics Demystified
Sales Management Demystified
Signals and Systems Demystified
Six Sigma Demystified
Spanish Demystified
SQL Demystified
Statics and Dynamics Demystified
Statistics Demystified
Technical Analysis Demystified
Technical Math Demystified
Trigonometry Demystified
UML Demystified
Visual Basic 2005 Demystified
Visual C# 2005 Demystified
Vitamins and Minerals Demystified
XML Demystified

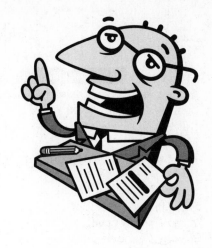

Medical-Surgical Nursing Demystified

Mary DiGiulio, RN, MSN, APRN
Donna Jackson, RN, MSN, APRN
Jim Keogh

New York Chicago San Francisco Lisbon London Madrid
Mexico City Milan New Delhi San Juan Seoul
Singapore Sydney Toronto

Sponsoring Editor
 Judy Bass

Editing Supervisor
 Maureen B. Walker

Project Manager
 Joanna V. Pomeranz

Copy Editor
 Matthew Kushinka

Proofreader
 D & P Editorial Services, LLC

Indexer
 Seth Maislin

Production Supervisor
 Pamela A. Pelton

Composition
 D & P Editorial Services, LLC

Art Director, Cover
 Jeff Weeks

To the memory of Jim, Rose, and Margot
who always believed in me

To Dave
Who means more than he sometimes knows

To Kathleen and Jacqueline
who have the world in front of them

Mary DiGiulio, RN, MSN

To Ken
Thank you for loving me, believing in me, encouraging me, and running the race
with me. I'm glad I have you.
Love, Donna

Donna Jackson, RN, MSN

This book is dedicated to Anne, Sandy, Joanne, Amber-Leigh Christine, and Shawn,
without whose help and support this book couldn't have been written.

Jim Keogh

CONTENTS

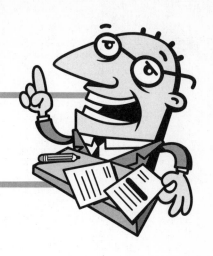

Contents

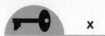

Contents

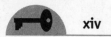

INTRODUCTION

Every patient knows to seek medical help when his or her aches and pains become too much to bear, but how does the healthcare provider determine what is wrong and what to do to restore the patient to good health? The answer depends on the patient's signs and symptoms and the results from medical tests. In this book you will learn to identify these signs and symptoms, interpret the medical test results, and perform the nursing interventions that will assist in solving or alleviating the patient's medical problem.

Medical-Surgical Nursing Demystified contains 15 chapters, each providing a description of a major body system and the diseases and disorders which can affect that system. The discussion of each disease or disorder is divided into the following sections:

- What Went Wrong?
- Prognosis
- Hallmark Signs and Symptoms
- Interpreting Test Results
- Treatment
- Nursing Diagnoses
- Nursing Intervention
- Crucial Diagnostic Tests

The "What Went Wrong?" section presents a brief description of how the body is affected when the particular disease or disorder occurs. The "Prognosis" section discusses the possibilities of curing this disease and permanent damage which can occur. The remaining sections present the information as lists of symptoms, diagnoses, etc. that make it easy for you to learn and that also serve as a useful tool for later reference.

A Look Inside

Since Medical-Surgical Nursing can be challenging for the beginner, this book was written to provide an organized, outline approach to learning about major diseases

and the part the nurse can play in the treatment process. The following paragraphs provide a thumbnail description of each chapter.

CHAPTER 1 CARDIOVASCULAR SYSTEM

The mere mention of the cardiovascular system brings all sorts of images to mind; however, these impressions are based on our experience as patients. Healthcare providers have a different view because they see it as a system that distributes nutrients and oxygen throughout the body and delivers carbon dioxide and metabolic by-products to various organs for removal from the body. Failure of the cardiovascular system has a compound effect because it interacts with the body's other systems causing a chain reaction of events. Healthcare providers need a thorough understanding of what can go wrong with the cardiovascular system; in this chapter you will earn to recognize cardiovascular system disorders and to perform the interventions that can assist in restoring its function.

CHAPTER 2 RESPIRATORY SYSTEM

The respiratory system interacts with cells in the body to exchange oxygen and carbon dioxide, enabling the oxygenation of all cells in the body. In this chapter you will learn which diseases and disorders can disrupt the respiratory system, how to recognize these conditions, and what steps you can take to assist in curing the respiratory system problems.

CHAPTER 3 IMMUNE SYSTEM

Remember the last time you experienced a bad cut. The site of the injury became swollen and red and you might have felt feverish. This happened because your immune system was trying to heal the wound by attacking the microorganisms that were invading your body. However, the abilities to fight off disease and to heal a wound are compromised when the immune system malfunctions. In this chapter you will learn about immune system disorders and what actions the nurse can perform to assist in the patient's recovery,

CHAPTER 4 HEMATOLOGIC SYSTEM

The hematologic system produces and circulates blood cells throughout the body. Any disorder of this system jeopardizes the functioning of every organ in the body. This chapter explores the hematologic system and its common disorders and discusses how to care for patients who experience them.

CHAPTER 5 NERVOUS SYSTEM

The nervous system is the body's command center that receives impulses and sends an appropriate response. In this chapter you will learn about the disorders that cause the malfunctioning of the nervous system and the interventions that mitigate neurological problems.

CHAPTER 6 MUSCULOSKELETAL SYSTEM

The musculoskeletal system is the body's superstructure that provides strength and movement. In this chapter you will learn about disorders of the musculoskeletal system and the treatments for restoring its functions.

CHAPTER 7 GASTROINTESTINAL SYSTEM

The body receives nourishment and excretes waste through the gastrointestinal system. Any disorder of the GI tract might disrupt the body's ability to store carbohydrates, lipids, and protein, all of which are used to energize cells. You will learn about these disorders and what to do about them in this chapter.

CHAPTER 8 ENDOCRINE SYSTEM

The endocrine system is the body's messenger. It turns on and off messages that direct the action of organs. Endocrine disorders cause chaos, as messages become misdirected. Endocrine system disorders and what to do about them are presented in this chapter.

CHAPTER 9 GENITOURINARY SYSTEM

Reproductive organs and the urinary system come from the same embryological origin, which is why they are combined in the genitourinary system. Disruptions of the genitourinary system are caused by a variety of disorders, some associated more with one gender than the other. In this chapter you will learn about these disorders and the treatments which can correct them.

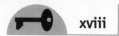

CHAPTER 10 INTEGUMENTARY SYSTEM

Diseases and disorders of the Integumentary system expose the body to invasion of viruses, bacteria and other microorganisms because the primary defense—the skin—is disrupted. In this chapter, you will learn about these diseases and disorders and discover ways to mitigate them.

CHAPTER 11 FLUIDS AND ELECTROLYTES

Fluids and electrolytes must be in balance for the body to properly function. An imbalance causes the body to compensate in ways that can have a rippling effect throughout other systems. In this chapter you will learn about fluids and electrolyte disorders and how to intervene to restore their balance.

CHAPTER 12 MENTAL HEALTH

Disorders that affect the mind can interfere with daily activities and lead to self-destructive behaviors. In this chapter, you will learn about mental health disorders, how to recognize them, and steps that can be taken to minimize their influence on the patient.

CHAPTER 13 PERIOPERATIVE

Surgical intervention is a radical but, at times, necessary treatment for a patient's condition. However, surgery can expose the patient to a set of disorders that would otherwise be avoided if no surgery had occurred. You will learn about these disorders and how to handle them in this chapter.

CHAPTER 14 WOMEN'S HEALTH

The women's health chapter covers a multitude of conditions that affect women. Here you will learn how to recognize these conditions, the medication used to treat them, and the interventions that can mitigate their ill effects on the patient.

CHAPTER 15 PAIN MANAGEMENT

Pain is associated with many disorders and must be successfully managed to reduce its disruptive affect on the patient's well-being. You will learn the techniques for managing pain in this chapter.

ABOUT THE AUTHORS

Mary DiGiulio is an Adult Nurse Practitioner on the faculty in the School of Nursing at UMDNJ in Newark, NJ and in practice in Teaneck, NJ. She has taught nursing at the graduate, baccalaureate and pre-licensure levels and presented for RN and PN review courses and nurse refresher courses.

Donna Jackson is an Adult Nurse Practitioner currently in practice in Teaneck, NJ. She is on the Advisory Board of the nursing program at Saint Peter's College in Jersey City, NJ. She has taught nursing courses at the graduate, baccalaureate and pre-licensure levels.

Jim Keogh is on the faculty of Saint Peter's College in Jersey City and New York University. He is the author of more than 70 books including Pharmacology Demystified, Microbiology Demystified, Nurse Management Demystified, Medical Billing and Coding Demystified, and Charting Demystified.

ACKNOWLEDGMENTS

Mary, Donna, and Jim are indebted to the dedication and work of Judy Bass, Maureen B. Walker, Pamela A. Pelton, Joanna V. Pomeranz, Nancy W. Dimitry, Gabriella Kadar, Don Pomeranz, and Don Dimitry who made this book possible.

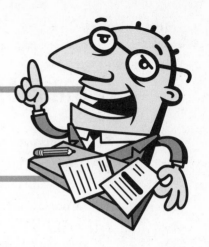

CHAPTER 1

Cardiovascular System

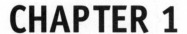

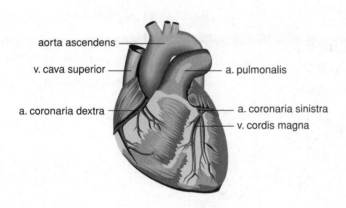

- aorta ascendens
- v. cava superior
- a. pulmonalis
- a. coronaria dextra
- a. coronaria sinistra
- v. cordis magna

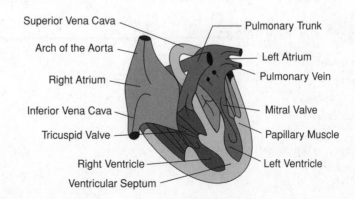

- Superior Vena Cava
- Arch of the Aorta
- Right Atrium
- Inferior Vena Cava
- Tricuspid Valve
- Right Ventricle
- Ventricular Septum
- Pulmonary Trunk
- Left Atrium
- Pulmonary Vein
- Mitral Valve
- Papillary Muscle
- Left Ventricle

Learning Objectives

1 Aortic aneurysm
2 Angina (Angina pectoris)
3 Myocardial infarction (MI)
4 Coronary artery disease (CAD)
5 Peripheral arterial disease (PAD)
6 Cardiac tamponade
7 Cardiogenic shock
8 Cardiomyopathy
9 Endocarditis
10 Heart failure [Congestive heart failure (CHF)]
11 Hypertension (HTN)
12 Hypovolemic shock
13 Myocarditis

14 Pericarditis
15 Pulmonary edema
16 Raynaud's disease
17 Rheumatic heart disease
18 Thrombophlebitis
19 Atrial fibrillation
20 Asystole
21 Ventricular fibrillation
22 Ventricular tachycardia
23 Aortic insufficiency (AI)
24 Mitral insufficiency
25 Mitral stenosis
26 Mitral valve prolapse (MVP)
27 Tricuspid insufficiency

Key Terms

Aneurysm
Angina
Aortic valve
Atherosclerosis
Atria
Atrioventricular (AV) valves
Cholesterol
Diastolic

Embolism
Infarction
Ischemia
Mitral valve
Necrosis
Occlusion
Pericardium
Pulmonic valve

Septal wall
Stenosis
Systolic
Tamponade
Tricuspid valve
Ventricle

How the Cardiovascular System Works

The cardiovascular system is responsible for delivery of blood, which carries oxygen and other nutrients, to the tissues of the body. The heart pumps the blood to the body where it delivers nutrients and oxygen, picks up waste products, and then returns to the heart.

The heart has four chambers. The upper chambers are the atria; the lower chambers are the ventricles. In the middle, there is a septum, a wall that separates the right side of the heart from the left side of the heart. Atrioventricular (AV) valves control the blood flow between the upper and lower chambers of the heart. The tricuspid valve is on the right side, while the mitral valve is on the left side between the atria and the ventricle. The pulmonic valve controls the flow between the right ventricle and the pulmonary artery, while the aortic valve controls the flow between the left ventricle and the aorta.

Unoxygenated blood empties into the right atrium from the systemic circulation via the inferior vena cava and superior vena cava. As the right atrium contracts, the tricuspid valve opens, allowing the blood to flow into the right ventricle. With contraction of the right ventricle, the pulmonic valve opens, allowing the unoxygenated blood to enter the pulmonary artery to go to the lungs to pick up oxygen. Once oxygenated, the blood returns to the heart via the pulmonary vein and enters the left atrium. As the left atrium contracts, the mitral valve opens, allowing the blood to flow into the left ventricle. As the left ventricle contracts, the aortic valve opens, allowing the blood to flow into the aorta and systemic circulation. The blood will return to the heart from the lower body via the inferior vena cava and from the upper body via the super vena cava. The actions on the right side and left side of the heart happen simultaneously. So when we listen to a normal heartbeat, the sounds we hear are the sounds of the valves closing. The mitral and tricuspid valves create the first heart sound (S1), while aortic and pulmonic valves create the second heart sound (S2).

The electrical conduction system of the heart starts at the sino-atrial (SA) node, which is located in the right atrium. It initiates the heart beat, ranging between 60 to 100 beats per minute, every day, for a lifetime. The electrical current travels across both atria, then converges on the atrio-ventricular (AV) node, where the current slows, allowing the atria to repolarize. The AV node is located in the superior portion of the ventricular septum. In the bottom portion are located the right and left Bundle of His, which is a group of special cardiac muscles that sends an electrical impulse to the ventricle to begin cardiac contractions. These end in the Purkinje fibers and spread out through the ventricles. The current passing through these fibers causes ventricular contraction, forcing the blood from the right ventricle to the lungs and from the left ventricle to the aorta, and thus, the systemic circulation.

Just the Facts

1 *Aortic Aneurysm*

WHAT WENT WRONG?

A weakening in the wall of a portion of the aorta results in a balloon-like bulge as blood flows through the aorta. The blood flow within this bulging area of the aorta becomes very turbulent. Over time this turbulence can cause the dilated area to increase in size, creating an aneurysm. The aneurysm can rupture causing a disruption in blood flow to everything below the affected area, and may even result in death.

This is commonly due to atherosclerosis where fatty substances, cholesterol, calcium and the clotting material fibrin, referred to as plaque, build up in the inner lining of an artery resulting in thickening and hardening of the arteries. It may also be caused by degeneration of the smooth muscle layer (middle) of the aorta, trauma, congenital defect, or infection. The aneurysm may be found incidentally on radiographic studies done for other reasons, or the patient may have developed symptoms indicating that something was wrong, such as severe back or abdominal pain, or a pulsating mass. Severe hypotension and syncope (fainting caused by insufficient blood supply to the brain) may indicate rupture.

PROGNOSIS

Outcome will vary depending on size and location of aneurysm. Some patients have aneurysms for months before a diagnosis is made, because they are asymptomatic. Treatment decisions will depend on the size and location of the aneurysm. Some patients with an aneurysm will have watchful waiting with periodic imaging to monitor the size of the aneurysm while other patients may need emergent surgery.

HALLMARK SIGNS AND SYMPTOMS

- Asymptomatic
- Abdominal pain
- Back pain that may radiate to posterior legs
- Abdominal pulsation

- Diminished femoral pulses
- Anxiety
- Restlessness
- Decreased pulse pressure
- Increased thready pulse

INTERPRETING TEST RESULTS

- An aneurysm will be displayed in a chest x-ray, abdominal ultrasound, CT scan, or MRI.
- Swishing sound over the abdominal aorta or iliac or femoral arteries because the natural flow of blood is disturbed (bruit).

TREATMENT

- Surgery to resect the aortic aneurysm by removing the section containing the aneurysm and replacing it with a graft.
- Administer antihypertensives, reducing the force of the pressure within the aorta to decrease the likelihood of rupture.
- Administer analgestics to treat patients who may be having pain from pressure on nearby structures (nerves, etc.) or tearing of the vessel.
- Administer oxycodone, morphine sulfate as needed to decrease oxygen demand.

NURSING DIAGNOSES

- Ineffective peripheral tissue perfusion
- Risk for deficient fluid volume
- Acute pain
- Anxiety

NURSING INTERVENTION

- Monitor vital signs—look for changes in blood pressure or elevated pulse and respiratory rates. During aortic dissection the blood pressure (BP) may initially increase due to severity of pain. It may then become difficult to impossible to obtain both the BP and pulse in one or both arms because of blood flow disruption to the arm(s). The patient may go into shock quickly if the aneurysm ruptures.

- Monitor cardiovascular system by checking heart sounds, peripheral pulses (upper and lower extremities), and checking for abdominal bruits, swishing sounds heard over the blood vessel when flow is disturbed.
- Measure intake and output.
- Hypovolemia is suspected if there is a low urine output and high specific gravity of urine.
- Palpate abdomen for distention or pulsatile mass.
- Abdominal distention, which is an enlarged abdomen, may signify imminent rupture of the aneurysm.
- Check for signs of severe decrease in blood or fluid (hypovolemic shock). The BP decreases as less blood circulates. Pulse rate increases as the heart tries to pump the blood faster to meet the oxygen demands of the body. Respiratory rate increases to meet oxygen needs while peripheral pulse sites are harder to find as BP lowers. The further away the pulse is from the heart, the more difficult it will be to find; it will be harder to locate the dorsalis pedis and posterior tibialis pulses earlier than the radial pulses.
- Pale, clammy skin will be present as circulation decreases.
- Severe back pain due to rupture or dissection.
- Anxiety due to uncertainty of what is happening.
- Restlessness due to anxiety, discomfort, and decreased oxygenation.
- Decreased pulse pressure due to less circulating volume, increased heart rate, and less filling time between heartbeats.
- Increased thready pulse.
- Limit patient's activity to a prescribed exercise and rest regimen.
- Be alert for decreased peripheral circulation.
  - Numbness.
  - Tingling.
  - Decrease in temperature of extremities.
  - Change in skin color in extremities.
  - Absence of peripheral pulses.
- Reduce patient anxiety.
- Maintain a quiet place.
- Have the patient express his or her feelings.

Angina (Angina Pectoris)

WHAT WENT WRONG?

A narrowing of blood vessels to the coronary artery, secondary to arteriosclerosis, results in inadequate blood flow through blood vessels of the heart muscle, causing chest pain. An episode of angina is typically precipitated by physical activity, excitement, or emotional stress. There are three categories of angina.

- Stable angina—pain is relieved by rest or nitrates and symptoms are consistent.
- Unstable angina—pain occurs at rest; is of new onset; is of increasing intensity, force, or duration; isn't relieved by rest; and is slow to subside in response to nitroglycerin.
- Prinzmetal's or vasospastic angina—usually occurs at rest or with minimal formal exercise or exertion; often occurs at night.

Atherosclerotic heart disease occurs when there is a buildup of plaque within the coronary arteries. Angina is often the first symptom that heart disease exists. When the demand for oxygen by the heart muscle exceeds the available supply, chest pain occurs.

PROGNOSIS

Patients can often be managed with lifestyle modifications and medications to control symptoms of angina. The most important factor is patient education. Patients need to understand the importance of their symptoms and when to seek medical attention. The pain must be evaluated initially and whenever a change in pattern or lack of response to treatment occurs.

HALLMARK SIGNS AND SYMPTOMS

- Chest pain lasting 3 to 5 minutes—not all patients get substernal pain; it may be described as pressure, heaviness, squeezing, or tightness. Use the patient's words.
- Can occur at rest or after exertion, excitement, or exposure to cold—due to increased oxygen demands or vasospasm.
- Usually relieved by rest—a chance to re-establish oxygen needs.

- Pain may radiate to other parts of the body such as the jaw, back, or arms—angina pain is not always felt in the chest. Ask if the patient has had similar pain in the past.
- Sweating (diaphoresis)—increased work of body to meet basic physiologic needs; anxiety.
- Tachycardia—heart pumping faster trying to meet oxygen needs as anxiety increases.
- Difficulty breathing, shortness of breath (dyspnea)—increased heart rate increases respiratory rate and increases oxygenation.
- Anxiety—not getting enough oxygen to heart muscle, the patient becomes nervous.

INTERPRETING TEST RESULTS

- Electrocardiogram during episode:
  - T-wave inverted with initial ischemia, which is reduced blood flow due to an obstructed vessel, usually first sign.
  - ST-segment changes occur with injury to the myocardium (heart muscle).
  - Abnormal Q-waves due to infarction of myocardium.
- Labs: troponins, CK-MB, which is an enzyme released by damaged cardiac tissue 2 to 6 hours following an infarction, electrolytes.
- Chest x-ray to determine signs of heart failure.
- Holter monitoring: a portable EKG which the patient wears for 24 to 48 hours, giving that many hours of continuous cardiac monitoring.
- Coronary arteriography to determine plaque build-up in coronary arteries.
- Cardiac PET (positron emission tomography) to determine plaque build-up in coronary arteries.
- Stress testing to determine symptoms when at exercise or under pharmacologic stress.
- Echocardiogram or stress-echo to determine any abnormality of wall motion due to ischemia.
- Cardiology consult.
- Nonemergent labs: Complete Blood Count (CBC) used to determine the general health status of the patient, chemistry (provides information about the status of eletrolytes, kidneys, acid/base balance, blood sugar and calcium levels), Prothrombin Time (PT/INR), Activated Partial Throboplastin Time

(PTT) (helps to detect and diagnose bleeding disorders and the effectiveness of anticoagulants), proBNP (BNP) measures the presence and severity of heart failure.

- Cholesterol panel to evaluate risk.
  - Increased risk for coronary artery disease with increased total cholesterol, increased low-density lipoproteins (LDL), increased triglycerides and decreased high-density lipoproteins. (HDL).

TREATMENT

The goal of treatment is to deliver sufficient oxygen to the heart muscle to meet its need. When suspecting chest pain, always give oxygen as the first line of defense. Medications are used initially to treat symptoms and increase blood flow to the heart muscle. Medications are used for symptom control and cholesterol management in the long term. Cardiovascular interventions are used to maintain adequate blood flow through the coronary arteries.

- 2 to 4 liters of oxygen.
- Administer beta-adrenergic blocker—this class has a cardioprotective effect, decreasing cardiac workload and likelihood of arrhythmia.
  - Drugs like propranolol, nadolol, atenolol, metoprolol.
- Administer nitrates—aids in getting oxygenated blood to heart muscle.
  - Nitroglycerin—sublingual tablets or spray; timed-release tablets.
  - Topical nitroglycerin—paste or timed-released patch.
- Aspirin for antiplatelet effect.
- Analgesic—typically morphine intravenously during acute pain. The medicine is very fast-acting when given this way and will decrease myocardial oxygen demand as well as decrease pain.

The following should be watched separately.

- Percutaneous transluminal coronary angioplasty. This is a nonsurgical procedure in which a long tube with a small balloon is passed through blood vessels into the narrowed artery. The balloon is inflated, causing the artery to expand.
- Coronary artery stent. This is a small, stainless steel mesh tube that is placed within the coronary artery to keep it open.
- Coronary artery bypass graph (CABG). This is a surgical procedure in which a vein from a leg or an artery from an arm or the chest is removed and

graphed to coronary arteries, bypassing the blockage and restoring free flow of blood to heart muscles.

- Low-cholesterol, low-sodium, and low-fat diet.

NURSING DIAGNOSES

- Anxiety
- Decreased cardiac output
- Acute pain

NURSING INTERVENTION

- Monitor vital signs—look for change in BP, P, R; irregular pulse; pulse deficit; when a discrepancy is found between an atrial rate and a radial rate, when measured simultaneously; pulse oximetry.
- Notify physician if systolic blood pressure is less than 90 mmHg. Nitrates dilate arteries to the heart and increase blood flow. You may have an order to hold nitrates if SBP <90 mmHg to reduce risk of patient passing out from lack of blood flow to brain.
- Notify physician if heart rate is less than 60 beats per minute. Beta-adrenergic blockers slow conduction through the AV node and reduce the heart rate and contractility. You may have an order to hold beta blockers if heart rate goes below 60; you should continuously monitor the patient's pulse rate.
- Assess chest pain each time the patient reports it.
  - Remember PQRST (an acronym for a method of pain assessment) as follows.

Determine the *p*lace, *q*uality (describe the pain—stabbing, squeezing, etc.), *r*adiation (does the pain travel anywhere else?), *s*everity (on a scale of 1 to 10), and *t*iming (when it started and how long it lasts and what preceded the pain).

- Monitor cardiac status using a 12-lead electrocardiogram (EKG) while the patient is experiencing an angina attack. Each time the patient has pain, a new 12-lead EKG is done to assess for changes, even if one was already done that day.
- Record fluid intake and output. Assess for renal function.
- Place patient in a semi-Fowler's position (semi-sitting with knees flexed).

- Explain to patient:
  - Rest when pain begins to decrease oxygen demands.
  - Take nitroglycerin when any pain begins—it helps dilate coronary arteries and get more oxygen to heart muscle.
  - Avoid stress and activities that bring on an angina attack.
  - Call 911 if the pain continues for more than 10 minutes or as the patient is taking the third nitroglycerine dose (1 sublingual dose every 5 minutes, if BP allows, for maximum of 3 doses).
  - Stop smoking! Smoking is associated with heart disease.
  - Adhere to the prescribed diet and exercise plan. Lower cholesterol and fat intake to decrease further plaque build-up, and decrease excess salt intake to help BP control. Slowly increase exercise to build up activity tolerance. Possibly exercise with cardiac rehabilitation.
  - How to recognize the symptoms of a myocardial infarction: Pay attention to chest pains as well as changes in patterns of pain and response to treatment. Be aware of changes in respiratory patterns, increase in shortness of breath, swelling, and general feelings of malaise.

3 *Myocardial Infarction (MI)*

WHAT WENT WRONG?

Blood supply to the myocardium is interrupted for a prolonged time due to the blockage of coronary arteries. This results in insufficient oxygen reaching cardiac muscle, causing cardiac muscles to die (necrosis). MI is commonly known as a heart attack.

The area of infarction is often due to build-up of plaque over time (atherosclerosis). It may also be due to a clot that develops in association with the atherosclerosis within the vessel. Patients are typically (not always) symptomatic, but some patients will not be aware of the event; they will have what is called a silent MI.

PROGNOSIS

The outcome depends on the coronary artery that is affected. The earlier the person enters the healthcare system, the better the prognosis is, because emergency measures will be available for otherwise fatal arrhythmias.

There is a better outcome for patients who receive adequate medical attention and make appropriate lifestyle changes post-myocardial infarction. Cardiac rehabilitation can help patients make these changes safely.

HALLMARK SIGNS AND SYMPTOMS

- Chest pain that is unrelieved by rest or nitroglycerin, unlike angina
- Pain that radiates to arms, jaw, back and/or neck
- Shortness of breath, especially in the elderly or women
- Nausea or vomiting possible
- Maybe asymptomatic, known as a silent MI, which is more common in diabetic patients
- Heart rate >100 (tachycardia) because of sympathetic stimulation, pain, or low cardiac output
- Variable blood pressure
- Anxiety
- Restlessness
- Feeling of impending doom
- Pale, cool, clammy skin; sweating (diaphoresis)
- Sudden death due to arrhythmia usually occurs within first hour

INTERPRETING TEST RESULTS

- EKG.
  - T-wave inversion—sign of ischemia.
  - ST-segment elevated or depressed—sign of injury.
  - Significant Q-waves—sign of infarction.
- Decreased pulse pressure because of diminished cardiac output.
- Increased white blood count (WBC) due to inflammatory response to injury.
- Blood chemistry:
  - Elevated creatine kinase MB (CK-MB)—usually done serially, the numbers will rise along a predetermined curve to signify myocardial damage and resolution.
  - Elevated troponin I- and troponin T-proteins elevated within one hour of myocardial damage.
- Less than 25 ml/hr of urine output due to lack of renal blood flow.

TREATMENT

Treatment is focused on reversing and preventing further damage to the myocardium. Early intervention is needed to have the best possible outcome. Thrombolytic therapy is instrumental in reducing mortality. A three-hour time window is ideal for maximizing benefit. Medications are used to enhance blood flow to the heart muscle while reducing the workload of the heart. Supplemental oxygen is used to help meet myocardial oxygen demand. Data from coronary angioplasty and percutaneous coronary intervention (stenting) of an occluded artery have been impressive. Following the acute management, the patient will have to make lifestyle changes—altering diet and exercise, stopping smoking, and so on.

- Administer oxygen, aspirin.
- Administer antiarrhythmics because arrhythmias are common as are conduction disturbances.
  - Amiodarone.
  - Lidocaine.
  - Procainamide.
- Electrical cardioversion for unstable ventricular tachycardia. In cardioversion, an initial shock is administered to the heart to re-establish sinus rhythm.
- Administer antihypertensive to keep blood pressure low.
  - Hydralazine.
- Percutaneous revascularization.
- Administer thrombolytic therapy within 3 to 12 hours of onset because it can re-establish blood flow in an occluded artery, reduce mortality, and halt the size of the infarction.
  - Alteplase.
  - Streptokinase.
  - Anistreplase.
  - Reteplase.
  - Heparin following thrombolytic therapy.
- Administer calcium channel blockers as they appear to prevent reinfarction and ischemia, only in non–Q-wave infarctions.
  - Verapamil.
  - Diltiazem.
- Administer beta-adrenergic blockers because they reduce the duration of ischemic pain and the incidence of ventricular fibrillation; decreases mortality.

- Propranolol.
- Nadolol.
- Metroprolol.
- Administer analgesics to relieve pain, reduce pulmonary congestion, and decrease myocardial oxygen consumption.
  - Morphine.
- Administer nitrates to reduce ischemic pain by dilation of blood vessels; helps to lower BP.
  - Nitroglycerin.
- Place patient on bed rest in CCU.
- No bathroom privileges. Bedside commode only.
- Low-fat, low-caloric, low-cholesterol diet.

NURSING DIAGNOSES

- Ineffective tissue perfusion
- Decreased cardiac output

NURSING INTERVENTION

- Monitor:
  - Cardiovascular—look for changes or instability in pulse, heart sounds, murmur.
  - Respiration—look for changes, fluid in lung fields, shortness of breath.
  - EKG during attack—12-lead during any episode of pain.
  - EKG continuous monitoring for arrhythmias.
  - Vital signs—check for changes in BP, pulse quality, peripheral pulses.
  - Pulse-oximetry monitoring.
- Explain to the patient:
  - Change to a low-fat, low-cholesterol, low-sodium diet.
  - The difference between angina pain and myocardial infarction pain.
  - When to take nitroglycerin.
  - Medication.
  - When to call 911.

- Smoking cessation.
- Limit activities.
- Need for cardiac rehabilitation.
- Stress reduction.
- Lifestyle changes such as increase in exercise, diet changes.

4 *Coronary Artery Disease (CAD)*

WHAT WENT WRONG?

Cholesterol, calcium and other elements carried by the blood are deposited on the wall of the coronary artery resulting in the narrowing of the artery and the reduction of blood flow through the vessel. This impedes blood supply to the heart muscle. These deposits start out as fatty streaks and eventually develop into plaque that inhibits blood flow through the artery. Elevated cholesterol levels and fat intake can contribute to this plaque build-up, as can hypertension, diabetes, and smoking. When the plaque builds up within the artery, the heart muscle is deprived of oxygen and nutrients ultimately damaging the heart muscle.

PROGNOSIS

Lifestyle changes and medications can significantly impact the risks of the individual. Dietary modification, activity, and medications can help to alter the disease process. Patients who continue with prior bad habits will continue with disease progression. Risk factors include age, male gender, and family history.

HALLMARK SIGNS AND SYMPTOMS

- Asymptomatic.
- Chest pain (angina) because of decreased blood flow to heart muscle and/or increase in myocardial oxygen demand resulting from stress.
- Pain may radiate to the arms, back, and jaw.
- Chest pain occurs after exertion, excitement, or when the patient is exposed to cold temperatures because there is an increase in blood flow throughout the body, raising the rate.

- Chest pain lasts between 3 to 5 minutes.
- Chest pain can occur when the patient is resting.

INTERPRETING TEST RESULTS

- Blood chemistry:
  - Increased total cholesterol.
  - Decreased high-density lipoproteins (HDL)—helps with reverse transport of cholesterol.
  - Increased low-density lipoproteins (LDL).
- Electrocardiogram during chest pain:
  - T-wave inversion—sign of ischemia.
  - ST-segment depressed—sign of injury to muscle.
  - The waves are depressed because of tissue injury.

TREATMENT

Treatment consists of risk factor modification, life style changes, medications, and revascularization.

- Weight loss.
- Diet change: lower sodium, lower cholesterol and fat, decreased calorie intake, increased dietary fiber.
- Administer low doses of aspirin.
- Administer beta-adrenergic blockers to reduce workload of heart:
  - metroprolol, propranolol, nadolol.
- Administer calcium channel blockers to reduce heart rate, blood pressure, and muscle contractility; helps with coronary vasodilation; slows AV node conduction.
- Administer nitrate if patient has symptomatic chest pains to reduce discomfort and enhance blood flow to myocardium.
- Platelet inhibitors:
  - dipyridamole
  - clopidogrel
  - ticlopidine

- Administer HMG CoA reductase inhibitors (statins)—lowers cholesterol:
  - lovastatin
  - simvastatin
  - atorvastatin
  - fluvastatin
  - pravastatin
  - rosuvastatin
- Fibric acid derivatives reduce synthesis and increase breakdown of VLDL particles:
  - gemfibrozil
- Bile acid binding resins binds bile acid in the intestine:
  - colestipol
- Nicotinic acid reduces production of VLDL:
  - niacin

NURSING DIAGNOSES

- Acute pain
- Activity intolerance
- Impaired gas exchange

NURSING INTERVENTION

- Monitor vital signs—signs of hypertension, irregular heart rate
- Monitor electrocardiogram—look for end organ damage, signs of heart disease
- Monitor labs—periodic lipid panel, liver function for patients on statins
- Monitor for myalgias (muscle aches)
- Explain to the patient:
  - Stop smoking
  - Reduce alcohol consumption
  - Change to a lower-fat, lower-cholesterol diet, as well as increased dietary fiber intake
  - Increase daily activity
  - Weight reduction

- Stress management
- Hospital-based cardiac rehabilitation programs

5 *Peripheral Arterial Disease (PAD)*

WHAT WENT WRONG?

Large peripheral arteries become narrowed and restricted (stenosis) leading to the temporary (acute) or permanent (chronic) reduction of blood flow to tissues (ischemia). This is most commonly due to atherosclerosis (plaque on the inner walls of arteries), but may also be caused by a blood clot (embolism), or from an inflammatory process. Severe peripheral arterial occlusive disease can lead to skin ulceration and gangrene. Peripheral arterial occlusive disease is more common in patients with diabetes or hypertension, in older adults, in those with hyperlipidemia, and in those who smoke, as these conditions can predispose to diminished circulation. Vascular disease that happens in one area of the body, e.g. coronary arteries, is not an isolated process. The plaque build-up caused by long-term elevated cholesterol levels will happen throughout the body. The most common area of involvement is the lower extremities.

PROGNOSIS

Patients typically have progressive disease. It is a chronic problem, getting worse with age. Symptoms may not be present until there is a 50 percent or greater occlusion of the vessel. Suspect disease in patients who have risk for other cardiovascular diseases. Medications can help to improve blood flow to the area and increased activity will improve exercise tolerance and quality of life. Vascular intervention may be necessary as the disease progresses.

HALLMARK SIGNS AND SYMPTOMS

- Femoral, popliteal arteries.
  - Sudden pain in the affected area because of spontaneous muscle contractions due to the reduced oxygenation of tissue.
  - Intermittent claudication—pain, numbness, and/or weakness with walking due to increased oxygen demand of the muscle during activity.

- Weak or absence of pulse in affected area because blood flow is reduced or blocked.
- Decreased temperature distal to the blockage because of restricted blood flow.
- Pallor or patchy coloring (mottling) of affected area because of reduced tissue oxygenation.
- Dependent rubor (increased redness when legs are lower).
- Hair loss on extremities.

INTERPRETING TEST RESULTS

- Doppler ultrasonography of affected area.
- Arteriography. Dye is injected into the affected artery enabling an outline of the artery and blockage to be seen in an x-ray.
- Ankle brachial index (ABI) helps to determine the amount of arterial insufficiency.

TREATMENT

The goal of treatment is to maintain adequate blood flow to the area and avoid tissue damage. Patients are encouraged to maintain activity and reduce risks for disease, such as smoking, as well as to control blood pressure and monitoring diabetes.

Medical treatment:

- Exercise.
- Smoking cessation.
- Decrease in lipids, depending on what the labwork shows.

Surgical treatment:

- Femoropopliteal bypass graft: A vessel from another part of the body is removed and grafted to the affected artery, permitting blood to bypass the blockage.
- Percutaneous transluminal angioplasty: A catheter containing a balloon is inserted into the affected artery. The balloon is inflated, stretching the artery; this causes a healing response that breaks up plaque on the artery wall.

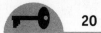

- Atherectomy: A catheter containing a grinding tool is inserted into the affected artery and is used to grind plaque from the artery wall.
- Embolectomy: Surgical removal of a blood clot from the affected artery.
- Thromboendarterectomy: Surgical removal of atherosclerotic tissue from the affected artery.
- Laser angioplasty: A laser-tipped catheter is inserted into the affected artery to remove the blockage.
- Stent: A metal mesh tube is inserted into the affected artery to keep the artery open.
- Amputation: Surgical removal of the affected limb that contains gangrene caused by low blood flow or complete blockage of blood to the affected limb.
- Administer antiplatelets medication to enhance blood flow to the lower extremities. This helps to get blood through the vessels and alleviates symptoms.
  - penoxifylline
  - cilostazol
  - aspirin
  - clopidogrel
  - dipyridamole
  - ticlopidine

NURSING DIAGNOSES

- Fear
- Ineffective tissue perfusion
- Risk for injury

NURSING INTERVENTION

- Monitor most distal pulse to assure circulation exists.
- Compare bilateral pulses.
- Monitor temperature, color of affected area indicating tissue perfusion.
- Support hose.
- Check capillary refill.
- Administer anticoagulant (such as heparin, warfarin) as directed.
- Administer pain medication as directed.

- Don't elevate leg or apply heat if occlusion affects the femoral or popliteal arteries.
- Elevation of the lower extremities makes it harder for the blood flow to get to the tissues.
- Avoid prolonged sitting, which increases the risk of compression to vessels (impeding blood flow to lower extremities) and increases risk of clot formation in lower extremities.
- Explain to the patient:
  - How to check pulses in the affected area if there is an absence of a pulse.
  - Call the physician if the patient experiences numbness, paralysis, or pain.
  - Don't wear tight clothes; avoid tight knee-high hose, which constricts at the popliteal space; avoid tight waist bands; ensure wide shoe box.
  - Change his/her lifestyle to reduce the risk of peripheral arterial occlusive disease.
  - The importance of regular examinations.
  - Foot check daily for open wounds, redness.
  - Regular visits to podiatrist.
  - Regular consults to vascular MD.

6 *Cardiac Tamponade*

WHAT WENT WRONG?

A large amount of liquid accumulates in the sack around the heart (pericardium), creating pressure on the heart that reduces the filling of ventricles with blood. This results in a low volume of blood being pumped with each contraction. The accumulating pressure within the pericardium may be due to fluid, pus, or blood. The end result is decreased stroke volume and cardiac output.

The cause of tamponade may be trauma, postoperative, post-MI, uremia, or cancer. The fluid may develop rapidly or over time, depending on cause. Tamponade is a life-threatening condition. The seriousness is related to the amount of pressure within the heart and the resulting decrease in ventricular filling.

PROGNOSIS

Cardiac tamponade is a medical emergency requiring immediate intervention, such as drainage of the fluids. Stabilization occurs quickly once the fluid is removed and pressure is alleviated. If fluid recurs, surgery may be necessary. The prognosis depends on the etiology of the tamponade.

HALLMARK SIGNS AND SYMPTOMS

- Neck vein distention—accumulation of fluid within the pericardium causes pressure on the heart, which prevents the venous return from the jugular veins. This causes distention, more pronounced on inspiration.
- Restlessness due to decreased oxygen to the brain.
- Muffled (dull) heart sounds on auscultation because it's harder to hear through fluid.
- Pulsus paradoxus—decrease of 10 mmHg or more in SBP during inspiration—change in pressure within the chest during inspiration, resulting in decreased ventricular filling, decreased output, fall in SBP.
- Sweating (diaphoresis).
- Difficulty breathing (dyspnea).
- Tachycardia.
- Hypotension.
- Fatigue.

INTERPRETING TEST RESULTS

- Echocardiograph: Ultrasound image of the heart to assess the heart's position, structure, and motion. Ventricle and atria are compressed. Fluid found within pericardial sac.
- Cardiac catheterization.
- Chest x-ray shows an enlarged heart if large effusion present.
- Electrocardiogram used to rule out other cardiac problems.

TREATMENT

Treatment is directed at reducing the pressure on the heart from the accumulating fluids in the pericardial sac. The following may be necessary to support and stabilize the patient.

- Pericardiocentesis: A needle is inserted into the pericardium and fluid is aspirated or drained.
- Administer adrenergic agent—increases heart rate and blood pressure.

NURSING DIAGNOSES

- Anxiety
- Ineffective tissue perfusion
- Decreased cardiac output

NURSING INTERVENTION

- Monitor vital signs.
- Assure adequate oxygenation.

Cardiogenic Shock

WHAT WENT WRONG?

A drop in blood pressure and blood flow caused by the heart's inability to pump blood as a result of a cardiac emergency, such as cardiac tamponade, myocardial ischemia, myocarditis, or cardiomyopathy (a disease of the heart that deteriorates the heart muscle). Blood pools in the left ventricle, which causes a back up of blood into the lungs, resulting in pulmonary edema. Contractions increase to compensate for the decreased cardiac output, causing an increase in demand for oxygen by the heart. However, the lungs are not oxygenating the blood sufficiently due to decreased blood flow; and therefore heart muscles are starved for oxygen.

PROGNOSIS

Treatment needs to find a balance between improving cardiac output and reducing oxygen needs and cardiac workload of the myocardium. This balance must be achieved while maintaining perfusion of the heart muscle. Prognosis depends on finding and treating the underlying cause. Cardiogenic shock requires immediate treatment, often before the cause is known.

HALLMARK SIGNS AND SYMPTOMS

- Hypotension, because blood flow decreases below normal.
- Tachycardia, because the heart is trying to pump faster to maintain adequate blood flow to the body, or occasionally bradycardia, where the heart rate is less than 60 beats per minute due to myocardial damage.
- Arrhythmias—when the heart muscle does not have enough oxygen it becomes irritable, making arrhythmias more likely.
- Clammy skin, because oxygenation to tissues is reduced.
- Drop in skin temperature because of reduced circulation as a result of hypotension.
- Urine output less than 30 ml per hour (oliguria) because the kidneys are not being perfused.
- Crackles heard in the lungs secondary to pulmonary edema, meaning fluid is building up in lungs.
- Confusion due to poor perfusion.
- Distended jugular veins—sign of fluid overload, inability of heart to manage fluid coming into heart.
- Cyanosis of lips, peripheral extremities due to poor perfusion.

INTERPRETING TEST RESULTS

- Chemistry—check electrolytes, kidney function to ascertain kidney perfusion; calcium level is increased or decreased secondary to muscle contractility.
- Echocardiogram—to look for ventricular rupture, pericarditis, or valve dysfunction.
- Electrocardiogram:
  - Q-wave enlarged due to heart failure.
  - Elevation of ST-waves is a sign of ischemia.

TREATMENT

Treatment is based on medical support for the heart until etiology (cause) can be determined. In cardiogenic stroke, the stroke volume and the heart rate must be increased to keep the organs perfused. The effects of the following medications should accomplish this.

- Administer vasodilator—dilates blood vessels (arterial and venous) to decrease the venous return to the heart and reduces the peripheral arterial resistance (what the heart has to pump against).
  - Nitroprusside; nitroglycerin.
- Administer adrenergic agent—to increase the heart rate and blood pressure:
  - epinephrine.
- Administer inotropes strengthens the heart beat, improves contractions, produces peripheral vasoconstriction:
  - dopamine
  - dobutamine
  - inammone
  - milrinone
- Administer vasopressor decreases blood flow to all organs except the heart and brain:
  - norepinephrine
- Provide supplemental oxygen—may need to be via intubation.

NURSING DIAGNOSES

- Ineffective tissue perfusion
- Decreased cardiac output

NURSING INTERVENTION

- Monitor vital signs—look for changes in BP, P, R.
- Monitor heart sounds.
- Monitor Swanz Ganz catheter is a catheter placed into the pulmonary artery to check for pressures in the heart, vessels, and lungs.
- Test capillary refill.
- Monitor arterial blood gas to learn pH, acidosis or alkalosis, bicarb level.
- Monitor respiratory status—due to poor perfusion, these patients are in respiratory distress; mechanical ventilation may be needed.
- Place the patient on bed rest.

- Monitor intake and output of fluids—look for adequate renal perfusion. Without sufficient cardiac function, the patient will not have enough blood flow to the kidneys to get adequate filtration.
- Explain to the patient:
  - Which symptoms to be aware of and when to call the doctor.
  - Take rest periods.
  - Call the physician if there are signs of fluid overload—weight increase, shortness of breath, fatigue, dependent edema.
  - Record weight each day and call the physician, nurse practitioner, or physician assistant if there is an increase of 3 lbs (1.4 kg).
  - Change to a low-sodium, low-fat diet.

8 *Cardiomyopathy*

WHAT WENT WRONG?

The middle layer of the heart wall that contains cardiac muscle (myocardium) weakens and stretches, causing the heart to lose its pumping strength and become enlarged. The heart remains functional; however, contractions are weak, resulting in decreased cardiac output. Most are idiopathic and not related to the major causes of heart disease. The three types of cardiomyopathy are:

1. Dilated cardiomyopathy (common): The heart muscle thins and enlarges, which leads to congestive heart failure. Progressive hypertrophy and dilatation result in problems with pumping action of ventricles.
2. Hypertrophic cardiomyopathy: The ventricular heart muscle thickens, resulting in outflow obstruction or restriction. There is some blood flow present.
3. Restrictive cardiomyopathy (rare): The heart muscle becomes stiff and restricts blood from filling ventricles, usually as a result of amyloidosis, radiation, or myocardial fibrosis after open-heart surgery.

PROGNOSIS

Prognosis is variable. Sudden cardiac death is a possible outcome in dilated or hypertrophic cardiomyopathy; arrhythmia is often a precursor to sudden death.

HALLMARK SIGNS AND SYMPTOMS

- Asymptomatic—Many clients with hypertrophic cardiomyopathy (HCM) are asymptomatic. Those with signs do not present until their mid-twenties.
- Dyspnea—The most frequent symptom is shortness of breath due to increase pressure in the lungs. The heart may not sufficiently relax resulting in higher pressure and a backup of blood into the lungs.
- Angina—Clients experience chest pain related to increase oxygen demand of the extra heart muscle and due to thick, narrowing coronary blood vessels within the heart's wall
- Syncope—Fainting is caused by heart arrhythmias related to the inability of the cardiac muscle to conduct electrical impulses.
- Sudden death—Young adults are at risk of sudden death during physical exercise resulting from ventricular fibrillation, which is a cardiac arrhythmia.
- Abnormal heart sounds
  - Murmur, which is the sound of turbulence results from abnormal blood flow
  - S3, which is a third heart sound commonly heard in heart failure. S3 is a soft sound made by the vibration of the ventricular wall when the ventricle fills too rapidly. S3 is heard after the S2 heart sound and is best found over the apex of the left ventricle, which is the fourth intercostal space along the mid-clavicular line
  - S4, which is the heart sound heard before the S1 heart sound is the result of the heart being too stiff. This is vibration of the valves and the ventricular walls when the atria contracts and the ventricles fill.

INTERPRETING TEST RESULTS

- Chest x-ray (CXR) shows enlarged heart, pulmonary congestion.
- Echocardiography shows left ventricular hypertrophy (LVH) and dysfunction in dilated and hypertrophic cardiomyopathy; small ventricular size and function in restrictive cardiomyopathy.
- Electrocardiogram: ST changes, conduction abnormalities, LVH.
  - Left ventricular hypertrophy shows as a broad QRS wave, usually in leads 4, 5, and 6 because of high voltage.
- Cardiac catheterization—to measure chamber pressures, cardiac output, ventricular function, but is often unable to add to information that has already been received from echocardiogram.

- Exercise testing may show poor cardiac function not evident in a resting state.

TREATMENT

Treatment is based on the specific cause. Avoiding the offending drug/treatment is imperative. Manage the underlying disease and provide cardiac support; however, few therapies can halt the process of cardiomyopathy.

- Change to a low-sodium diet.
- Beta adrenergic blockers—cause the heart to beat slowly, allowing more time for ventricular filling and improve contractile function:
  - propranolol, nadolol, metoprolol (for hypertropic cardiomyopathy)
- Angiotensin-converting enzyme (ACE) inhibitors—to decrease left ventricular filling pressures.
- Calcium channel blockers—reduced cardiac workload by increasing contractile ability:
  - verapamil (for hypertrophic cardiomyopathy)
- Diuretics reduce fluid retention:
  - furosemide, bumetanide, metolazone (for dilated cardiomyopathy)
  - spironolactone (aldosterone antagonist)
- Administer inotropic agent to enable the heart to have greater contractile force:
  - dobutamine
  - milrinone
  - digoxin (for dilated cardiomyopathy)
- Administer oral anticoagulant to reduce the coagulation of blood:
  - warfarin (for dilated and hypertrophic cardiomyopathy)
- Implantable cardioverter-defibrillator for high risk.
- Myectomy—incision into septum and removal of tissue.

NURSING DIAGNOSES

- Activity intolerance
- Impaired gas exchange
- Decreased cardiac output

NURSING INTERVENTION

- Place patient in a semi-Fowler's position for comfort, which eases respiratory effort.
- Record intake and output of fluids.
- Monitor vital signs to assess for increased respiratory rate, arrythmias.
- Monitor electrocardiogram to look for changes from previous tracing.
- Explain to the patient: fluids restriction may be necessary as heart failure is a concurrent disease with dilated cardiomyopathy.
  - Record daily weight and call physician if weight increases 3 lbs (1.4 kg).
  - No smoking or drinking alcohol.
  - No straining during bowel movements.
  - Increase exercise.

9 *Endocarditis*

WHAT WENT WRONG?

Microorganisms, usually bacteria, enter the blood stream and attach to the inner lining of the heart (endocardium) and heart valves, resulting in inflammation. Ulceration and necrosis occur when microorganisms cover the heart valves. This usually occurs in patients with rheumatic heart disease or degenerative heart disease; those with recent instrumentation (IV, GU, and respiratory procedures) or dental procedures; and IV drug users.

PROGNOSIS

The prognosis depends on both the organism (as some are more virulent than others) and the degree of damage to the heart. Myocarditis may recur.

HALLMARK SIGNS AND SYMPTOMS

- Chills/fever—due to infectious process.
- Petecchiae on the palate, beneath the fingernails, osler nodes (painful, discolored, raised areas on fingers and feet), Janeway lesions (painful lesions on palms and soles).

- Fatigue—due to infectious process.
- Murmurs—new or changing.

INTERPRETING TEST RESULTS

- Blood culture and sensitivity test.
  - Three sets of cultures one hour apart to determine the specific organism so treatment can be started.
- Echocardiogram is used to detect vegetation on valves or heart valves damaged by the microorganism, and also to determine which valves are involved.
- Transesophageal echocardiogram offers a view to detect vegetation on heart valves or view heart valves damaged by a microorganism.
- Chest x-ray to look for underlying cardiac abnormality and pulmonary infiltrate.

TREATMENT

Treatment depends on the underlying infectious agent. Empiric treatment should be started while waiting for culture results. Outcomes are affected by possible valvular destruction, emboli, and growth of bacteria on the valves or endocardium.

- Administer antibiotics based on the result of culture and sensitivity test.
- Valve replacement may be necessary if damage to valves is significant.
- Bed rest to decrease demand on heart.

NURSING DIAGNOSES

- Decrease cardiac output
- Risk for injury
- Activity intolerance

NURSING INTERVENTION

- Monitor for signs of heart failure due to increased stress on heart due to altered valve function.
  - Breathing difficulties (dyspnea).

- Heat rate >100 beats per minute (tachycardia).
- Crackles in lungs.
- Neck vein distention.
- Edema, usually of extremities; may also be of sacrum in bed-bound patients.
- Weight gain.
- Monitor for embolism—a piece of vegetation from valve may have broken off into circulation.
  - Blood in the urine (hematuria).
  - Pain with each breath due to pulmonary embolism.
- Monitor renal function.
  - Increased BUN (blood urea nitrogen).
  - Increased creatinine clearance.
  - Decreased urine output.
- Prophylatic antibiotics before, during, and after medical procedures that expose the patient's blood to microorganisms—otherwise it is easy for micro-organisms to enter bloodstream and colonize the heart valves.
- Explain to the patient:
  - Need to complete antibiotic course.
  - Can have a relapse.
  - Call the physician, nurse practitioner, or physician assistant if the patient develops fever, chills, night sweats.

10 *Heart Failure [Congestive Heart Failure (CHF)]*

WHAT WENT WRONG?

In congestive heart failure, the heart is unable to pump sufficient blood to maintain adequate circulation. This results in a backup of blood and the extra pressure may cause accumulation of fluid into the lungs. Heart failure is primarily due to problems with ventricular pumping action of the cardiac muscle, which may be caused by diseases such as myocardial infarctions (heart attacks), endocarditis (infection in the heart), hypertension (high blood pressure), or valvular insufficiency.

When disease affects primarily the left side of the heart, the blood will back up into the lungs. When disease affects primarily the right side of the heart, the systemic circulation may be overloaded. When the heart failure becomes significant, the whole circulatory system may be compromised.

HALLMARK SIGNS AND SYMPTOMS

- Extra heart sounds (normal heart sounds were described in the beginning):
  - S3: Soft sound caused by vibration of the ventricular wall caused by rapid filling. Heard after S2 heart sound. Heard over the apex of the left ventricle, fourth intercostal space along the mid-clavicular line. Best heard when patient lies on left side. Usually indicates heart failure.
  - S4: Vibration of valves and the ventricular walls during the second phase of ventricular filling when the atria contract. Heard before S1, in the same location as S3, usually due to a "stiff heart."
  - Murmur: Sounds of turbulence caused by blood flow. Heard anywhere around the heart.
- Congestive heart failure
- Fatigue
- Syncope
- Chest pain

PROGNOSIS

Medications can help the heart to pump more efficiently. Some medications are used for disease management; others are used for symptom control. Monitoring dietary intake of sodium and fluids can also help with symptom control.

Heart failure is the main complication of heart disease, produced by an abnormality of pumping function. The heart is unable to carry blood effectively to meet metabolic needs. The resulting problems include acute left ventricular dysfunction usually due to arrhythmias and myocardial infarction, and chronic failure due to fluid overload, usually in valvular heart disease.

Heart failure is a compromise of any of the following:

- Contractility of the muscle
- Heart rate
- Ventricular preload
- Ventricular afterload

While most hearts can tolerate some changes in the above items, some diseased, older hearts may not be able to do so; heart failure results.

Treatment results of early disease are usually good. Long-term prognosis can be variable, depending on the severity of the disease and associated conditions.

HALLMARK SIGNS AND SYMPTOMS

- Early:
  - Basilar rales from fluid overload
  - Nocturia
  - Exertional dyspnea
  - Fatigue
  - Positive hepatojuglar reflux from liver congestion
  - S3 heart sound
- Mid:
  - Cough
  - Orthopnea
  - Discomfort in right upper abdomen due to hepatomegaly
  - Cardiac rales
  - Edema
  - Cardiomegaly
- Late:
  - Anasarca—generalized edema from ineffective pump function
  - Frothy or pink sputum from capillary permeability

INTERPRETING TEST RESULTS

- B-type natriuretic peptide—elevated levels in CHF; produced when the ventricles are stretched.
- EKG may show signs of ischemia (T-wave inversion), tachycardia, or extra-systole (extra beats).
- CBC may show anemia—Hgb less than 12 in female, less than 14 in male; HCT; less than 3 times the Hgb.
- Chemistry may show renal problems, electrolyte disturbance.

- Chest x-ray.
  - Left-sided heart failure:
    - Pulmonary congestion because of accumulation of fluid in the lungs.
    - Enlarged left ventricle (LVH) because of the increased stress on the heart to pump blood.
  - Right-sided heart failure:
    - Pulmonary congestion because of accumulation of fluid in the lungs.
    - Accumulation of fluid in the pleural cavity (pleural effusion).
    - Enlarged heart (cardiomegaly) because of the increased stress on the heart to pump blood.

TREATMENT

Treatment is aimed at the underlying disease, i.e. ischemia, valve defects, arrhythmias. Excreting volume with diuretics, supplemental oxygen, use of medications to reduce workload of heart muscle, peripheral vascular resistance (afterload), and venous return to the heart (preload) may all be used. Dietary indiscretions may be a contributing factor, i.e. too much salt, too many calories.

- Administer diuretics for symptom control resulting in patient comfort by reducing blood volume.
  - Furosemide, bumetanide, metolazone, hydrochlorothiazide, spironolactone —be aware of electrolyte imbalance—these medications may alter the K+ level.
- Administer ACE inhibitors to decrease afterload.
  - Captopril, enalapril, lisinopril.
- Administer beta blockers, which help to raise ejection fraction, and decrease ventricular size.
- Administer inotrope to strengthen myocardial contractility:
  - Digoxin.
- Administer vasodilator to reduce preload, relieve dyspnea:
  - nitroprusside, nitroglycerin ointment.
- Administer anticoagulants in patients with severe heart failure, as they have a propensity to develop thrombus and emboli; those with concurrent atrial fibrillation will also need anticoagulation.
- Reduce fluids as fluid overload is a causative factor in CHF.

- High Fowler's position to ease breathing and enhance diaphragmatic excursion.
- Supplemental oxygen to meet increased demand of myocardium.
- Low-sodium diet to prevent additional fluid retention.

NURSING DIAGNOSES

- Impaired gas exchange
- Decreased cardiac output
- Excess fluid volume

NURSING INTERVENTION

- Monitor vital signs and look for changes.
- Record fluid intake and output—weigh daily to assess for fluid overload.
- Position patient in semi-Fowler's position to ease breathing.
- Administer oxygen as ordered because it helps to decrease workload of heart.
- Tell the patient:
  - Eat foods low in sodium to avoid fluid retention. (For these patients, there is no such thing as "low-salt" cold cuts.)
  - Raise legs when sitting to lessen dependent edema.
  - Call the physician, nurse practitioner, or physician assistant if experiencing fluid retention, such as a weight gain of several pounds in 1 to 2 days.

11 *Hypertension (HTN)*

WHAT WENT WRONG?

Pressure inside blood vessels exceeds 140 mmHg systolic and 90 mmHg diastolic on more than one occasion resulting from a primary disease or no known cause. These are the classifications of hypertension:

- Normal <120 mmHg systolic / <80 mmHg diastolic
- Prehypertension: 120–139 mmHg systolic / 80–89 mmHg diastolic
- Stage 1 hypertension: 140–159 mmHg systolic / 90–99 mmHg diastolic

- Stage 2 hypertension: ≥ 160 mmHg / systolic ≥ 100 mmHg diastolic
- In diabetic patients: hypertension is defined as 130/80 or higher

PROGNOSIS

The vast majority of patients have primary hypertension, or high blood pressure, that is not caused by other disease. Patients are typically asymptomatic and need to understand the importance of treatment to avoid long-term complications. End organ damage can affect the heart, kidneys, brain, or eyes. Adequate control of blood pressure is possible with medications and lifestyle modification, but these need to be maintained for the long term, often for the rest of the patient's life. Many patients will ultimately need to be on multiple medications to achieve adequate blood pressure control.

HALLMARK SIGNS AND SYMPTOMS

- Asymptomatic
- Headache
- Dizziness

INTERPRETING TEST RESULTS

- Blood pressure readings higher than 140/90 mmHg on at least three occasions.
- Ventricular hypertrophy depicted on EKG or chest x-ray.
- Blood test to look for associated cardiovascular risks.
  - High cholesterol—often associated with hypertension.
  - Check electrolytes for imbalance—sodium, potassium, chloride, CO_2.
  - Monitor BUN and creatinine for renal function, a sign of impaired organ damage.
  - Chemistry to check for diabetes mellitus.

TREATMENT

Treatment is aimed at decreasing the risk of CVA, CAD, heart failure, renal disease, and other long-term sequelae of hypertension. Risk factors need to be assessed:

- Smoking
- Dyslipidemia—elevated cholesterol, LDL, triglycerides, low HDL
- Diabetes
- Age greater than 60
- Men and postmenopausal females
- Family history

Non-pharmacologic interventions are tried first, then medications are prescribed.

There is a four-step treatment plan:

- Step 1:
  - Lifestyle changes
  - Reduce caloric intake and exercise to reduce weight
  - Low-sodium diet
  - No smoking
  - Reduce alcohol intake
  - Reduce caffeine intake
- Step 2: Begin medication
  - Administer diuretics to reduce circulating blood volume:
    - furosemide, spironolactone, hydrochlorothazide, bumetanide
  - Beta-adrenergic blockers to lower heart rate and cardiac output:
    - propranolol, metroprolol, atenolol
  - Calcium channel blockers to cause peripheral vasodilation, less tachycardia:
    - verapamil, diltiazem, nicardipine
  - Administer ACE to inhibit the rennin angiotensin aldosterone system. In diabetes, ACE inhibitors also delay the progression of renal disease.
    - enalapril, lisinopril, benazepril, captopril, fosinopril, quinapril, perindopril
- Step 3:
  - Increase dosages of currently administered medication
- Step 4:
  - Combination of agents in above classes
  - Multiple drugs may be needed to control blood pressure

NURSING DIAGNOSES

- Imbalanced nutrition: more than the body requires.
- Knowledge deficit
- Excess fluid volume

NURSING INTERVENTION

- Monitor blood pressure with multiple readings—lying, sitting, and standing, bilateral both arms.
- Record fluid intake and output.

  Reduce stress by providing a quiet environment.
- Explain to the patient:
  - No smoking—smoking contributes to cardiovascular disease, raising blood pressure.
  - Change to a low-sodium and low-cholesterol diet—salt adds to elevated blood pressure in some patients by contributing to fluid retention; lower cholesterol intake lowers risk for associated hyperlipidemia.
  - Reduce alcohol intake—reduces risk for end organ damage from alcohol intake.
  - Reduce weight—decreased risk for obesity, better BP control with better weight control.
  - Exercise.
  - Call physician when BP is elevated.
  - Side effects of medications.

12 *Hypovolemic Shock*

WHAT WENT WRONG?

Rapid fluid loss causes inadequate circulation resulting in inadequate perfusion of organs. Hypovolemic shock can be caused by external hemorrhage, fluids moving in the body from vessels into tissue (third spacing), or dehydration. External hemorrhage is loss of blood, plasma, fluids and electrolytes, due to trauma, GI bleed, vomiting, or diarrhea. Third spacing can result from ascites or pancreatitis.

PROGNOSIS

Prognosis depends on the etiology of the low volume; there may occasionally be more than one reason.

HALLMARK SIGNS AND SYMPTOMS

- Hypotension because blood volume in the body is decreased
- Urine output less than 25 ml/hour because less blood is perfusing the kidneys, causing decreased urinary output
- Heart rate >100 (tachycardia), because the heart attempts to compensate for the decreased volume
- Cold skin, because of peripheral vasoconstriction due to decreased volume
- Restlessness, agitation; may be seen due to poor perfusion of the brain

INTERPRETING TEST RESULTS

- Blood tests.
  - CBC anemia.
  - Chemistry to look at volume as depicted by the creatinine and BUN.
  - Coagulation studies.
  - Type and cross-match for blood transfusion.
- Arterial Blood Gas (ABG)
  - Decrease pH—if not perfusing well, acidosis will occur.
  - Metabolic acidosis—byproducts of metabolism will accumulate.
  - Increase partial pressure of arterial carbon dioxide and decrease partial pressure of arterial oxygen due to poor perfusion.

TREATMENT

Treatment depends on severity of symptoms. As always, maintaining open airway, breathing, circulation, and fluid resuscitation is of vital importance. After stabilization, the focus is on determining and treating the cause of the shock.

- Control bleeding—CBC, stool guaiac test, [to find hidden (occult) blood in stool], assess for bleeding.
- Replace fluid—proper fluid replacement depends on the etiology of the shock; IV fluid and/or blood products are the choices.

NURSING DIAGNOSES

- Deficient fluid volume
- Ineffective tissue perfusion
- Decreased cardiac output

NURSING INTERVENTION

- IV using 14G catheter (16 or 18 gauge also adequate if not able to obtain 14; use largest possible):
  - Lactated Ringer's solution (which contains electrolytes) or normal saline (0.9 percent).
  - Blood replacement—type-specific or type O negative, which is the universal donor type.
- Monitor every 15 minutes:
  - Blood pressure. If systolic lower than 80 mmHg, then increase oxygen flow rate.
  - Vital Signs every 15 minutes.
- Measure urine output each hour with indwelling urinary catheter. Increase fluid rate if urine output is less than 30 ml/hour. Be alert for signs of fluid overflow. These include, but are not limited to, crackles in the lungs and dyspnea.
- Assess for cool, pale, clammy skin, indicating hypovolemic shock.
- Explain to the patient:
  - What caused the hypovolemia and how to avoid a recurrence.
  - The purpose of the treatment.

13 *Myocarditis*

WHAT WENT WRONG?

Inflammation of the heart muscle is usually caused by infection, most often viral. Infection can also be caused by alcohol poisoning from chronic alcohol abuse, drugs, or diseases that can result in the degeneration of heart muscle. This reduces the ability of the heart to pump blood efficiently, leading to congestive heart failure.

PROGNOSIS

Outcomes vary depending on the etiology. Improvement depends on the stresses of the causative disease. Some resolve spontaneously; others develop dilated cardiomyopathy, CHF.

HALLMARK SIGNS AND SYMPTOMS

- Fever because of infectious process
- Tachycardia
- Difficulty breathing (dyspnea) because left side dysfunction leads to CHF
- Chest pain
- Hear sounds:
  - S3 gallop due to fluid overload

INTERPRETING TEST RESULTS

- EKG.
  - ST-segment changes due to inflammatory changes in the heart due to the irritability of the myocardium from an infectious process.
- Endomyocardial biopsy to determine a specific organism and the presence of inflammation after infection has resolved.
- CXR—cardiomegaly.
- Echocardiogram to assess cardiac size and function.
- Labs—CK, MB, and troponins because of cell injury and death.

TREATMENT

Treatment is directed at the causative factor(s). Occasionally treatment may include support for CHF and antiarrhythmics, if needed.

- Administer antiarrhythmics to stabilize an irritable heart:
  - quinidine
  - procainamide

NURSING DIAGNOSES

- Hyperthermia
- Decreased cardiac output
- Activity intolerance

NURSING INTERVENTION

- Temporarily limit the patient's activities to decrease stress on the heart.
- Provide bedside commode.
- Monitor for:
  - Difficulty breathing (dyspnea) because fluid overload.
  - Heart rate >100 beats per minute (tachycardia) because infection or inflammation may increase the heart rate.
- No competitive sports.
- Return to normal activities slowly once physician approves.

14 *Pericarditis*

WHAT WENT WRONG?

The membrane that encloses the heart (pericardium) is inflamed. Pericarditis is either acute or chronic.

Acute pericarditis is most commonly associated with viral infections. Upper respiratory symptoms are not uncommon and can occur a few weeks prior to the onset of pericarditis. Pericarditis may be caused by any infectious agent, AMI, malignancy, autoimmune diseases, or drug reaction.

PROGNOSIS

Outcome of acute pericarditis is often self-limited, resolving in two to six weeks. Patients are typically treated with nonsteroidal anti-inflammatories (NSAIDs) to decrease the inflammation of the pericardium.

HALLMARK SIGNS AND SYMPTOMS

- Acute:
  - A grating heart sound heard (pericardial friction rub) due to friction from inflammation between the layers surrounding the heart
  - Sudden sharp pain over the precordium (mid- to lower sternum area) radiating to the neck, shoulders, back, and arm
  - Pain decreases when the patient leans forward, sits up
  - Teeth pain, anxiety, myalgias
  - Difficulty breathing (dyspnea), rapid breathing (tachypnea)
  - Arrhythmias
- Chronic:
  - Enlarged liver (hepatomegaly), ascites because of liver congestion
  - Increased fluid retention due to ineffective pumping
  - Pericardial friction rub

INTERPRETING TEST RESULTS

- Increase WBC and sed rate (the rate at which red blood cells settle in a test tube. A high rate indicates inflammation), thyroid studies, renal function, Rh factor, ANA complement.
- May see increased CK (creatine kinase), LDH (lactate dehydrogenase), liver enzymes levels.
- EKG.
  - Sinus tachycardia.

- ST-segment elevation.
- Echocardiogram shows echo-free space between pericardium and the ventricular wall due to effusion; also shows fluid in the pericardial space.
- CXR may show fluid in spaces.

TREATMENT

Treatment is directed at resolving the underlying etiology.

Pericardiocentesis is done to remove fluid from the pericardial sac to relieve pressure on the heart or for diagnostic testing. A long cardiac needle is inserted near the xiphoid process and fluid is aspirated during careful cardiac monitoring.

Pericardial biopsy

- Administer corticosteroids to decrease inflammation of pericardium.
  - Methylprednisolone.
- Administer nonsteroidal anti-inflammatory (NSAID) drugs to decrease inflammation of the pericardium and provide for pain relief.
  - Aspirin, indomethacin.

NURSING DIAGNOSES

- Acute pain
- Decreased cardiac output
- Risk for activity intolerance

NURSING INTERVENTION

- Place the patient in full Fowler's position to ease breathing.
- Explain to the patient:
  - He/she will recover.
  - Slowly resume daily activities.
  - Plan for rest periods during the day due to fatigue.
  - Perform coughing and deep breathing exercises—patient may have been avoiding deep breathing due to discomfort.

15 *Pulmonary Edema*

WHAT WENT WRONG?

Fluid builds up in the lungs as a result of ineffective pumping of blood by the heart as a result of left-sided heart failure, AMI, worsening of heart failure, or volume overload. The patient experiences hypoxia, which is insufficient oxygen supply to tissues, caused by decreased oxygenation of the blood. Several noncardiac issues may lead to pulmonary embolism.

PROGNOSIS

Poor heart function results in fluid overload, which results in further diminished cardiac function, causing marked dyspnea.

HALLMARK SIGNS AND SYMPTOMS

- Difficulty breathing even when sitting upright (because of the fluid in the lungs)
- Rapid breathing: greater than 20 breaths per minute (tachypnea), because the body is trying to get more oxygen
- Frothy sputum with a tinge of blood due to capillary permeability
- Cyanosis
- Cool, clammy skin because the body is diverting blood flow from the periphery
- Restlessness and fear due to lack of oxygenation
- Distended jugular vein due to increased pressure within chest
- Crackles, wheezing heard in the lungs as the air moves through the fluid

INTERPRETING TEST RESULTS

- Oxygen saturation under 90 percent.
- CXR: aleveolar fluid, large heart.
- Echocardiogram to determine ejection fraction percentages in the heart.

TREATMENT

Treatment may continue at home unless a worsening change in condition merits hospitalization. Immediate treatment of heart failure, while searching for underlying correctable conditions, is necessary.

- Administer supplemental oxygen, which increases arterial pO_2. Mechanical ventilation may be necessary.
- Administer morphine, which lowers left atrial pressure, decreases myocardial oxygen demand, lowers anxiety, and relieves pain.
- Administer diuretics to remove excess fluid:
  - furosemide, bumetanide, meolazone
- Administer cardiac glycosides to increase contractions of the heart:
  - digoxin
- Administer cardiac inotropics to strengthen the heart:
  - dobutamine
  - inamrinone
  - milrinone
- Administer nitrates to decrease BP, and left ventricular filling pressures:
  - isosorbide dinitrate

NURSING DIAGNOSES

- Impaired gas exchange
- Anxiety
- Excess fluid volume

NURSING INTERVENTION

- Place the patient in full Fowler's position to enhance air exchange and diaphragmatic movement, sitting with legs dangling over sides of bed.
- Monitor cardiovascular function for changes in heart sounds, extra sounds, murmurs.
- Monitor respirations for changes in lung sounds, chest expansion.

- Check oxygen saturation (pulse oximetry).
- Record fluid intake and output.
- Weigh the patient daily. Call physician if patient gains 2 lbs daily.
- Call physician if BUN and creatinine increase.
- Record characteristics of sputum.
- Explain to the patient:
  - Call the physician, nurse practitioner, or physician assistant if the patient detects fluid overload: weight gain, shortness of breath, fatigue, chest pains.
  - Call 911 if in respiratory distress.
  - Decrease sodium in diet.
  - Sleep with head elevated i.e. three pillows, or blocks under head of bed frame.

16 Raynaud's Disease

WHAT WENT WRONG?

Blood flow to the extremities decreases as peripheral arteries narrow from vasospasm when exposed to cold or emotional stress. This results in the fingers, toes, nose, and ears blanching to a pale shade and/or turning blue and red as blood flow decreases. It usually occurs bilaterally, often sparing the thumbs, and begins to resolve with warming of affected areas. Raynaud's is a benign condition usually controlled by avoidance of underlying factors, i.e., cold and stress. Secondary Raynaud's can be seen with other disorders, mostly inflammatory and/or connective tissue diseases. This is more common in older men, usually involves the hands, and can have other complications.

PROGNOSIS

Prognosis for primary Raynaud's is good. Symptoms may be controlled by avoidance or by medications. In secondary Raynaud's, long-term ischemic complications may develop, such as loss of fat pads of fingers, gangrene due to diminished sensation, and propensity to develop frostbite.

HALLMARK SIGNS AND SYMPTOMS

- Discoloration of extremities progressing from pale, to blue, and then red because of decreased blood flow
- Tingling and numbness in the extremities because of poor perfusion

INTERPRETING TEST RESULTS

- Vasospasm is detected in an arteriograph.
- Labwork to look for underlying disease process—CBC may show anemia; sed rate (ESR), rheumatoid arthritis (RA), antinuclear antibody (ANA) (these autoimmune tests will be positive).

TREATMENT

Treatment is outpatient and consists of avoidance of aggravating factors and may need medication for primary, and treatment of underlying disorders and ischemia in secondary.

- Administer calcium channel blockers to ameliorate symptoms:
  - diltiazem
  - nifedipine
- Administer vasodilators to aid in blood flow.
- Avoid cold and stress because this may causes vasospasms.
- Avoid smoking because it causes vasoconstriction.
- Surgical removal of a part of a sympathetic nerve (sympathectomy) because it can eliminate symptoms.

NURSING DIAGNOSES

- Risk for injury
- Risk for peripheral neurovascular dysfunction
- Ineffective tissue perfusion

NURSING INTERVENTION

- Teach patient to wear mittens rather than gloves when exposed to the cold because it allows for air flow around fingers to hold body heat.

- Explain to the patient:
  - Stop smoking.
  - Avoid cold.
  - Inspect skin regularly for cracks and treat immediately to prevent infections.
  - Moisturizers.

17   *Rheumatic Heart Disease*

WHAT WENT WRONG?

Rheumatic fever usually results from a prior upper respiratory infection with group A streptococcus. It may lead to permanent valve disease and cardiac damage, with the mitral valve being more commonly affected.

PROGNOSIS

Prognosis of rheumatic heart disease (RHD) depends on the amount of damage done to the valves. When progressive valve disease occurs in the mitral valve, it is imperative to recognize the early onset of atrial fibrillation, to ensure early initiation of anticoagulation to prevent emboli.

HALLMARK SIGNS AND SYMPTOMS

- A new murmur of insufficiency S3
- Joint pain because of the inflammation
- Increased temperature greater than 100.3°F because it may signify infection
- Carditis—chest pain, heart failure, friction rub

INTERPRETING TEST RESULTS

- Increase in cardiac enzymes to look for other causes of chest pain
- Positive C-reactive protein, ESR which are elevated in inflammation
- Increase in WBC because it may be of infectious origin
- Echocardiogram to assess for damage to valves

TREATMENT

Treatment of RHD is based on the severity of the valve damage. Valve replacement may be necessary. If a fibrillation (contracting of the heart) is present, ensure adequate anticoagulation with an International Normalized Ratio between 2 and 3. Rheumatic fever prophylaxis may be required; antibiotics are recommended for prevention of recurrent episodes.

- Administer nonsteroidal anti-inflammatory medication to decrease inflammation and pain:
  - aspirin
  - indomethacin
- Administer antibiotics if an infectious process is confirmed:
  - erythromycin
  - penicillin
- Repair or replacement of heart valves due to irreparable damage.
- Antibiotic prophylaxis for unsterile procedures—usually penicillin; if allergic to penicillin, clindamycin is usually the drug of choice.
- Anticoagulation if atrial fibrillation.

NURSING DIAGNOSES

- Decrease cardiac output
- Activity intolerance
- Risk for infection

NURSING INTERVENTION

- Monitor for difficulty breathing (dyspnea) and hacking, nonproductive cough, because these are signs of heart failure.
- Determine if patient is allergic to penicillin.
- Monitor for infection because rheumatic fever may recur:
  - Red, sore throat with pain when swallowing.
  - Swollen cervical lymph glands.
  - Headache.
  - Temperature greater than 100°F.

- Explain to patient:
  - Anticoagulation use, interference with foods and medications, need for frequent lab monitoring.
  - Avoid contact with anyone who has a respiratory tract infection.
  - Maintain good dental hygiene.
  - Call the physician, nurse practitioner, or physician assistant if detect signs of heart failure: shortness of breath, weight gain, nonproductive cough.
  - Return to normal activities slowly.

18 *Thrombophlebitis*

WHAT WENT WRONG?

Throbmophlebitis is the inflammation of a vein as a result of the formation of one or more blood clots (thrombus). It is usually seen in the lower extremities, calves, or pelvis. This may be the result of injury to the area, may be precipitated by certain medications or poor blood flow, or may be the result of a coagulation disorder.

PROGNOSIS

Prognosis is usually good unless embolization, or moving of the clot, occurs. It may move to the lung or brain, which can be life-threatening.

HALLMARK SIGNS AND SYMPTOMS

- May be asymptomatic
- Edema, tenderness, and warmth in the affected area as part of an inflammatory response
- Palpable tender cord
- Positive Homan's sign—pain on dorsiflexion of the ipsalateral foot—is an unreliable sign
- Cramping because blood flow to the area is impaired due to the presence of the clot

- If the clot dislodges from the vein and travels to the lung, other symptoms will develop:
  - Difficulty breathing (dyspnea) when the clot has traveled to the lungs
  - Rapid breathing >20 breaths per minute (tachypnea) because of a clot in the lungs
  - Chest pain in the area of clot
  - Crackle sounds in lungs in the area of clot

INTERPRETING TEST RESULTS

- Ultrasound determines if blood is flowing to the affected area.
- Photoplethysmography depicts any defects in venous filling in the affected area.
- Lab work to look for clotting disorders.

TREATMENT

Patients with large deep vein thrombosis (DVT), or with comorbidities (a disease coexisting with, and often impacting on, another disease present), and/or advanced age should be managed in the hospital. Treatment consists of anticoagulation to prevent further occurrences.

- Administer anti-inflammatory medication to decrease the inflammation within the vessel
  - aspirin, indomethacin
- Administer anticoagulant medication to prevent the clot from becoming larger:
  - heparin, warfarin, dalteparin, enoxaparin
- Limit activity initially to diminish risk of moving clot—bedrest with bathroom priviledges

NURSING DIAGNOSES

- Ineffective tissue perfusion
- Acute pain
- Impaired skin integrity

NURSING INTERVENTION

- Monitor breathing because changes in respiratory status can signal that a clot has dislodged and moved to the lung.
- Monitor labs because the patient is receiving anticoagulants. Monitor for therapeutic effect.
- Apply warm moist compresses over affected area because it enhances blood flow to area.
- Explain to the patient:
  - Report signs of bleeding—anticoagulant may be too much.
  - Report signs of clotting—pain in affected area, shortness of breath—patient may have underlying clotting disorder.
  - Move about frequently when allowed—discourages chances of developing another clot.
  - Don't cross legs—avoid constriction of lower extremity vessels.
  - Don't use oral contraceptives—increases risk of clot formation.
  - Support hose.
  - Elevate affected area.

19 *Atrial Fibrillation*

WHAT WENT WRONG?

Uncoordinated firing of electrical impulses in the wall of the atria (upper chambers of the heart) causes the heart to quiver instead of beating regularly, resulting in ineffective contractions. This is usually due to an abnormality in the electrical system of the heart. Blood is ineffectively pumped to the ventricles (lower chambers of the heart) and may result in not enough blood being pumped throughout the body. Usually the heart beats rapidly; however, this is not always the case. Atrial fibrillation (also called AF or "a fib") is the most common chronic arrhythmia and is not life-threatening on its own, but increases the patient's risk for blood clots and strokes.

PROGNOSIS

The arrhythmia usually goes away once the cause of atrial fibrillation is identified and treated. If left untreated or if it returns, there is a risk of stroke and other complications.

HALLMARK SIGNS AND SYMPTOMS

- Asymptomatic
- Irregular pulse
- Feeling faint (near syncope)
- Palpitations
- Lightheadedness
- Dyspnea

INTERPRETING TEST RESULTS

- Electrocardiogram will show irregularities characteristic of the disease:
  - QRS complexes are of irregular duration and structure.
  - PR interval barely noticeable.
  - Erratic, low-voltage, or absent P-waves.
- Echocardiogram to look for structural abnormalities.
- Thyroid function tests as hyperthyroidism can lead to atrial fibrillation.

TREATMENT

Treatment is directed towards restoring the regular heart rate and rhythm. If the atrial fibrillation is less than 72 hours old, chemical or electrocardioversion is endeavored. Electrocardioversion, or shocking the heart, often restores normal sinus rhythm. If greater than 72 hours, anticoagulation is begun as the risk of thromboembolism is great.

- Administer antiarrhythmics once patient stabilizes—these medications may be effective in restoring a regular rhythm and also for in long-term therapy:
  - amiodarone
  - digoxin
  - diltiazem
  - verapamil
- Unstable patient: Synchronized cardioversion is a treatment that involves an electrical shock delivered to the heart, which is synchronized with the R- or S-wave of the EKG, in an attempt to restore coordinated firing of electrical impulses.

- Install a pacemaker.
- If atrial fibrillation is the ongoing rhythm, warfarin therapy will be initiated to reduce the risk of emboli.

NURSING DIAGNOSES

- Impaired gas exchange
- Decreased cardiac output
- Ineffective tissue perfusion

NURSING INTERVENTION

- Monitor for signs of decreased blood flow to tissues or organs (hypoperfusion) because decreased cardiac output, as indicated by these symptoms, can occur as a result of atrial fibrillation:
  - Decreased pulse pressure.
  - Cool extremities.
  - Altered mental state.
  - Rapid resting heart rate.
  - Alternating breathing between deep and shallow.
  - Increased BUN.
- Prepare for synchronized cardioversion, if patient is unstable.
- Assess for life-threatening arrhythmias.
- Assess for signs of drug toxicity and withhold if the patient is toxic—i.e., seizures, respiratory arrest, arrhythmias.
- Limit patient's activities to reduce cardiac workload.
- Explain to the patient:
  - The need for warfarin therapy, as well as monitoring of INR, diet modifications, use of NSAIDs, and aspirin.
  - The importance of regular examinations to ascertain for any changes in rhythm.
  - Call the physician if the patient feels light-headed or dizzy, as this can be a symptom of a change in rhythm.
  - Avoid ethanol, caffeine, nicotine as they can trigger an arrhythmia.

- Proper care and restrictions if the patient has a pacemaker—frequent monitoring of the pacemaker battery, who will follow up with the cardiologist, and so on. Frequency depends on the type of pacemaker and the cardiologist.

20 *Asystole*

WHAT WENT WRONG?

Asystole is defined as no cardiac electrical activity. This causes ventricles to stop contractions, leading to no cardiac output and no blood flow. Cardiac standstill is a medical emergency. Treatment must be started immediately, while simultaneously attempting to understand the etiology of a non-beating heart. Asystole is a criterion for certifying that the patient is dead. Asystole may be caused by disruption in the electrical conduction system, causing life-threatening arrhythmias, sudden cardiac death, hypovolemia, cardiac tamponade, massive pulmonary embolism, acute myocardial infarction, metabolic disorder, or drug overdoses. In case of a drug overdose—usually PEA (pulseless electrical activity)—reverse overdose or treat.

PROGNOSIS

Prognosis is poor unless the heart can be started. The longer asystole continues, the more tissue is lost.

HALLMARK SIGNS AND SYMPTOMS

- No pulse
- Cyanosis
- Apnea
- No palpable blood pressure

INTERPRETING TEST RESULTS

- Electrocardiogram—P-, QRS–, T-waves are barely noticeable or absent.
- Arterial blood gases.

- Lab work—CBC, electrolytes, drug levels, coagulation studies.
- No atrial or ventricular rhythm on the electrocardiogram.

TREATMENT

Treatment consists of restarting the heart and, when that has occurred, determining the cause of the asystole. Basic Life Support (CPR) should optimally be started within two minutes (once asystole is established, CPR should be initiated immediately when asystole is detected, and Advanced Cardiac Life Support within eight minutes.

- Cardiopulmonary resuscitation.
- Advanced Cardiac Life Support.
- Oxygen.
- Start IVs to maintain access.
- Transcutaneous pacing, where electrodes are placed on the front and back of the chest while high current is delivered to the patient to pace the ventricles.
- Endotracheal intubation.
- Administer buffering agent to correct acidosis:
  - sodium bicarbonate
- Administer antiarrhythmics to control arrhythmia:
  - atropine
  - epinephrine

NURSING DIAGNOSES

- Impaired gas exchange
- Decreased cardiac output
- Ineffective tissue perfusion

NURSING INTERVENTION

- Begin CPR.
- Prepare to administer medication per physician's order or protocol.

- Explain to the patient:
  - Note: If asytole exists, patient is not conscious. Talk to family members if they are present. Refer to Basic Life Support (BLS) protocol.
  - Call the physician, nurse practitioner, or physician assistant if the patient experiences dizziness.
  - The importance of regular examinations.

21 *Ventricular Fibrillation*

WHAT WENT WRONG?

Electrical impulses, that trigger the ventricles to contract, fire erratically. This causes the ventricles to quiver and prevents regular effective contractions, resulting in the disruption of blood flow to the body. The usual causes are ventricular tachycardia, electrolyte disturbances, myocardial infarction, electric shock, and drug toxicities.

PROGNOSIS

Prognosis depends on how long it takes to establish a beating heart.

HALLMARK SIGNS AND SYMPTOMS

- No pulse
- Breathing is stopped (apnea)
- No palpable blood pressure

INTERPRETING TEST RESULTS

- Electrocardiogram:
  - Chaotic ventricular rhythm.
  - QRS irregular and wide.
  - P-wave barely noticeable.

TREATMENT

- Cardiopulmonary resuscitation (CPR).
- Advanced Cardiac Life Support (ACLS).

- Defibrillation (refer to ACLS protocol).
- Endotracheal intubation to manually compress a bag to squeeze air (referred to as bag valve mask ventilation) and thus, oxygen, into the lungs.
- Administer buffering agent to correct acidosis:
  - sodium bicarbonate
- Administer antiarrhythmics to control arrhythmia:
  - lidocaine
  - epinephrine
  - bretylium
  - procainamide

NURSING DIAGNOSES

- Impaired gas exchange
- Decreased cardiac output
- Ineffective tissue perfusion

NURSING INTERVENTION

- Begin CPR (place on monitor, BP, P, R, pulse-oximetry).
- Perform defibrillation, if certified.
- Prepare to administer medications per physician's order or protocol.
- Explain to the patient:
  - Note: Patient is more than likely noncoherent. Speak to family.
  - Call the physician, nurse practitioner, or physician assistant if the patient experiences dizziness.
  - The importance of regular examinations.

22 *Ventricular Tachycardia*

WHAT WENT WRONG?

Abnormal electrical impulses within the ventricles cause the heart to contract more than 160 beats per minute. This results in inadequate filling of the ventricles with blood between beats; subsequently, less blood is pumped throughout the body than during normal contractions.

Ventricular tachycardia (called "V tach") often occurs after acute myocardial infarction and in cardiomyopathy, CAD, mitral valve prolapse, and other myocardial disease.

PROGNOSIS

Prognosis depends on the duration of the arrhythmia, and prompt response. Recurrent V tach signals a poor prognosis.

HALLMARK SIGNS AND SYMPTOMS

- Unconscious
- Apnea or diminished breathing
- Pale, diaphoretic skin
- Dizziness because less oxygen is reaching the brain
- Hypotension because blood flow is increased to a rate that reduces time available to oxygenate tissues
- Weak pulses due to poor perfusion

INTERPRETING TEST RESULTS

- Arterial Blood Gas (ABG).
- Electrolytes.
- CBC.
- Drug levels.
- Coagulation studies.
- Electrocardiogram:
  - Unusual QRS.
  - No P-wave.
- Ventricular tachycardia may suddenly start and stop depending on the irritability of the heart.
- Ventricle contractions greater than 160 beats per minute.

TREATMENT

Treatment consists of establishing a regular rate and rhythm.

- Cardiopulmonary resuscitation if pulse is absent (refer to ACLS: pulseless V tach requires defibrillation).
- Advanced Cardiac Life Support if pulse is absent.
- Endotracheal intubation.
- Oxygen.
- Administer antiarrhythmics to control arrhythmia:
  - lidocaine
  - epinephrine
  - bretylium
  - procainamide
  - amiodarone
- Synchronized cardioversion is an electrical discharge that is synchronized with the R- or S-wave of the QRS complex to restore coordinated firing of electrical impulses.

NURSING DIAGNOSES

- Impaired gas exchange
- Decreased cardiac output
- Ineffective tissue perfusion

NURSING INTERVENTION

- Begin CPR if pulse is absent.
- Prepare to administer medication per physician's order or protocol.
- Explain to the patient the necessity of follow-up.
  - Call the physician if the patient experiences dizziness.
  - The importance of regular examinations.

23 *Aortic Insufficiency (AI)*

WHAT WENT WRONG?

Leakage of the aortic valve causes blood to flow back into the left ventricle. This results in increased blood volume in the left ventricle, causing it to dilate and become hypertrophic, thus reducing blood flow from the heart. The usual cause is incompetent cusps or leaflets of the valve, from endocarditis, valve structural problems, connective tissue disorders, rheumatic heart disease, hypertension, arteriosclerosis, and other conditions.

PROGNOSIS

Prognosis depends on the severity of the valve damage and the acuteness of the symptoms in the patient.

HALLMARK SIGNS AND SYMPTOMS

- Difficulty breathing (dyspnea) because of ineffective pumping
- Fatigue
- Orthopnea
- Palpations because the heart is irritable due to improper blood flow

INTERPRETING TEST RESULTS

- X-ray shows an enlarged left ventricle.
- Echocardiogram confirms the left ventricle is enlarged and the valve is working inefficiently.

TREATMENT

Treatment is based on the gravity of the symptoms of the patient.

- Aortic valve replacement or repair.
- Administer anticoagulant medication following surgery to prevent thrombus around the aortic valve:

- heparin
- warfarin
- enoxaparin

NURSING DIAGNOSES

- Anxiety
- Decreased cardiac output
- Activity intolerance

NURSING INTERVENTION

- Place patient in a high Fowler's position to facilitate breathing.
- Oxygen.
- Pain management.
- Monitor for:
  - Pulmonary edema because of backflow to the lungs.
  - Thrombus because a foreign object (valve) is in place, and may cause clotting.
  - Arrhythmias because the heart may be irritable secondary to surgery.
- Weigh the patient daily to be aware of fluid overload.
- Explain to the patient:
  - Schedule rest periods during the day.
  - Restrict diet to low-sodium and low-fat foods.

24 *Mitral Insufficiency*

WHAT WENT WRONG?

Leakage of the mitral valve causes blood to flow back from the left ventricle into the left atrium. As a result, blood might flow back into the lungs. Mitral regurgitation is due to an incompetent valve, damaged from rheumatic fever, CAD, or endocarditis.

PROGNOSIS

The prognosis may be chronic with stabilization of symptoms, or acute, usually after myocardial infarction, leading to valve replacement.

HALLMARK SIGNS AND SYMPTOMS

- Orthopnea due to the pressure rising into the atria, causing backflow into the lungs.
- Fatigue because of an ineffective heart.
- Systolic murmur at the apex, S3 gallop.
- Left ventricular hypertrophy—the size of the ventricle can reflect the amount of regurgitation.

INTERPRETING TEST RESULTS

- Echocardiogram shows the underlying etiology of the insufficiency.
- Cardiac catheterization depicts the flow through the mitral valve; can measure amount of regurgitation as well as pressures in the chambers.

TREATMENT

Patients with chronic, stable disease may be managed for years without symptoms, or their symptoms may be under control with medication. Others may require surgery, again, based on the symptoms. Ventricular damage may occur before symptoms present, so frequent monitoring is indicated.

- Administer vasodilators to reduce flow by lowering systemic vascular resistance.
- Administer anticoagulant medication following surgery to prevent thrombus around the aortic valve:
  - heparin
  - warfarin
  - enoxaparin
- Mitral valve repair or replacement.

NURSING DIAGNOSES

- Anxiety
- Decreased cardiac output
- Activity intolerance

NURSING INTERVENTION

- Place patient in a high Fowler's position to facilitate breathing.
- Monitor for:
  - Pulmonary edema because of fluid overload.
  - Thrombus because of a prosthetic valve.
  - Arrhythmias because the heart may be irritable during and after surgery.
  - Intake and output to monitor fluid balance.
- Weigh the patient daily to check fluid overload.
- Explain to the patient:
  - Schedule rest periods during the day.
  - Restrict diet to low-salt and low-fat foods.

25 *Mitral Stenosis*

WHAT WENT WRONG?

In mitral stenosis, scar tissue secondary to rheumatic fever forms on the mitral valve. This causes it to narrow, increasing resistance to blood flow between the left ventricle and left atrium, which means the heart needs to pump harder to maintain blood flow.

PROGNOSIS

Mitral valve stenosis may be asymptomatic for years, never needing attention. However, eventually symptoms may occur and progress, necessitating intervention. Medication may be enough, or surgical intervention may be necessary.

HALLMARK SIGNS AND SYMPTOMS

- Murmur at apex
- Difficulty breathing (dyspnea) on exertion
- Fatigue because of a poorly functioning heart
- Weakness because the heart is working inefficiently
- Palpations because the heart needs to work harder to pump blood

INTERPRETING TEST RESULTS

- Cardiac catheterization depicts the flow through the mitral valve.
- X-ray shows enlarged left atrial and left ventricle.
- EKG depicts left atrial hypertrophy, exhibiting as broad, notched P-waves in lead II with negative deflection of the P-wave in lead V1.

TREATMENT

Mitral stenosis is generally a progressive disease and treatment is directed at maintaining function. When necessary, mitral replacement is indicated. Most of these patients need endocarditis antibiotic prophylaxis, which is administering antibiotics to prevent a bacterial infection occurring before invasive procedures and dental cleaning. If atrial fibrillation occurs, anticoagulation is indicated.

- Medication to stabilize symptoms.
- Administer anticoagulant medication following surgery to prevent thrombus around the aortic valve:
  - heparin
  - warfarin
  - dalteparin
  - enoxaparin
- Mitral valve repair or replacement.

NURSING DIAGNOSES

- Anxiety
- Decreased cardiac output
- Activity intolerance

NURSING INTERVENTION

- Place patient in a high Fowler's position to ease breathing.
- Monitor for:
  - Pulmonary edema because it may be a complication of surgery.
  - Thrombus because of a prosthetic valve.
  - Arrhythmias because of an irritated heart; patient may feel palpitations, anxiety.
  - Arterial Blood Gas (ABG) to monitor for oxygenation, acidosis, alkalosis.
- Weigh the patient daily to determine fluid balance.
- Explain to the patient:
  - Signs and symptoms to look for and to report changes in condition.
  - Schedule rest periods during the day.
  - Restrict diet to low-sodium and low-fat foods.

26 *Mitral Valve Prolapse (MVP)*

WHAT WENT WRONG?

The mitral valve bulges back into the left atrium, allowing blood to flow backwards from the left ventricle into the left atrium. This is a common problem and is not considered a serious condition. It is often congenital.

PROGNOSIS

Most patients with MVP are unaware they have it until symptoms start occurring. Often it is an incidental finding on an echocardiogram. A large majority of patients require no treatment other than endocarditis prophylaxis during dental and unsterile procedures. Some patients progress with their symptoms, developing arrhythmias and requiring medications. Severe MVP may require mitral valve repair or replacement.

HALLMARK SIGNS AND SYMPTOMS

- Asymptomatic because the valve leaflets do not bulge greatly
- Palpations because the valve is not operating properly

- Systolic click and/or late systolic murmur
- Chest pain
- Fatigue
- Syncope
- Dyspnea

INTERPRETING TEST RESULTS

- EKG may be normal or show an atrial arrhythmia (irregular P-waves), left atrial/ventricular enlargement (broad P-, QRS–waves).
- Chest x-ray is usually normal, unless left chambers are large (in late disease).

TREATMENT

Treatment of MVP is determined by the severity of the symptoms. Most patients require endocarditis antibiotic prophylaxis.

- Administer antiarrhythmic medications
- Administer anticoagulant medication after valve replacement to prevent thrombus around the aortic valve.
- Ensure patient understands the need for daily, life-long anticoagulation therapy once a mechanical valve is in place:
  - heparin
  - warfarin (Coumadin)—requires frequent labwork to monitor consistency of blood
  - dalteparin (Fragmin)
  - enoxaparin (Lovenox)
- Mitral valve repair or replacement.

NURSING DIAGNOSES

- Anxiety
- Decreased cardiac output
- Activity intolerance

NURSING INTERVENTION

- Place patient in a high Fowler's position to facilitate breathing.
- After surgery, monitor for:
  - Pulmonary edema to look for blood backflowing into lungs.
  - Heart failure to assess for a poorly functioning heart.
  - Thrombus because of a prosthetic valve.
  - Arrhythmias because the heart may be irritated after surgery.
  - Arterial Blood Gas (ABG) to check for adequate oxygenation and acid/base balance.
- Weigh the patient daily to assess for fluid overload.
- Explain to the patient proper recovery from major surgery:
  - Schedule rest periods during the day.
  - Restrict diet to low-sodium and low-fat.

27 *Tricuspid Insufficiency*

WHAT WENT WRONG?

Leakage in the tricuspid valve causes a backflow from the right ventricle into the right atrium. This results in increased pressure in the atrium and higher resistance to blood flowing from veins, resulting in enlargement of the right atrium. This may occur from an anatomic problem, but usually occurs from right ventricular overload (in turn caused by left ventricular overload). It may also occur due to an inferior myocardial infarction, or damage from endocarditis.

PROGNOSIS

If the underlying problem can be resolved, the insufficiency may subside. If resolution does not occur, tricuspid valve repair or replacement may be necessary.

HALLMARK SIGNS AND SYMPTOMS

- Difficulty breathing (dyspnea) due to backflow into the lungs
- Fatigue because the heart is working inefficiently

- Jugular venous distention due to overload in the right atria
- Hepatic congestion from backflow
- S3 murmur upon inspiration

INTERPRETING TEST RESULTS

- X-ray shows enlarged right ventricle and right atrium because of volume overload.
- Echocardiogram depicts prolapsed tricuspid valve and enlarged right side of the heart.
- EKG depicts enlarged right ventricle and right atrium, characterized by broad P- and QRS–waves.

TREATMENT

Correct any underlying heart disease to reduce pressure on the right atrium, ventricle, and thus, the valve.

- Administer anticoagulant medication following surgery to prevent thrombus around the tricuspid valve:
  - heparin
  - warfarin
  - dalteparin
  - enoxaparin
- Tricuspid valve repair or replacement.

NURSING DIAGNOSES

- Anxiety
- Decreased cardiac output
- Activity intolerance

NURSING INTERVENTION

- Place patient in a high Fowler's position to facilitate breathing.

- Monitor for:
  - Pulmonary edema because backflow to the lungs may occur.
  - Heart failure to assess cardiac function.
  - Thrombus because of a prosthetic valve.
  - Arrhythmias because the heart may be irritable.
  - Arterial Blood Gas (ABG)to assess for adequate oxygenation, acid/base balance.
- Weigh the patient daily to look for fluid overload.
- Explain to the patient what symptoms to look for.
  - Schedule rest periods during the day.
  - Restrict diet to low-sodium and low-fat foods.

Crucial Diagnostic Tests

Electrocardiograph (EKG, ECG)

WHY IS IT GIVEN?

The EKG is a graphic representation of the electrical activity of the heart in a non-invasive procedure. It shows a three-dimensional perspective of the electrical function of the heart. There are four common uses of an electrocardiograph. These are (1) to measure the heart for a short time period such as during a physical or an assessment; (2) ongoing monitoring using telemetry while the patient is an inpatient; (3) ambulatory (Holter) monitoring for a 24-hour period while the patient goes about normal daily activities; (4) stress test.

HOW DOES THE TEST WORK?

An electrical signal is generated each time the chambers of the heart contract. Small pads containing electrodes are placed on the surface of the skin to detect the hearts electrical signal. Each electrode is connected with wires to an electro-cardiograph, which draws up to 12 different graphical representation of the electrical signal. There are twelve electrodes used in a typical EKG: bipolar limb leads I, II, and III; augmented limb leads AVR, AVL, and AVF; and precordial chest leads V1 through V6.

WHAT TO DO?

Typically a technician will perform the electrocardiograph and a physician or a nurse with advanced training will interpret the results of the test.

The nurse should be able to recognize a normal sinus rhythm and abnormal rhythms that are life-threatening such as ventricular tachycardia and ventricular fibrillation. The nurse should be able to reattach electrodes.

Teach the patient the following:

- The patient will not experience an electrical shock.
- The patient must lie still for several minutes if the electrocardiograph is done during a physical or assessment.
- The patient can move about if the electrocardiograph of the patient is ambulatory or if the patient is an inpatient during monitoring.
- If ambulatory, the patient should keep an activity diary of his or her symptoms.
- If ambulatory, the patient should not operate machinery, including microwave ovens and electric shavers, nor should he or she bathe or shower while attached to the electrocardiograph.
- If it is a stress test, the patient should wear appropriate attire for exercise and report any discomfort during the test so proper assessment can be completed to determine the etiology of the discomfort.

Cardiac Catheterization (Angiography)

WHY IS IT GIVEN?

This is an invasive procedure used to examine the coronary arteries and intracardiac structures, as well as to measure cardiac output, intracardiac pressures, and oxygenation

HOW DOES THE TEST WORK?

A radiopaque dye, which makes structures visible on x-rays, is injected through a catheter into the femoral artery in the patient's left leg or in the antecubital fossa, which is the crease of the arm); it then flows to the coronary arteries. The flow of the radiopaque dye is viewed and recorded using a fluoroscope, enabling the physician to determine obstructions to the flow and the structures of the heart.

WHAT TO DO?

Before the test:

- Chemistry to assess creatinine, BUN and creatinine clearance. These are tests to determine kidney function.
- Determine if the patient is allergic to seafood or iodine. If so, notify the physician immediately because the patient might be also allergic to the radio-paque dye.
- Obtain written consent from the patient. Risks and benefits of the test need to be explained to the patient before commencing.
- Nothing by mouth (NPO) for 4 to 6 hours before the test to reduce the risk of aspiration.
- Explain the procedure to the patient and its possible side effects. These are flushing of the face, nausea, urge to urinate, and chest pain, which are usually reactions to the dye.
- Record baseline vital signs, so to assess for changes.

After the test:

- Assess for bleeding at the injection site since a major artery has been accessed. If there is bleeding, apply pressure until bleeding stops.
- Keep patient on bed rest for 8 hours, so as not to dislodge a clot from the artery used for the catheter.
- Keep pressure on injection site for 8 hours to ensure clotting at the site.
- If femoral artery is used, keep left leg straight for 8 hours to minimize risk of dislodging clot.
- If antecubital fossa used, keep arm straight for 3 hours to minimize risk of dislodging clot.
- Monitor vital signs to assess for changes.
- Increase fluid intake to assist the kidneys in excreting the dye.

Echocardiograph

WHY IS IT GIVEN?

An ultrasound of the heart provides a noninvasive examination of intracardiac structures and blood flow.

HOW DOES THE TEST WORK?

Sound waves are directed to and deflected by the heart, causing an echo that is detected by the echocardiograph, which is interpreted by a physician.

WHAT TO DO?

- Describe the procedure to the patient.
- The patient must lie still for 30 minutes during the test to ensure an accurate picture of the structures of the heart.

Nuclear Cardiology

WHY IS IT GIVEN?

These tests determine myocardial perfusion and contractility of the heart, ischemia, infarction, wall motion, and ejection fraction.

HOW DOES THE TEST WORK?

Radioisotopes are injected through the IV. The radiation detector monitors the flow of the radioisotope as it flows through the heart.

WHAT TO DO?

Before the test:

- Obtain written consent from the patient to ensure he or she understands the risks of the test.
- Explain the test to the patient, emphasizing that the patient must lie still during the test.

After the test:

- Determine if there is bleeding at the injection site.

Digital Subtraction Angiography

WHY IS IT GIVEN?

Digital Subtraction Angiography (DSA) enables the physician to view arterial blood supply to the heart using an injection of radiopaque contrast material.

HOW DOES THE TEST WORK?

The patient is injected with an intravascular contrast material containing iodine. Images of bone and soft tissue are viewed from fluoroscopy through the use of a computer, enabling the physician to view the cardiovascular system.

WHAT TO DO?

Before the test:

- Obtain written consent from the patient once risks and benefits have been explained.
- Explain the test to the patient, emphasizing that he or she must lie still during the test.

After the test:

- Determine if there is bleeding at the injection site.
- The patient must drink 1 liter (1 quart) of fluid to aid the kidneys in excreting the dye.
- Monitor the patient's vital signs to assess for changes.

Hemodynamic Monitoring

WHY IS IT GIVEN?

Hemodynamic monitoring measures cardiac output and intracardiac pressure.

HOW DOES THE TEST WORK?

A balloon-tipped catheter is inserted into the pulmonary artery, usually through the femoral artery. It is able to measure pressures in the heart's various chambers and vessels.

WHAT TO DO?

Before the test:

- Obtain written consent from the patient to ensure he or she understands risks and benefits.
- Explain the test to the patient.

After the test:

- Determine if there is bleeding at the injection site.
- Determine if there is infection at the injection site, redness, warmth, swelling, or discomfort.
- Examine for complications: air embolus, arrhythmia, and clots. Assess for decrease in respiratory effort, increase in respiratory rate, dyspnea.

Chest X-ray

WHY IS IT GIVEN?

Chest x-rays are done to detect size and position of the heart and structural abnormalities of the lungs.

HOW DOES THE TEST WORK?

An x-ray machine directs x-rays through the chest and onto film positioned behind the patient's back. As x-rays are directed to the patient, some are absorbed by the body and others pass through to the x-ray film. Areas of the body that absorb x-rays appear light on the x-ray film. Dark areas on the film represent x-rays that passed through the body.

WHAT TO DO?

- Explain the test to the patient and that the patient will be asked to hold his or her breath while the x-ray is taken.
- Before the test, remove all jewelry, zippers, hooks, and any metal on the part of the body being x-rayed.

Blood Chemistry

WHY IS IT GIVEN?

This provides a profile of the patient's health, including:

- Electrolyte balance (sodium, potassium, bicarbonate, magnesium, calcium, phosphorus).
- Kidney function (BUN, creatinine).
- Liver function: (AST/ALT). (These are enzymes released when the liver is damaged)
- Diabetes: (serum glucose)
- Cholesterol level: (cholesterol, LDL, HDL, triglycerides)
- Cardiac: [creatine kinase (CK) and CK isoenzymes (these are enzymes released if there is damage to the heart muscle), cardiac troponin levels (troponin is a protein in cardiac and skeletal muscles), myoglobin (an early indication of a myocardial infarction), lactate dehydrogenase (LDH), and LDH isoenzymes] These are enzymes released when cardiac tissue is damaged.

HOW DOES THE TEST WORK?

Three to five milliliters of blood is sampled. Different tests require different tubes. The abnormal results are:

- Electrolyte balance (sodium, potassium, bicarbonate, magnesium, calcium, phosphorus) will be abnormal in fluid imbalance, acid base imbalance.
- Kidney function (BUN, creatinine) will be elevated in kidney disease.
- Liver function: (AST/ALT) will be elevated in liver disease.
- Diabetes: (serum glucose) indicated when fasting glucose is above 125.

- Cholesterol level: (cholesterol, LDL, HDL, triglycerides). Numbers need to be low except for HDL; a higher number is better; abnormal numbers indicate risk for cardiovascular disease.
- Cardiac: [creatine kinase (CK), CK isoenzymes, cardiac troponin levels, myoglobin, lactate dehydrogenase (LD), and LD isoenzymes]. When elevated, these show injury to cardiac muscle.

WHAT TO DO?

- No exercise before sampling blood, as it may falsely elevate some numbers.
- NPO, if directed by the physician. Accurate measurements of triglycerides and glucose require a fasting state.
- No IM injections before sampling. If an injection is necessary, then note the name of the medication, time, and dose and send it along with the sample to the lab, as it may alter results.
- Check for bleeding at venipuncture site.
- Fast for 12 hours for serum glucose test.
- Fast for 12 hours for cholesterol tests to assure accurate triglyceride.

Hematologic Studies

WHY IS IT GIVEN?

This provides a profile of the patient's blood, including:

- CBC count—reports hemoglobin, hematocrit, and size and shape of red blood cells (RBC) that help in oxygen transport. Their average lifespan is 120 days and they are formed in the bone marrow. A test is often performed to assess anemia, shortness of breath, response to medication, hemorrhage, surgery, and trauma.
- WBC count—shows the level of white blood cells in the current circulation. WBCs are responsible for fighting infection in the body. There are five subtypes of WBCs: neutrophils, basophils, eosinophils, lymphocytes, and monocytes. WBCs are often drawn to determine infection, inflammation, allergic response, and parasitic infection.
- Erythrocyte sedimentation rate (ESR) is a nonspecific test to show infection and inflammation.

- Coagulation studies [prothrombin time (PT), INR (Internationalized Normalized Ratio), partial thromboplastin time (PTT), platelet count]. These are bleeding time tests to indicate the patient's clotting ability. Most interfere at some point in the clotting cascade. INR is used to monitor stable patients taking warfarin. PT is used to help screen patients taking warfarin. Since PT is made in the liver, this test is also useful to monitor liver functions. Abnormalities in the PTT indicate defects in the patient's coagulation status and with blood factors. Used to monitor heparin therapy.

HOW DOES THE TEST WORK?

Three to five milliliters is sampled. The abnormal results are:

- RBC count—usual indication is to look for anemia.
- WBC count—when elevated, it shows infection.
- Erythrocyte sedimentation rate (ESR)—shows inflammation when elevated.
- Bleeding (prothrombin time, INR, partial thromboplastin time, platelet count) —measure clotting of blood.
- Hemoblogin (Hgb) and hematocrit (Hct) show the level of iron- and oxygen-carrying capability of the blood.

WHAT TO DO?

- Check for bleeding at venipuncture site.

Arterial Blood Gas (ABG)

WHY IS IT BEING TESTED?

This determines the patient's ventilation, tissue oxygenation and acid-base status.

HOW DOES THE TEST WORK?

Three to five milliliters of blood is obtained from an artery. Usually the radial, brachial or femoral arteries are used. The abnormal results are:

- Increased pH shows metabolic alkalosis or respiratory alkalosis.
- Decreased pH shows metabolic acidosis or respiratory acidosis.

- Increased pCO_2 indicates COPD.
- Decreased pCO_2 indicates hypoxemia.
- Increased HCO_3 indicates dehydration, COPD.
- Decreased HCO_3 indicates fluid loss.
- Increased pO_2 shows hyperventilation.
- Decreased pO_2 shows anemia, respiratory difficulties.

WHAT TO DO?

Before the test:

- Explain to the patient that arterial sticks may be more uncomfortable than venous labwork performed by the phlebotomists.
- Provide the lab with information on whether or not the patient is receiving supplemental or mechanical ventilation as well as on the amount of oxygen received or the setting of the ventilator as it may alter the results.

After the test:

- Apply mechanical pressure to puncture site for 5 minutes.
- Apply pressure dressing to puncture site for 30 minutes once bleeding has stopped.
- Monitor the puncture site for bleeding.

Venogram

WHY IS IT GIVEN?

This x-ray test takes pictures of the blood flow through the veins. It is used to identify and locate blood clots and to determine the condition of the valves in the veins.

HOW DOES THE TEST WORK?

An iodine dye is injected into the vein, making the vein visible in a fluoroscope; this allows the physician to visualize the flow of venous blood.

WHAT TO DO?

Before the test:

- Assess latest chemistry to check on BUN, creatinine, and creatinine clearance.
- Determine if the patient is allergic to seafood or iodine. If so, notify the physician immediately because the patient might be also allergic to the dye.
- Obtain written consent from the patient to assure adequate knowledge of risks and benefits.

Explain the procedure to the patient and its possible effects. These are flushing of the face, nausea, urge to urinate, and chest pain, which may be a reaction to the dye.

After the test:

- Check for bleeding at the injection site to assess for hemorrhage. If bleeding, apply pressure until bleeding stops.
- Check for infection at the injection site. Look for redness, warmth, and oozing of purulent matter.
- Increase fluid intake to assist the kidneys in excreting the dye.

Pulse Oximetry

WHY IS IT GIVEN?

This determines the abbreviated arterial oxygen saturation of the blood. The full arterial oxygen saturation is determined by the arterial blood gas test.

HOW DOES THE TEST WORK?

An infrared light passes through the patient's nail bed or skin. The amount of infrared light passing through determines the amount of arterial oxygen saturation of the blood.

WHAT TO DO?

- Clamp the sensor on the patient's finger over the nail bed, toe, ear lobe, or bridge of the nose.
- Make sure that the site is clean. Nail polish or artificial nails may interfere with the reading.

Quiz

1. You are diagnosed with an aortic aneurysm and ask why the condition didn't show up on your annual physical examination. The best response is:

    (a) It did show and your physician did not want to alarm you.

    (b) Aortic aneurysms are asymptomatic.

    (c) You probably don't remember that your physician told you about your condition.

    (d) Aortic aneurysms are always symptomatic.

2. Your patient tells you that he sometimes has chest pains when he performs strenuous work. He sits waiting for his physician to call back and the pain goes away. What is the best explanation of his condition?

    (a) He is experiencing stable angina.

    (b) He is experiencing indigestion.

    (c) He is experiencing unstable angina.

    (d) He is experiencing Prinzmetal's angina.

3. The patient is experiencing chest pain and pain radiating to his arms, jaw and back. His physician diagnosed his condition as a myocardial infarction. The patient asks what happened to him. The best response is:

    (a) You had a heart attack.

    (b) Your aortic valve was malformed at birth causing a disruption in blood flow.

    (c) All patients who are as overweight as you will have a heart attack.

    (d) One or more arteries that supply blood to your heart is blocked, thereby preventing blood from flowing to your cardiac muscles.

4. A patient diagnosed with congestive heart failure asks you why fluid accumulates in his lungs. The best response is:

(a) Because of the excessive volume of IV fluid that is being administered.

(b) The left side of his heart is weak and is losing the capability to pump blood to his lungs.

(c) The right side of his heart is weak and is losing the capability to pump blood to his lungs.

(d) He stands too long at work.

5. Your patient is experiencing congestive heart failure. What medication would you expect to administer to strengthen myocardial contractility?

(a) nitroprusside

(b) digoxin

(c) nitroglycerin ointment

(d) furosemide

6. Upon hearing that he has acute pericarditis, the patient asks how he could have gotten the disease. The best response is:

(a) The upper respiratory viral infection that you experienced a couple of weeks ago could have led to acute pericarditis.

(b) It is a genetic condition that you received from your father.

(c) It is a genetic condition that you received from your mother.

(d) It is the weakening of the left side of your heart.

7. The patient has difficulty breathing, fatigue, orthopnea, and palpation. Her physician diagnosed her as having aortic insufficiency. She underwent aortic valve repair. What medication would you expect to administer?

(a) heparin

(b) ativan

(c) haldol

(d) thorazine

8. The patient asks you why she is being administered so many arterial blood gas tests. The best response is:

(a) This test determines if your liver and kidneys are functioning properly.

(b) This test determines if you have a sufficient WBC to fight infection.

(c) This test determines if you are hyperglycemic, which is a side effect of your medication.

(d) This test determines how well your tissues are oxygenated.

9. The patient asks you what the clip on his finger is for. The best response is:

(a) This is pulse oximetry and is used to gives us an idea of how much oxygen is in your blood.

(b) This is a cardiac monitor that alerts us to any arrhythmia that you might experience during the night.

(c) This measures your temperature.

(d) This tells us the number of red blood cells you have which are needed to provide oxygen throughout your body.

10. The patient is admitted to rule out cardiac disease and is scheduled for a chest x-ray. He asks you how a chest x-ray would help the physician examine his heart. The best response is:

(a) A chest x-ray is used to rule out that a fractured rib caused your pain.

(b) A chest x-ray is used to detect the size and position of the heart.

(c) The chest x-ray is an error. I'll cancel the order.

(d) All patients who are admitted must have a chest x-ray.

CHAPTER 2

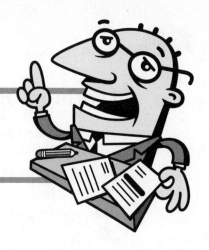

Respiratory System

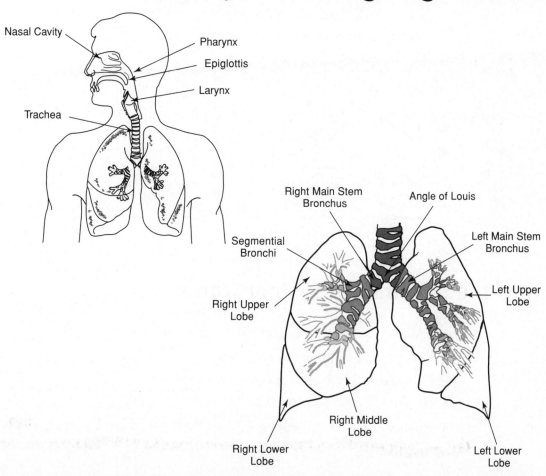

Nasal Cavity
Pharynx
Epiglottis
Larynx
Trachea

Right Main Stem Bronchus
Angle of Louis
Segmental Bronchi
Left Main Stem Bronchus
Right Upper Lobe
Left Upper Lobe
Right Middle Lobe
Right Lower Lobe
Left Lower Lobe

Learning Objectives

1. Acute Respiratory Distress Syndrome (ARDS)
2. Asbestosis
3. Asthma
4. Atelectasis
5. Bronchiectasis
6. Bronchitis
7. Cor pulmonale
8. Emphysema

9. Lung cancer
10. Pleural effusion
11. Pneumonia
12. Pneumothorax
13. Respiratory acidosis
14. Tuberculosis (TB)
15. Acute respiratory failure
16. Pulmonary embolism
17. Influenza

 Key Terms

Acid base balance
Alveoli
Bifurcates
Bronchi
Cilia
Crackles

Cyanosis
Dyspnea
Expiration
Fibrosis
Hypoxemia
Inspiration

Interstitium
Mesothelioma
Nasopharynx
Pulmonary edema
Rhonchi
Tachypnea

How the Respiratory System Works

The respiratory system has the following basic functions:

- Movement of air in and out of the lungs
- Exchange of oxygen and carbon dioxide
- Helping maintain acid-base balance

Ventilation moves air in (inspiration) and out (expiration) of the lungs. During inspiration, air flows in through the nose and passes into the nasopharynx.

Air is then drawn through the pharynx, larynx, trachea, and bronchi. The bronchi branches (bifurcates) right and left into smaller tubes called bronchioles that terminate in alveoli. The airways are lined with mucous membranes to add moisture to the inhaled air. There is a thin layer of mucous in the airways that helps to trap foreign particles, such as dust, pollen, or bacteria. Cilia—small, hair-like projections—help to move the mucous with the foreign material upward so it can be coughed out.

Alveoli are air-filled sacs containing membranes coated with surfactant. The surfactant helps the alveoli to expand evenly on inspiration and prevents collapse on exhalation. Carbon dioxide and oxygen are exchanged; a higher concentration of gas moves to the lower area of concentration. A higher concentration of carbon dioxide in the hemoglobin moves across the membrane into the alveoli and is expired by the lung. Higher concentration of oxygen in the alveoli crosses the membrane and attaches to the hemoglobin which is then distributed by the circulatory system throughout the body.

Lungs are contained within a pleural sac in the thoracic cavity and operate on negative pressure. The visceral pleura is close to the lungs and the parietal pleura is close to the chest wall. There is a pleural space between these two layers that contains a small amount of fluid to prevent friction with chest movement on inspiration and expiration.

Just the Facts

1 *Acute Respiratory Distress Syndrome (ARDS)*

WHAT WENT WRONG?

Patients develop acute respiratory failure. Lungs stiffen as a result of a build-up of fluid in the lungs. Fluid builds up in the tissue of the lungs (interstitium) and the alveoli. This fluid and stiffness impairs the lungs' ability to move air in and out (ventilation). There is an inflammatory response in the tissues of the lungs. Damage to the surfactant within the alveoli leads to alveolar collapse, further impairing gas exchange. An attempt to repair the alveolar damage may lead to fibrosis within the lung. Even as the respiratory rate increases, sufficient oxygen cannot enter the circulation (hypoxemia). Oxygen saturation decreases. Respiratory acidosis develops, and the patient appears to have respiratory distress.

This is most commonly due to shock, sepsis, or as a result of trauma or inhalation injury. Patients may have no history of pulmonary disorders, also known as Adult Respiratory Distress Syndrome.

PROGNOSIS

Early recognition and treatment is critical. Even with intensive treatment, ARDS has a mortality rate of 50 to 60 percent. Some patients will progress into a more chronic type of ARDS which has permanent lung changes. These patients may require long-term mechanical ventilation.

HALLMARK SIGNS AND SYMPTOMS

- Hypoxemia—insufficient level of oxygen in the blood, despite supplemental oxygen at 100 percent.
- Difficulty breathing (dyspnea)—increased need for oxygen to meet body's demand. The need for oxygen will increase as fluid builds up in the lungs and compliance worsens.
- Pulmonary edema—fluid build-up in the lungs.
- Breathing rate greater than 20 breaths per minute (tachypnea)—breathing becomes faster in an attempt to get oxygen into the body.
- Decreased breath sounds—harder to hear through fluid in alveoli; no air movement in collapsed alveoli.
- Anxiety—secondary to not getting enough oxygen.
- Rales (crackles) heard in the lungs—air moving through fluid in alveoli and small airways on inspiration and expiration (not heard initially).
- Wheezing (rhonchi)—inflammation develops or mucous is created. This narrows the airways, creating a sound as the air travels through the narrowed airway.
- Restlessness—due to decreased oxygen levels.
- Cyanosis—due to lack of oxygenation.
- Accessory muscle use for respirations—look for retractions between ribs (intercostal) and below the sternum (substernal).

INTERPRETING TEST RESULTS

- Pulse oximetry shows lowered oxygen levels below 90 percent.
- Arterial blood gases (ABGs) show respiratory acidosis—increased $PaCO_2$ (>45 mmHg), decreasing PaO_2 level even with supplemental oxygen.
- Chest x-ray—both lungs show infiltrates within lung fields; "whiteout" or ground glass appearance.
- Pulmonary capillary wedge pressure (PCWP) low to normal.

TREATMENT

- Bedrest.
- Endotracheal intubation.
- Mechanical ventilation with positive end-expiratory pressure (PEEP) or continuous positive airway pressure (CPAP).
- Administer anesthetic to ease comfort during insertion of endotracheal tube:
  - propofol
- Administer neuromuscular blocking agent—used when patients are on mechanical ventilation to avoid patient working against the action of the ventilator. These drugs allow respiratory muscles to rest:
  - pancuronium, vecuronium
- Administer diuretics to help decrease excess fluid in lungs:
  - furosemide, ethacrynic acid, bumetanide
- Administer H2 blocker or proton pump inhibitor to decrease gastric acid. This will decrease likelihood of a stress ulcer in the stomach or aspiration of gastric acid into the lung:
  - ranitidine, famotidine, nizatidine, omeprazole
- Administer anticoagulant—clotting may have been causative in disease; immobility contributory to clot formation:
  - heparin
- Administer analgesic—used for comfort and to decrease myocardial oxygen demand:
  - morphine
- Administer steroids to decrease inflammatory response in the lung tissue:
  - hydrocortisone, methylprednisolone

- Administer exogenous surfactant:
  - beractant
- Administer antibiotics for respiratory or systemic infections.
  - Ideally selected based on results of culture and sensitivity (C&S) of sputum.
  - May be given to cover likely infectious organism pending results of C&S.

NURSING DIAGNOSES

- Ineffective breathing pattern
- Impaired gas exchange
- Ineffective tissue perfusion

NURSING INTERVENTION

- Monitor WBC count:
  - Elevation of WBC with infection, inflammation.
  - Decrease in WBC in a patient who is immune-compromised or who has a viral infection.
- Monitor hemoglobin (Hgb) and hematocrit (Hct) for anemias.
- Monitor PT, PTT, and INR for coagulation abnormalities; monitor heparin dosing.
- Record intake and output of fluid:
  - Monitor for signs of renal insufficiency or failure (decrease in urinary output less than 30 ml/h) and monitor BUN and Creatinine.
  - Monitor for possible fluid overload—more fluid going in than coming out. Patient may end up in heart failure, compounding the fluid building up in the lungs.
- Weigh the patient daily—inability to handle excess fluids, causing third spacing of fluids into interstitial spaces, increasing weight and causing edema.
- Change position at least every 2 hours to prevent pressure build-up, causing skin breakdown.
- Avoid overexerting the patient during treatment—patient will tire easily and will have problems with increased oxygen demands. Also provide rest periods during activities.

- Explain to the patient:
  - The importance of doing coughing and deep-breathing exercises—after coming off the ventilator the patient needs to move adequate air in and out of the lungs. Coughing helps to rid the lungs of any remaining fluid.
  - How to identify the signs of respiratory distress, any sign that symptoms may be returning: shortness of breath, coughing, wheezing, rapid breathing, cyanosis, restlessness, or anxiety.

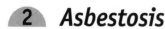 **Asbestosis**

WHAT WENT WRONG?

Asbestos fibers enter the lungs, causing inflammation in the bronchioles and in the walls of the alveoli. After inhalation, the fibers settle into the lung tissue. Fibrosis develops and ultimately pleural plaques form. The changes within the lung result in a restrictive lung disease. The damage to the lung causes impairment in breathing and air exchange.

PROGNOSIS

It may take a decade or longer from the time of exposure before symptoms begin to develop. Some patients have worked in occupations known for asbestosis exposure (mining, shipyards, fireproofing, and construction before the mid-1970s), for 10 or 15 years prior to symptom development. There is an increased risk of lung cancer (mesothelioma) in patients with history of asbestosis exposure, especially if the patient has also smoked. Mesothelioma may develop 2 to 4 decades postexposure.

HALLMARK SIGNS AND SYMPTOMS

- Difficulty breathing (dyspnea) on exertion and at rest due to changes in the lung tissue
- Chest pain or tightness due to changes within the lung tissue and restrictive air movement

- Dry cough due to irritation within the lungs
- Frequent respiratory infections due to changes within the lung, increasing susceptibility to infection
- Respiration greater than 20 breaths per minute (tachypnea) due to decreased vital capacity
- Rales or crackles when listening to breath sounds

INTERPRETING TEST RESULTS

- Chest x-ray to reduce chance of illness. Lungs show linear opacities, irregular opacities. Opacities are increased tissue density on the lung indicating fibrosis or pleural plaque.
- CT scan shows opacities indicating increased tissue density of fibrosis or pleural plaque.
- Arterial blood gas shows decreased oxygen due to restrictive pattern of respiration.
- Pulse oximetry shows decreased pattern.
- Pulmonary Function Test (PFT) shows a restrictive pattern, decreased vital capacity.

TREATMENT

There is no specific treatment for asbestosis, nor is there a cure.

- Flu vaccine and pneumoccocal vaccine to reduce chance of illness.
- Oxygen therapy (1 to 2 liters per minute) to ease breathing discomfort by increasing available oxygen to meet body's needs.
- Administer antibiotics for exacerbations of respiratory symptoms—to treat infectious process based on results of culture and sensitivity study or empirically.

NURSING DIAGNOSES

- Fatigue
- Impaired gas exchange
- Imbalanced nutrition: less than the body requires

NURSING INTERVENTION

- Administer chest percussion and vibration to loosen and expel secretions.
- Explain to patient:
  - How to avoid infections (reduced exposure to others with an infection and vaccines administered according to physician's orders).
  - Proper use of oxygen therapy.

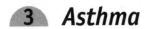 ## 3 *Asthma*

WHAT WENT WRONG?

The airways become obstructed from either inflammation of the lining of the airways or constriction of the bronchial smooth muscles (bronchospasm). A known allergen, for example, pollen—is inhaled, causing activation of antibodies that recognize the allergen. Mast cells and histamine are activated, initiating a local inflammatory response. Prostaglandins enhance the effect of histamine. Leukotrienes also respond, enhancing the inflammatory response. White blood cells responding to the area release inflammatory mediators.

A stimulus causes an inflammatory reaction, increasing the size of the bronchial linings; this results in restriction of the airways. There may be a bronchial smooth muscle reaction at the same time. There are two kinds of asthma:

- Extrinsic asthma, also known as atopic, caused by allergens such as pollen, animal dander, mold, or dust. Often accompanied by allergic rhinitis and eczema; this may run in families.
- Intrinsic asthma, also known as nonatopic, caused by a nonallergic factor such as following a respiratory tract infection, exposure to cold air, changes in air humidity, or respiratory irritants.

PROGNOSIS

Triggers for the asthmatic patient can often be identified and avoided. Patients can learn to check peak flow levels and manage symptoms in conjunction with their caregiver. Well controlled asthma typically has temporary, reversible exacerbations that can be controlled with medications, often in an outpatient setting. With

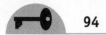

frequent attacks, a mild exposure to a known trigger will often be sufficient to exacerbate an attack. Patients who do not respond to medications or who use medications improperly may die during an asthma attack.

HALLMARK SIGNS AND SYMPTOMS

- Wheezing initially present on expiration continues throughout respiratory cycle as inflammation progresses. Air has difficulty moving through the narrowed airways, making noise. Not all asthmatics will have wheezing.
- Asymptomatic between asthma attacks. Symptoms resolve when there is no inflammation present.
- Difficulty breathing (dyspnea) as airways narrow due to inflammation. This is typically progressive as inflammation increases.
- Respiration greater than 20 breaths per minute (tachypnea) as the body attempts to get more oxygen into the lungs to meet physiologic needs.
- Use of accessory muscles to breathe as the body tries harder to get more air into the lungs.
- Tightness in the chest due to narrowing of the airways (bronchoconstriction).
- Cough.
- Tachycardia—heart rate greater than 100, as the body attempts to get more oxygen to the tissues.

INTERPRETING TEST RESULTS

- Decreased oxygen and increased carbon dioxide present in arterial blood gas due to inability to move adequate air, which results in inadequate gas exchange.
- Decreased force on expiration [either forced expiratory volume in the first second (FEV_1) or peak expiratory rate flow (PERF)] during attack shown in pulmonary function test. Narrowed airways make it more difficult for the patient to exhale, prolonging time of exhalation and decreasing force of exhalation. Patients can check expiratory effort at home on a peak flow meter.
- Hyperinflated lungs shown in chest x-ray due to air trapping.
- Pulse oximetry shows diminished oxygen saturation.
- CBC—elevated eosinophils.
- Sputum—positive for eosinophils.

TREATMENT

The focus of treatment is to return the respiratory status to normal, deliver adequate oxygen, and limit the number of recurrences. Patient education should focus on understanding the disease, its management, and when emergency care may be necessary.

- Administer supplemental oxygen to help meet body's needs.
- Identify and remove allergens and known triggers to avoid causing an asthma attack.
- Give patient 3 liters/day of fluid to help liquefy any secretions.
- Administer short-acting beta$_2$-adrenergic drugs to bronchodilate:
  - albuterol, pirbuterol, metaproterenol, terbutaline, levalbuterol
- Administer long-acting beta$_2$-adrenergic drugs to manage symptoms day to day; keep airways open, not for acute symptoms:
  - salmeterol, formoterol
- Administer leukotriene modulators to reduce local inflammatory response in lung to reduce exacerbations; does not have immediate effect on symptoms:
  - zafirlukast, zileuton, montelukast
- Administer anticholinergic drugs
  - ipratropium inhaler, tiotropium handihaler
- Administer antacid, H2 blocker, or proton pump inhibitor to decrease the amount of acid in the stomach, reducing the possibility of ulcers due to stress of disease or medication effects.
  - Antacids: aluminum hydroxide/magnesium hydroxide, calcium carbonate
  - H2 blockers: ranitidine, famotidine, nizatidine, cimetidine
  - Proton pump inhibitors: omeprazole, lansoprazole, esomeprazole, rabeprazole, pantoprazole
- Administer mast cell stabilizer to retain an early component of the initial response to allergens, which will prevent further reactions from occurring; this is not for acute symptoms. This is useful for pretreatment for allergen exposure or chronic use to improve control of symptoms.
  - cromolyn, nedocromil
- Administer steroids to decrease inflammation, which will help open airways; these are not for acute symptoms:
  - hydrocortisone, methylprednisolone intravenously

- beclomethasone, triamcinolone, fluticasone, budesonide, flunisolide, mo-metasone inhalers
- prednisolone, prednisone orally
- Administer methylxanthines to assist with bronchodilation, often used when other medications not effective:
  - aminophylline, theophylline

NURSING DIAGNOSES

- Impaired gas exchange
- Ineffective airway clearance
- Ineffective tissue perfusion

NURSING INTERVENTION

- Monitor respiration: patient's respiratory status can continue to deteriorate; look at respiratory rate, effort, use of accessory muscles, skin color, breath sounds.
- Place patient in high Fowler's position to ease respirations.
- Monitor vital signs, look for changes in BP, tachycardia, tachypnea.
- Explain to the patient:
  - How to use a peak flow meter.
  - How to use the metered dose inhaler or dry powder and in which order to take inhaled medication.
  - Avoid exposure to allergen.
  - How to recognize the early signs of asthma.
  - How to perform coughing and deep-breathing exercises.

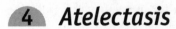 Atelectasis

WHAT WENT WRONG?

A portion of the lung does not expand completely, decreasing the lung's capacity to exchange gases, which results in decreased oxygenation of blood. Obstruction of part of the airway will cause collapse distal to the area that is blocked. Obstruction can be from a mucous plug inside the airway, or a tumor or fluid within the pleural space may be pressing on the airway from the outside. Postoperatively, patients are at risk for atelectasis due to pain, immobility, medications for pain or anesthesia, and lack of deep breathing.

PROGNOSIS

Prognosis depends on the cause and the size of the involved area.

HALLMARK SIGNS AND SYMPTOMS

- Difficulty breathing (dyspnea) due to the lack of expansion of part of the lung
- Anxiety due to decrease in oxygenation
- Increased respiratory rate (tachypnea) in an attempt to increase available oxygen
- Heart rate above 100 beats per minute (tachycardia) as body tries to increase available oxygen
- Sweating (diaphoresis) as a result of increased work of respirations
- Cyanosis due to decreased oxygen level
- Hypoxemia due to lack of gas exchange in the affected area
- Decreased breath sounds due to lack of air movement in the area of collapse
- Accessory muscle use with respiration as the body tries to get more oxygen

INTERPRETING TEST RESULTS

- Shadows on chest x-ray indicate collapsed area of the lung. The airless state in this area of the lung creates a more dense appearance on the x-ray.
- CT scan will show an area of atelectasis.

TREATMENT

Treatment is focused on re-inflation of the involved area of the lung, removing the cause of obstruction, and the delivery of adequate oxygen. The extent of the treatment depends on the area of the lung involved and the cause.

- Administer oxygen to meet body's demand.
- Administer mucolytics to help loosen or thin secretions:
  - acetylcystine, inhaled
  - guaifenesin, oral
- Administer bronchodilators to open airways:
  - albuterol
  - levalbuterol

NURSING DIAGNOSES

- Impaired gas exchange
- Risk for infection
- Ineffective tissue perfusion

NURSING INTERVENTION

- Cough and deep-breathing exercise every 2 hours to prevent a further area of atelectasis.
- Instruct the patient to use the incentive spirometer every 2 hours to encourage deep breathing and monitor progress.
- Provide humidified air.
- Monitor breath sounds for abnormalities such as diminished sounds.
- Monitor mechanical ventilation if needed. If a large area of the lung is affected, respiratory support may be needed.
- Explain to the patient:
  - How to perform coughing and deep-breathing exercises.
  - Proper use of incentive spirometer.

5 *Bronchiectasis*

WHAT WENT WRONG?

Bronchi and bronchioles become abnormally and permanently dilated, caused by infection and inflammation. This results in excessive production of mucous that obstructs the bronchi. There is some obstruction of the airways and a chronic infection. The changes within the lung can be localized or generalized. The lung may develop areas of atelectasis where thick mucous obstructs the smaller airways, making the mucous difficult to expel. This results in inflammation and infection of the airways and leads to bronchiectasis.

PROGNOSIS

Early diagnosis and appropriate treatment of infections are essential for management. Postural drainage and chest physical therapy aid in movement of mucous from the airways. The difficulty in breathing is caused by excess mucus similar to patients with Chronic Obstructive Pulmonary Disease (COPD) (emphysema or chronic bronchitis).

HALLMARK SIGNS AND SYMPTOMS

- Difficult breathing (dyspnea) due to the mucous production and irritation within the airways.
- Productive, foul-smelling odorous cough, due to thick, difficult-to-expel, tenacious mucous, often with bacterial colonization.
- Cough may be worse when lying down.
- Recurrent bronchial infections.
- Hemoptysis (blood-tinged or bloody mucous).
- Loss of weight because patients are not eating well, due to respiratory changes and foul-smelling mucous with cough. Increased respiratory effort requires more calories to meet normal requirements.
- Crackles or rhonchi on inspiration due to mucous build-up.
- Anemia of chronic disease.

- Cyanosis.
- Clubbing of the fingers.

INTERPRETING TEST RESULTS

- Culture and sensitivity of sputum to identify bacteria and appropriate antibiotics.
- Shadows in affected area of the lungs on the chest x-ray.
- CT scan or high-resolution CT will show areas of bronchiectasis.
- Decreased lung vital capacity on pulmonary function test.

TREATMENT

Treatment is focused on getting enough oxygen to meet current needs of the patient, expel mucous, and treat infections.

- Supplemental oxygen to help meet body's needs.
- Postural drainage to assist with drainage of secretions.
- Chest PT to loosen secretions.
- Remove excessive secretions during a bronchoscopy.
- Administer bronchodilators to help keep airways open:
  - albuterol, levalbuterol
- Administer antibiotics to treat infection:
  - selected based on the results of a culture and sensitivity study

NURSING DIAGNOSES

- Ineffective airway clearance
- Imbalanced nutrition: less than what the body requires
- Impaired gas exchange

NURSING INTERVENTION

- Monitor respiratory rate, effort, breath sounds, skin color, and use of accessory muscles.

- Perform chest percussion to help loosen secretions.
- Explain to the patient:
  - That family member can perform chest PT.
  - How to do postural drainage.
  - How to administer oxygen.
  - How to properly administer medications.

6 *Bronchitis*

WHAT WENT WRONG?

Increased mucus production, caused by infection and airborne irritants that block airways in the lungs, results in the decreased ability to exchange gases. There are two forms of bronchitis: acute bronchitis, where blockage of the airways is reversible, and chronic bronchitis, where blockage is not reversible. Patients with acute bronchitis are symptomatic typically for 7 to 10 days often due to viral (but sometimes bacterial) infection. Patients with chronic bronchitis will have symptoms of a chronic productive cough for at least 3 consecutive months in 2 consecutive years. There is increased mucous production, inflammatory changes, and, ultimately, fibrosis in the airway walls. The patient with chronic bronchitis has an increased incidence of respiratory infection.

PROGNOSIS

Patients with acute bronchitis who have a resolution of symptoms and respiratory status will return to normal condition. Chronic bronchitis is classified as a chronic obstructive pulmonary disease (COPD), which is often linked to smoking and has a progressive pattern. Shortness of breath is initially present only with exertion, and eventually is present even at rest. Patients with chronic bronchitis often develop right-sided heart failure and peripheral or dependent edema. Patients will have acute exacerbations of chronic bronchitis.

HALLMARK SIGNS AND SYMPTOMS

- Cough due to mucous production and irritation of airways.
- Shortness of breath.

- Fever in acute episodes due to infection.
- Accessory muscles are used for breathing—as respiratory effort increases, additional muscles are necessary to assist.
- Productive cough due to irritation of airways. Mucous is a protective reaction of the respiratory system.
- Weight gain secondary to edema in chronic bronchitis is due to right-sided heart failure.
- Wheezing due to inflammation within the airways.

INTERPRETING TEST RESULTS

- Shadows in affected area of the lungs on the chest x-ray during infection.
- Pulmonary function testing shows:
  - Forced vital capacity (FVC) changes because more time is needed to forcibly exhale an amount of air after a maximal inhalation.
  - FEV_1 is decreased because more time is needed for exhalation.
  - Residual volume (RV) is increased due to air trapping.
- Decreased oxygen and increased carbon dioxide in arterial blood gas.

TREATMENT

Acute bronchitis is treated in the short term with symptomatic treatment and antibiotics when a bacterial infection is present. Chronic bronchitis is treated with a combination of medications to keep the airways open, reduce inflammation within airways, and prevent complications or exacerbations.

- Administer $beta_2$-agonists by inhaler or nebulizer to dilate the bronchi:
  - terbutaline, albuterol, levalbuterol
  - formoterol, salmeterol
- Administer anticholinergics which allow for relaxation of bronchial smooth muscle:
  - ipratropium, tiotropium inhaler
- Administer steroids to decrease inflammation within the airways
  - hydrocortisone, methylprednisolone systemically
  - beclomethasone, triamcinolone, fluticasone, budesonide, flunisolide inhalers
  - prednisolone, prednisone orally

- Administer methylxanthines to enhance bronchodilation:
  - aminophylline
  - theophylline (Theo-Dur)
- Administer diuretics to reduce fluid retention in patients who develop right-sided heart failure:
  - furosemide, bumetanide
- Administer expectorant to help liquefy secretions:
  - guaifenesin
- Administer antibiotics in acute exacerbation of chronic bronchitis:
  - selected by culture and sensitivity study or given empirically
- Administer antacid, H2 blocker, or proton pump inhibitor to decrease the amount of acid in stomach, reducing possible ulcer formation due to stress of disease or medication effects.
  - antacids: aluminum hydroxide/magnesium hydroxide, calcium carbonate
  - H2 blockers: ranitidine, famotidine, nizatidine, cimetidine
  - proton pump inhibitors: omeprazole, lansoprazole, esomeprazole, rabeprazole, pantoprazole
- Administer vaccines—to decrease chances of infection:
  - influenza
  - pneumonia
- Give 3 liters of fluid per day to help liquefy secretions
- Oxygen: 2 liters per minute via nasal canula to help meet body's needs; low flow rates help reduce dyspnea while avoiding CO_2 retention.
- Increase protein, calories, and vitamin C in diet to meet body's needs.
- Administer the incentive spirometer or flutter valve to encourage coughing and expelling of mucous.
- Nocturnal negative pressure ventilation used for hypercapnic (elevated CO_2 levels) patients.

NURSING DIAGNOSES

- Ineffective airway clearance
- Activity intolerance
- Ineffective breathing pattern

NURSING INTERVENTION

- Monitor respirations looking at rate, effort, use of accessory muscles, skin color; listen to breath sounds.
- Place patient in high Fowler's position to ease respiration.
- Weigh the patient daily. Excess fluid due to heart failure will increase weight. Notify physician, NP, or PA of weight gain of 2 pounds in 24 hours.
- Have the patient perform the turning, coughing, and deep-breathing exercises to enhance lung expansion and expel mucous.
- Monitor sputum for changes in color or amount, which may signal infection in patients with chronic bronchitis.
- Monitor intake and output.
- Increase fluids to keep mucous thinner and easier to expel.
- Explain to the patient:
  - How to administer oxygen.

7 *Cor Pulmonale*

WHAT WENT WRONG?

In Cor Pulmonale, the structure and function of the right ventricle are compromised by chronic obstructive pulmonary disease (COPD), obstruction of the airflow into and out of the lungs. The heart tries to compensate, resulting in right-sided heart failure.

The patient has heart failure due to a primary lung disorder, which causes pulmonary hypertension and enlargement of the right ventricle. Patients will have symptoms of both the underlying pulmonary disorder and the right-sided heart failure. COPD includes chronic bronchitis and emphysema.

PROGNOSIS

Management of both the underlying lung disease and the heart failure is necessary to alleviate the symptoms for the patient. Medical management may provide significant relief of symptoms for the patient. Exacerbations of the underlying disease process are still likely. Progression of the disease state is possible, requiring adjustment in medications or further lifestyle modifications.

HALLMARK SIGNS AND SYMPTOMS

- Cyanosis
- Fatigue due to hypoxia and heart failure
- Wheezing due to underlying lung condition such as COPD or emphysema
- Difficulty breathing (dyspnea) on exertion and when lying down (orthopnea) due to increased oxygen needs with movement and increased respiratory effort of the diaphragm when lying down
- Productive cough due to underlying respiratory condition
- Edema due to right-sided failure; fluid build-up will be in dependent areas
- Weight gain due to fluid retention
- Respiration greater than 20 breaths per minute (tachypnea); rate increases to meet body's oxygen needs
- Increased heart rate above 100 beats per minute (tachycardia) as the body attempts to compensate for hypoxia and carry more oxygen

INTERPRETING TEST RESULTS

- Enlarged pulmonary arteries and right ventricle shown on a chest x-ray.
- Enlarged right ventricle shown on echocardiography as a result of pulmonary hypertension.
- Increased right ventricular and pulmonary artery pressures in a pulmonary artery catheterization. The right ventricle is pumping against greater-than-normal resistance within the pulmonary artery when sending blood to the lungs.
- Decreased oxygen and increased carbon dioxide in arterial blood gas due to underlying lung disease.
- Pulse oximetry shows decreased oxygen saturation.
- Increased hemoglobin to compensate for hypoxia.

TREATMENT

- Bedrest or decreased activity.
- Oxygen therapy at 2 liters/minute (low flow rate) to help meet body's needs. The COPD patient cannot tolerate a high flow of oxygen.
- Administer calcium channel blockers to vasodilate:

- diltiazem, nifedipine, nicardipine, amlodipine
- Administer medications to vasodilate the pulmonary artery:
  - diazoxide, hydralazine, nitroprusside
- Administer angiotensin-converting enzyme inhibitor:
  - captopril, enalapril
- Administer anticoagulant to reduce risk of clot formation:
  - heparin
- Administer diuretic to remove excess fluid:
  - furosemide, bumetanide
- Administer cardiac glycoside for symptom relief of heart failure:
  - digoxin
- Reduce sodium in the diet to reduce fluid retention.
- Reduce fluid intake to reduce fluid retention.

NURSING DIAGNOSES

- Excessive fluid volume
- Impaired gas exchange
- Activity intolerance

NURSING INTERVENTION

- Limit fluid to 2 liters per day.
- Monitor digoxin level to avoid toxic effect.
- Check pulse before administering cardiac glycoside. A side effect of the drug is slowing of the heart rate. Hold medication and contact the physician as needed.
- Monitor serum potassium levels; ACE inhibitors and some diuretics can cause potassium retention.
- Monitor respiratory status for rate, effort, use of accessory muscle, skin color, and breath sounds.
- Explain to the patient:
  - How to administer oxygen therapy.
  - Medication management.

8 *Emphysema*

WHAT WENT WRONG?

Chronic inflammation reduces the flexibility of the walls of alveoli, resulting in over-distention of the alveolar walls. This causes air to be trapped in the lungs, impeding gas exchange. Smoking is often linked to development of emphysema. A less frequent cause is an inherited alpha$_1$-antitrypsan deficiency.

PROGNOSIS

Symptoms often begin insidiously and are progressive. Shortness of breath is initially associated with exertion, then presents at rest. These patients are more susceptible to lung infections. Supplemental oxygen becomes necessary at first for exacerbations, then for daily use. Periodic exacerbations requiring hospitalization are not unusual.

HALLMARK SIGNS AND SYMPTOMS

- Difficulty breathing (dyspnea) due to air trapping, which retains carbon dioxide and reduces alveolar gas exchange.
- Barrel chest develops over time as more air is trapped within the distal airways. The anteroposterior diameter (distance between front and back of the chest) increases, giving the chest a more barrel-like appearance.
- Use of accessory muscles to breathe as the respiratory effort increases. The number of muscles used to inhale will increase in an effort to get enough oxygen into the body.
- Loss of weight as extra calories are needed to maintain respiration. Increased effort of breathing also detracts from eating.
- Patients prefer a seated position which allows for greater chest expansion.

INTERPRETING TEST RESULTS

- Increased residual volume shown in pulmonary function test due to air trapping.

- Decreased oxygen and increased carbon dioxide in arterial blood gas as gas exchange is impaired due to air trapping; more pronounced as disease progresses.
- Chest x-ray shows overinflation of lungs and flattening of the diaphragm.

TREATMENT

Treatment will vary depending on the stage of the emphysema. As the disease progresses the treatment will change. Medications to control symptoms and keep airways open, use of supplemental oxygen, and smoking cessation are the mainstays of treatment.

- Administer beta$_2$-agonists to bronchodilate by inhaler or nebulizer:
  - terbutaline, albuterol, levalbuterol
- Administer long-acting bronchodilating medications by metered dose inhaler or dry powder inhaler:
  - formoterol, salmeterol
- Administer anticholinergics which allow for relaxation of bronchial smooth muscle:
  - ipratropium, tiotropium inhaler
- Administer methylxanthines to dilate the bronchi. These are typically used in conjunction with other medications, not for acute effect:
  - aminophylline
  - theophylline
- Administer steroids to decrease inflammation within the airways:
  - hydrocortisone, methylprednisolone systemically
  - beclomethasone, triamcinolone, fluticasone, budesonide, flunisolide inhalers
  - prednisolone, prednisone orally
- Administer antacid, H2 blocker, or proton pump inhibitor to decrease the amount of acid in stomach, reducing possible ulcer formation due to stress of the disease or medication effects:
  - antacids: aluminum hydroxide/magnesium hydroxide, calcium carbonate
  - H2 blockers: ranitidine, famotidine, nizatidine, cimetidine
  - Proton pump inhibitors: omeprazole, lansoprazole, esomeprazole, rabeprazole, pantoprazole

- Administer expectorant—to loosen secretions:
  - guaifenesin
- Administer diuretics to decrease fluid retention in patients that are developing right-sided heart failure secondary to lung disease:
  - furosemide, bumetanide
- Administer vaccines—to prevent respiratory infections:
  - influenza
  - pneumonia
- Administer antibiotics:
  - selected based on results of culture and sensitivity study or given empirically
- Administer alpha$_1$-antitrypsin therapy for patients with deficiency.
- Administer oxygen, 2 liters per minute, to help meet body's oxygen needs while avoiding CO_2 retention.
- Give patient 3 liters of fluids per day to help liquefy secretions.
- Nocturnal negative pressure ventilation for hypercapnic (elevated CO_2 levels) patients.
- Teach patient how to use:
  - the incentive spirometer to encourage deep breathing and enhance coughing and expelling of mucous.
  - the flutter valve to increase expiration force.

NURSING DIAGNOSES

- Impaired gas exchange
- Fatigue
- Risk for infection

NURSING INTERVENTION

- Monitor the patient's sputum for color, amount, or changes in characteristics, which may indicate infection.
- Place patient in high Fowler's position, which eases respiratory effort.
- Administer low-flow oxygen, which increases oxygen delivered to patient without compromising respiratory drive.

- Monitor intake and output fluids.
- Explain to the patient:
  - The importance of turning, coughing, and deep-breathing exercises.
  - How to administer oxygen therapy.
  - Avoid exposure to irritants and people with infections.

9   *Lung Cancer*

WHAT WENT WRONG?

Lung cancer is the abnormal, uncontrolled cell growth in lung tissues, resulting in a tumor. A tumor in the lung may be primary when it develops in lung tissue. It may be secondary when it spreads (metastasizes) from cancer in other areas of the body, such as the liver, brain, or kidneys. There are two major categories of lung cancer—small cell and non-small cell. Repetitive exposure to inhaled irritants increases a person's risk for lung cancer. Cigarette smoke, occupational exposures, air pollution containing benzopyrenes, and hydrocarbons have all been shown to increase risk.

- Small cell:
  - Oat cell—fast-growing, early metastasis
- Non-small cell:
  - Adenocarcinoma—moderate growth rate, early metastasis
  - Squamous cell—slow-growing, late metastasis
  - Large cell—fast-growing, early metastasis

PROGNOSIS

Lung cancer is the leading cause of cancer death. Many patients with lung cancer are diagnosed at a later stage, leading to the long-term (5-year) survival rate of less than 20 percent. Earlier diagnosis is more beneficial for treatment and outcome. The longer the cancer has been in the lungs, the greater the likelihood of metastasis to other areas.

HALLMARK SIGNS AND SYMPTOMS

- Coughing due to irritation from mass. Presence of mucous or exudate may not be until later in disease.
- Coughing up blood (hemoptysis).
- Fatigue.
- Weight loss due to the caloric needs of the tumor, taking away from the needs of the body.
- Anorexia.
- Difficulty breathing (dyspnea) caused by damaged lung tissue. The patient begins to have respiratory problems later in the disease.
- Chest pains as mass presses on surrounding tissue; may not be until late in disease.
- Sputum production.
- Pleural effusion.

INTERPRETING TEST RESULTS

- Mass in lung shown on chest x-ray.
- CT scan shows mass, lymph node involvement.
- Bronchoscopy may show cancer cells on bronchoscopic washings; may reveal tumor site.
- Cancer cells seen in sputum.
- Biopsy will show cell type:
  - Needle biopsy through chest wall for peripheral tumors.
  - Tissue biopsy from lung for deeper tumors.
- Bone scan or CT scans shows metastasis of the disease.

TREATMENT

Treatment is focused on resolution of the tumor. Surgical removal is appropriate for some patients, but not always necessary. Chemotherapy and radiation are both methods that are used to destroy the cancerous cells. Oxygen therapy is used to aid in meeting the current needs of the body, but not all patients will require supplemental oxygen therapy. Attention to nutrition is important to meet the demands of the body. Pain control is an integral component of care in any type of cancer treatment. Appropriate pain management needs to be individualized for the patient.

- Surgical removal of affected area of the lung (wedge resection, segmental resection, lobectomy) or total lung (pneumonectomy).
- Radiation therapy to decrease tumor size.
- Chemotherapy often with a combination of drugs:
  - cyclophosphamide, doxorubicin, vincristine, etoposide, cisplatin
  - may see relapse after treatment
- Oxygen therapy to supplement the needs of the body.
- High-protein, high-calorie diet to meet the needs of the body.
- Administer antiemetics to combat side effects of chemotherapy:
  - ondansetron, prochlorperazine
- Administer analgesics for pain control:
  - morphine, fentanyl

NURSING DIAGNOSES

- Anxiety
- Activity intolerance
- Impaired gas exchange

NURSING INTERVENTION

- Monitor respiratory status, looking at rate, effort, use of accessory muscles, and skin color; auscultate breath sounds.
- Monitor pain and administer analgesics appropriately.
- Monitor vital signs for changes, elevated pulse, elevated respiration, change in BP, and elevated temperature, which may signal infection.
- Monitor pulse oximetry for decrease in oxygenation levels.
- Assist patient with turning, coughing, and deep-breathing exercises.
- Place patient in semi-Fowler's position to ease respiratory effort.
- Explain to the patient:
  - The importance of taking rest periods.

10 *Pleural Effusion*

WHAT WENT WRONG?

Abnormal accumulation of fluid within the pleural space between the parietal and visceral pleura covering the lungs. The fluid may be serous fluid, blood (hemothorax), or pus (empyema). Fluid builds up when the development of the fluid exceeds the body's ability to remove the fluid. Excess fluid inhibits full expansion of the lung. A large area of fluid build-up will displace the lung tissue, compromising air exchange in the area. As fluid builds up and takes the place of lung tissue, it may push the collapsing lung past the middle (mediastinum) of the chest. This displaces the central structures, compromising the air exchange of the other lung as well. Causes of pleural effusion are varied and include congestive heart failure, renal failure, malignancy, lupus erythematosis, pulmonary infarction, infection, or trauma. It can also occur as a postoperative complication.

PROGNOSIS

Prognosis varies depending on cause and amount of fluid present. Once fluid is removed, patient is monitored to see if fluid builds up again. The fluid may need to be removed periodically, depending on the cause.

HALLMARK SIGNS AND SYMPTOMS

- Chest pain due to presence of inflammation of the pleura in the area; not always present.
- Difficulty breathing (dyspnea) due to diminished chest expansion in the area.
- Decreased breath sounds on auscultation over the area due to presence of fluid.
- Dullness on percussion over the affected area due to the presence of fluid.
- Fever due to infection with empyema.
- Increased pulse and respirations; decreased BP due to blood loss with hemothorax.
- Low oxygen saturation on pulse oximeter.

INTERPRETING TEST RESULTS

- Chest x-ray shows pleural effusion.
- Chest CT scan shows pleural effusion.
- Chest ultrasound shows pleural effusion.
- Thoracentesis (removal of fluid with a needle from the pleural space) shows type of fluid.

TREATMENT

Fluid removal is performed either as a one-time procedure or with a chest tube, to continuously allow for drainage of the fluid until the tube is removed. Supplemental oxygen may be needed to help meet the body's needs.

- Thoracentesis to remove the fluid.
- Chest tube to remove larger amounts of drainage over time.
- Oxygen as needed.
- Administer antibiotics for empyema:
  - Selected according to results of culture and sensitivity study

NURSING DIAGNOSES

- Impaired gas exchange
- Risk for infection
- Pain

NURSING INTERVENTION

- Administer supplemental oxygen therapy to help meet body's needs.
- Monitor for changes in vital signs.
- Have the patient perform turning, coughing, deep-breathing exercises to enhance lung expansion.
- Monitor chest tube drainage for color, amount, and changes in drainage.
- Assure patency of chest tube to make sure the tube is draining properly.

- Explain to the patient:
  - Disease process.
  - Need for coughing and deep breathing.

11 *Pneumonia*

WHAT WENT WRONG?

Infectious pneumonia may be due to a variety of microorganisms and can be community-acquired or hospital-acquired (nosocomial). A patient can inhale bacteria, viruses, parasites, or irritating agents, or a patient can aspirate liquids or foods. He or she can also develop increased mucous production and thickening alveolar fluid as a result of impaired gas exchange. All of these can lead to inflammation of the lower airways.

Organisms commonly associated with infection include *Staphylococcus aureus, Streptococcus pneumoniae, Haemophilus influenza, Mycoplasma pneumoniae, Legionella pneumonia, Chlamydia pneumoniae* (parasite), and *Pseudomonas aeruginosa.*

PROGNOSIS

Prognosis will vary depending on patient's age, preexisting lung disease, infecting organism and response to antibiotics. Patients at risk for pneumonia are: older patients; those with respiratory disease; patients with comorbid conditions such as heart, liver, or kidney disease; and patients who develop complications (such as atelectasis or pleural effusion). Patients at greater risk for complications from pneumonia will be treated within the hospital, while those at lower risk may be treated at home. Patients with respiratory rates over 30, tachycardia, altered mental status, or hypotension also are considered higher-risk.

Patients without other coexisting conditions, who do not appear to have the higher-risk symptoms listed above, can usually be safely treated as outpatients. Patients with comorbidities (higher-risk coexisting symptoms) or who appear ill are usually treated in the hospital. Some require critical care treatments and must be closely monitored. There is still a significant mortality rate from pneumonia, despite the recognition of pneumonia and use of antibiotics.

HALLMARK SIGNS AND SYMPTOMS

- Shortness of breath due to inflammation within the lungs, impairing gas exchange
- Difficulty breathing (dyspnea) due to inflammation and mucus within the lungs
- Fever due to infectious process
- Chills due to increased temperature
- Cough due to mucous production and irritation of the airways
- Crackles due to fluid within the alveolar space and smaller airways
- Rhonchi due to mucus in airways; wheezing due to inflammation within the larger airways
- Discolored, possibly blood-tinged, sputum due to irritation in the airways or microorganisms causing infection
- Tachycardia and tachypnea as the body attempts to meet the demand for oxygen
- Pain on respiration due to pleuritic inflammation, pleural effusion, or atelectasis development
- Headache, muscle aches (myalgia), joint pains, or nausea may be present depending on the infecting organism

INTERPRETING TEST RESULTS

- Shadows on chest x-ray, indicating infiltration, may be in a lobar or segmental pattern or more scattered.
- Culture and sensitivity of the sputum to identify the infective agent and the appropriate antibiotics.
- Elevated WBC (leukocytosis) showing sign of infection.
- Low oxygen saturation on pulse oximetry.
- Arterial blood gas may show low oxygen and elevated carbon dioxide levels.

TREATMENT

Supplemental oxygen is given to help meet the body's needs. Antibiotics are given for the most likely organism (empirically) until the sputum culture results are returned. Patients may need bronchodilators to help open the airways.

- Administer oxygen as needed.
- For bacterial infections, administer antibiotics such as macrolides (azithromycin, clarithromycin), fluoroquinolones (levofloxacin, moxifloxacin), beta-lactams (amoxicillin/clavulanate, cefotaxime, ceftriaxone, cefuroxime axetil, cefpodoxime, ampicillin/sulbactam), or ketolide (telithromycin).
- Administer antipyretics when fever >101 for patient comfort:
  - acetaminophen, ibuprofen
- Administer brochodilators to keep airways open, enhance airflow if needed:
  - albuterol, metaproterenol, levalbuterol via nebulizer or metered dose inhaler
- Increase fluid intake to help loosen secretions and prevent dehydration.
- Instruct the patient on how to use the incentive spirometer to encourage deep breathing; monitor progress.

NURSING DIAGNOSES

- Risk for aspiration
- Impaired ventilation
- Ineffective airway clearance

NURSING INTERVENTION

- Monitor respiration for rate, effort, use of accessory muscles, skin color, and breath sounds.
- Record fluid intake and output for differences, signs of dehydration.
- Record sputum characteristics for changes in color, amount, and consistency.
- Properly dispose of sputum.
- Explain to the patient:
  - Take adequate fluids—3 liters per day—to prevent excess fluid loss through the respiratory system with exhalation.
  - Use of incentive spirometer.

12 *Pneumothorax*

WHAT WENT WRONG?

The pleural sac surrounding the lung normally contains a small amount of fluid to prevent friction as the lungs expand and relax during the respiratory cycle. When air is allowed to enter the pleural space between the lung and the chest wall, a pnuemothorax develops. This air pocket takes up space that is normally occupied by lung tissue, causing an area of the lung to partially collapse. If there is a penetrating chest wound, the patient may have an open pneumothorax, also known as a sucking chest wound (for the sound it makes during breathing). A closed pneumothorax may be caused by blunt trauma, post-central line insertion, or post-thoracentesis. Spontaneous pneumothorax may be secondary to another disease or occur on its own. As the air accumulates, there may be a partial or complete collapse of the lung—the more air that accumulates, the greater the area of collapse. If there is a large enough amount of air trapped between the pleural layers, the tension within the area increases. This increase in tension results in pushing the mediastinum toward the unaffected lung, causing it to partially collapse and compromising venous return to the heart. This is a tension pneumothorax.

PROGNOSIS

Prognosis will vary depending on causes and size of pneumothorax. Any pneumothorax that enlarges or progresses to a tension pneumothorax is a greater risk for the patient. Tension pneumothorax presents a life-threatening situation. A small area of pneumothorax may be monitored without intervention while a larger area requires treatment for resolution of the problem.

HALLMARK SIGNS AND SYMPTOMS

- Sharp chest pain, made worse by activity, moving, coughing, and breathing
- Shortness of breath due to inability to fully expand the lungs during inspiration
- Absent breath sounds over the affected area due to presence of air between lungs and chest wall
- Subcutaneous emphysema (presence of air in the tissue beneath the skin)—a crackling feeling beneath the skin on palpation over the area
- Tachycardia (increased heart rate) and tachypnea (increased respiratory rate) as body attempts to meet needs

- Mediastinal shift and tracheal deviation toward the unaffected side with tension pneumothorax

INTERPRETING TEST RESULTS

- Shadows on chest x-ray, indicating a collapsed lung.
- Increased carbon dioxide shown in arterial blood gas.
- Low oxygen saturation on pulse oximetry.

TREATMENT

Once identified, a pneumothorax can be treated and completely resolved. A tension pneumothorax can become a life-threatening condition. Careful monitoring and early intervention is critical for these patients. A small area may resolve without intervention, but the patient will still be monitored until resolution.

- Bedrest.
- Supplemental oxygen if needed.
- Chest tube connected to suction to re-expand lung if needed.
- Administer analgesic if needed:
    - morphine

NURSING DIAGNOSES

- Acute pain
- Ineffective breathing
- Impaired gas exchange

NURSING INTERVENTION

- Place patient in high Fowler's or semi-Fowler's position to ease respiratory effort.
- Monitor drainage of the chest tube for amount and characteristics of output. Note changes.
- Monitor vital signs for changes.

- Monitor respirations for rate, effort, use of accessory muscles, skin color, and breath sounds.
- Teach turning, coughing, and deep-breathing exercises.
- Explain to the patient:
  - Disease process.
  - Importance of coughing and deep breathing.

13 *Respiratory Acidosis*

WHAT WENT WRONG?

Hypoventilation, asphyxia, or central nervous system disorders cause a disturbance in the acid-base balance of the patient's blood, resulting in increased carbon dioxide in the blood (hypercapnia). The increase in carbon dioxide in the blood combines with water; this combination releases hydrogen and bicarbonate ions. The brain stem is stimulated and increases the respiratory drive to blow off carbon dioxide. Over time, the sustained elevated arterial carbon dioxide level causes the kidneys to attempt to compensate by retaining bicarbonate and sodium and excreting hydrogen ions.

PROGNOSIS

Respiratory acidosis may be due to an acute or chronic respiratory condition. Respiratory failure results in severe acidosis. The more rapid onset of acidosis does not allow time for the kidneys to compensate. Healthy patients usually can increase the amount of CO_2 that the lungs are getting rid of to assist in lowering the blood levels of CO_2. Patients with underlying respiratory disorders will not be able to rid the body of the excess CO_2 in this way.

HALLMARK SIGNS AND SYMPTOMS

- Hypoxemia
- Cardiac arrhythmia or tachycardia due to hypoxemia from hypoventilation
- BP changes depending on underlying cause
- Headache due to hypoxemia
- Difficulty breathing (dyspnea) due to hypoxemia

- Confusion and restlessness due to hypoxemia
- Irritability due to hypoxemia

INTERPRETING TEST RESULTS

- Carbon dioxide (CO_2) >50 mmHg shown in arterial blood gas
- pH of blood <7.35 shows acidosis in arterial blood gas

TREATMENT

Treatment is focused on restoring appropriate ventilation, returning carbon dioxide levels to normal, and returning pH levels to normal.

- Give supplemental oxygen, monitoring flow rate to avoid excess oxygen to those who have chronic pulmonary conditions. The chronic nature of the respiratory acidosis in these patients may have caused the internal respiratory control to adjust in response to a decrease in oxygen level rather than an increase in carbon dioxide level, which is always higher than normal.
- Administer bronchodilators to open constricted airways:
  - albuterol, metaproterenol, levalbuterol
- Administer medications as necessary to correct underlying disorder.
- Administer antibiotics as ordered as a result of the sensitivity test.
- Mechanical ventilation if necessary to support breathing.
- Treat underlying cause.

NURSING DIAGNOSES

- Ineffective breathing
- Fear
- Impaired gas exchange

NURSING INTERVENTION

- Monitor respiration for rate, effort, use of accessory muscles, skin color, mucous production, and breath sounds.
- Monitor blood chemistry—potassium, CO_2, chloride

- Explain to the patient:
  - How to administer oxygen therapy.
  - How to perform turning, coughing, and deep-breathing exercises.

14 *Tuberculosis (TB)*

WHAT WENT WRONG?

An infectious disease spread by airborne route. Infection is caused by inhalation of droplets that contain the tuberculosis bacteria (*Mycobacterium tuberculosis*). An infected person can spread the small airborne particles through coughing, sneezing, or talking. Close contact with those affected increases the chances of transmission. Once inhaled, the organism typically settles into the lung, but can infect any organ in the body. The organism has an outer capsule.

Primary TB occurs when the patient is initially infected with the mycobacterium. After being inhaled into the lung, the organism causes a localized reaction. As the macrophages and sensitized T-lymphocytes attempt to isolate and kill off the mycobacterium within the lung, damage is also caused to the surrounding lung tissue. A well-defined granulomatous lesion develops that contains the mycobacterium, macrophages and other cells. Necrotic changes occur within this lesion. Caseous granulomas develop along lymph node channels during the same time. These areas create a Ghon's complex which is a combination of the area initially infected by the airborne bacillus called the Ghon's focus and a lymphatic lesion. The majority of people with newly acquired infections and an adequate immune system will develop latent infection, as the body walls off the infecting organism within these granulomas. Disease is not active in these patients at this point and will not be transmitted until there is some manifestation of the disease. In patients with inadequate immune response, the tuberculosis will be progressive, lung tissue destruction will continue, and other areas of the lung will also become involved.

In secondary TB, the disease is reactivated at a later stage. The patient may be reinfected from droplets, or from a prior primary lesion. Since the patient has previously been infected with TB, the immune response is to rapidly wall off the infection. Cavitation of these areas occurs as the organism travels along the airways.

Exposure to TB occurs when a person has had recent contact with a person suspected or confirmed having TB. These patients do not have positive skin test, signs or symptoms of disease, or chest x-ray changes. They may or may not have disease.

Latent TB infection occurs when a person has a positive tuberculin skin test but no symptoms of disease. Chest x-ray may show granuloma or calcification.

TB disease is confirmed when a person has signs and symptoms of tuberculosis. The chest x-ray typically has abnormalities in the apical aspects of the lung fields. In HIV patients other areas may also be affected.

PROGNOSIS

Some patients develop drug-resistant TB, making treatment more difficult. The drug-resistant TB may be resistant at the time of initial infection, or may develop as a result of medications during treatment. This occurs either because the treatment was not adequate or not taken appropriately.

HALLMARK SIGNS AND SYMPTOMS

- Weight loss and anorexia
- Night sweats
- Fever, possibly low-grade, due to infection
- Productive cough with discolored, blood-tinged sputum
- Shortness of breath due to lung changes
- Malaise and fatigue due to active illness affecting lungs

INTERPRETING TEST RESULTS

- Positive Mantoux (PPD) skin test shows exposure to tuberculosis due to development of cell-mediated immunity; typically takes between 2 and 10 weeks from time of exposure.
- Chest x-ray may show areas of granuloma or cavitation.
- Sputum test identifies *M. tuberculosis* bacteria:
  - Acid fast-staining done to initially screen for TB—bacillus will hold stain
  - Culture confirms the diagnosis but is slow-growing.

TREATMENT

Patients with active TB are initially placed on respiratory isolation as inpatients to reduce the risk of spreading the organism by droplet infection or aerosolization. Medications are initiated to treat TB and prevent transmission to others. Treatment may be initiated for active disease or for those without active disease who have had recent exposure. Combination therapy is typically used to decrease the likelihood

of drug-resistant organisms. Initial treatment times generally range from 6 to 12 months. Longer treatment plans may be necessary for those with HIV infection or drug-resistant strains of TB. Some patient populations are monitored closely for compliance with direct observation of drug treatment. Patient teaching is important for medication protocol compliance and monitoring for side effects. Repeat sputum cultures are typically taken to see that the treatment for active disease is effective.

- Administer antitubercular medications to treat and prevent transmission:
  - isoniazid, rifampin, pyrazinamide, ethambutol, streptomycin
- Respiratory isolation for in-hospital care—the bacteria is spread by droplet.
- Increase protein, carbohydrates, and vitamin C diet for patients.

NURSING DIAGNOSES

- Fatigue
- Ineffective airway clearance

NURSING INTERVENTION

- Monitor respiration for rate, effort, use of accessory muscles, and skin color changes.
- Increase fluid intake to help liquefy any secretions.
- Record fluid intake and output.
- Explain to the patient:
  - How to prevent spreading the disease.
  - The importance of finishing all prescribed medication.
  - Plan for rest periods during the day.

15　*Acute Respiratory Failure*

WHAT WENT WRONG?

The lungs are unable to adequately exchange oxygen and carbon dioxide because of insufficient ventilation. The body is not able to maintain enough oxygen or the body may not get rid of enough carbon dioxide. A respiratory illness can deteriorate into acute respiratory failure. Central nervous system depression (due to trauma or medication) or disease can also lead to acute respiratory failure.

PROGNOSIS

Patients with respiratory failure are not getting enough oxygen. This may be a sudden event or a decompensation of a chronic respiratory condition such as emphysema or chronic bronchitis. Supplemental oxygen and bronchodilating medications are used to enhance airflow to the lungs. The underlying cause needs to be identified and corrected to reverse the problem and return the patient to normal respiratory status.

HALLMARK SIGNS AND SYMPTOMS

- Accessory muscles used to breathe as body works harder to move air
- Difficulty breathing (dyspnea) due to lack of oxygen
- Difficulty breathing when lying down (orthopnea) due to increased work of breathing in this position; diaphragm has to work harder; posterior chest wall does not expand well
- Fatigue due to work of breathing and lack of oxygenation
- Coughing may be due to inflammation, bronchospasm, fluid, or underlying lung condition
- Blood in sputum (hemoptysis) due to irritation of airways
- Respiration greater than 20 breaths per minute (tachypnea) in attempt to get more air and oxygen into lungs
- Sweating (diaphoresis) as body works harder to move air, using more muscles
- Cyanosis due to hypoxemia
- Anxiety due to air hunger and lack of oxygenation
- Rales (crackles) heard in the lungs if fluid builds up in alveoli and smaller airways
- Wheezing (rhonchi) due to inflammation within airways
- Diminished breath sounds due to decreased air movement

INTERPRETING TEST RESULTS

- Arterial blood gas:
  - decreased oxygen PaO_2 <60 mmHg without underlying lung disease

- elevated carbon dioxide ($PaCO_2$) >50 mmHg without underlying lung disease
- arterial oxygen saturation (SaO_2) <90 percent
- pH <7.30 (respiratory acidosis)
- Pulse oximetry shows low oxygen saturation.
- Increased WBC count due to infection.

TREATMENT

- Oxygen therapy to meet body's needs via nasal canula or mask.
- Administer bronchodilators to enhance airflow through airways in lungs:
  - albuterol, levalbuterol, metaproterenol, terbutaline
- Administer anticholinergics to treat bronchospasm:
  - ipratropium
- Intubation to maintain patent airway and assist mechanical ventilation.
- Administer anesthetic to ease intubation:
  - propofol
- Mechanical ventilation to support respiratory effort.
- Administer neuromuscular blocking agent to ease mechanical ventilation so the patient won't fight ventilator:
  - pancuronium, vecuronium, atracurium
- Administer steroids to decrease inflammatory response within lungs:
  - hydrocortisone, methylprednisolone, prednisone
- Administer anticoagulant to reduce risk of clot formation:
  - heparin, warfarin
- Administer analgesic for discomfort and to decrease myocardial oxygen demand:
  - morphine
- Administer histamine-2 blockers or proton pump inhibitors to reduce chances of stress-induced gastric ulcer:
  - famotidine, ranitidine, nizatidine, cimetidine
  - omeprazole, esomeprazole, lansoprazole, rabeprazole, pantoprazole
- Administer antibiotics to treat infection (or may be preventative):
  - selected according to results of culture and sensitivity study

NURSING DIAGNOSES

- Ineffective breathing pattern
- Ineffective airway clearance
- Anxiety

NURSING INTERVENTION

- Monitor respiratory status for rate, effort, use of accessory muscles, sputum production, and breath sounds.
- Monitor pulse oximetry to check oxygen saturation levels.
- Monitor sputum for changes in color and amount.
- Monitor vital signs for changes.
- Place patient in high Fowler's or semi-Fowler's position on bedrest to ease respiratory effort by allowing optimal diaphragmatic excursion.
- Monitor ventilator settings if appropriate.
- Change patient position every 2 hours to decrease chance of skin breakdown.
- Monitor intake and output of fluids to check for balance.
- Explain to the patient:
  - The importance of doing coughing and deep-breathing exercises to fully expand lungs and enhance the expelling of mucous.
  - How to identify the signs of respiratory distress.

16 *Pulmonary Embolism*

WHAT WENT WRONG?

Blood flow is obstructed in the lungs caused by thrombus (blood clot), air, or fat emboli that become stuck in an artery, causing impaired gas exchange. Patients may be predisposed to clot formation, have pooling of blood, or damage to vessel walls, or take certain medications that increase the risk of thrombus formation. Thrombus are commonly found in vessels in lower extremities. When a thrombus loosens and travels in the peripheral circulation, it is called an embolus. The embolus travels through the right side of the heart and is sent to the lungs where it lodges in one of the arteries. Depending on the size of the artery that the embolus lodges in, a section of lung will have no blood supply and alveolar function will suffer. As blood supply to an area of the lung diminishes, alveoli collapse, causing atelectasis.

PROGNOSIS

A small area of atelectasis will allow for resolution and return to normal function of the rest of the lung tissue. A large embolus at or near the main pulmonary artery may be fatal. Patients may need to take ongoing anticoagulants if they have repeat episodes or emboli or have an underlying clotting disorder.

HALLMARK SIGNS AND SYMPTOMS

- Sudden difficulty breathing (dyspnea) happens when the clot suddenly lodges in the artery
- Heart rate greater than 100 beats per minute (tachycardia)
- Respiration greater than 20 breaths per minutes (tachypnea) as the body attempts to get more oxygen
- Chest pain due to clot presence and area of atelectasis
- Coughing with blood-tinged sputum (hemoptysis)
- Crackles (rales) heard near area of clot

INTERPRETING TEST RESULTS

- Chest x-ray may show dilated pulmonary artery or pleural effusion.
- Lung scan shows ventilation-perfusion mismatch.
- Helical CT scan will show clot in pulmonary arteries.
- Pulmonary angiography will show presence of clot.
- Arterial blood gases may show decreased oxygen (PaO_2) and carbon dioxide ($PaCO_2$), depending on the size of the clot.
- D-dimer will be positive when a thromboembolic event has occurred.
- Lower extremity ultrasound is often done to test for presence of thrombus.

TREATMENT

Treatment is aimed at meeting the body's oxygen needs, preventing the clot from enlarging or moving, and preventing other clots from forming.

- Supplemental oxygen therapy.
- Administer thrombolytics to enhance breakdown of existing clot:
  - urokinase, alteplase
- Administer anticoagulants to prevent further clot formation:
  - heparin, warfarin
- Administer analgesic for pain control and to decrease myocardial oxygen demand:
  - morphine
- Surgical insertion of a vena cava filter in select patients to catch clots that travel from lower extremities up through inferior vena cava toward lung.
- Bed rest to prevent thrombus from breaking free from lower extremities.
- Surgical removal of the embolus may be necessary in some cases.

NURSING DIAGNOSES

- Impaired gas exchange
- Ineffective tissue perfusion
- Anxiety

NURSING INTERVENTION

- Monitor cardiovascular status for heart rate, rhythm, heart sounds, and pulse deficit.
- Monitor arterial blood gas for changes and decrease in oxygenation.
- Monitor pulse oximetry for oxygen saturation.
- Place patient in high Fowler's position.
- Have the patient perform turning, coughing, and deep-breathing exercises to enhance air movement.
- Monitor respiration for rate, effort, use of accessory muscles, skin color, and lung sounds.

- Explain to the patient:
  - To avoid sitting and standing for too long to decrease chance of clot formation.
  - Not to cross legs to avoid constriction of vessels in the lower extremities, decreasing the chances of clot formation.
  - How to identify side effects from using anticoagulants, such as bleeding or bruising.
  - That pulmonary embolism is an adverse effect from using hormonal contraceptives and a different form of birth control needs to be used in the future.

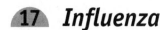 **17　*Influenza***

WHAT WENT WRONG?

A viral infection affecting the respiratory tract that spreads through droplets. The virus can be inhaled or picked up from surfaces through direct contact. Infection can settle into either the upper or lower respiratory tract. The virus causes damage to the upper layers of cells. The natural defenses of the respiratory tract are compromised and it is easier for bacteria to attach to the underlying respiratory tissues.

PROGNOSIS

Influenza symptoms typically run their course within about a week. Current medications help to decrease the length and severity of symptoms associated with influenza. Some patients will develop secondary infections, such as sinusitis or viral or bacterial pneumonia following influenza. Patients with pneumonia have an increased risk of mortality from influenza.

HALLMARK SIGNS AND SYMPTOMS

- Symptoms have an abrupt onset
- Nonproductive cough
- Chills and sweats
- Fatigue and malaise

- Fever over 101°F
- Headache
- Muscle aches (myalgia)
- Watery, nasal discharge
- Sore throat

INTERPRETING TEST RESULTS

- Nasopharyngeal viral culture.
- Rapid diagnostic kit.

TREATMENT

Symptomatic treatment to increase patient comfort and medications to shorten the duration and intensity of symptoms are the focus of patient management. Medications need to be started early in the symptoms.

- Administer antipyretics for comfort:
  - acetaminophen
- Administer antiviral medications:
  - zanamivir, oseltamivir
  - amantadine, rimantadine

NURSING DIAGNOSES

- Risk for injury
- Impaired gas exchange
- Hyperthermia

NURSING INTERVENTION

- Administer fluids and electrolytes to replace what is being lost due to sweating and insensible loss from elevated temperature.
- Monitor vital signs.

- Monitor respiratory status for rate, effort, use of accessory muscles, skin color, and breath sounds.

Crucial Diagnostic Tests

Bronchoscopy

WHY IS IT DONE?

Bronchoscopy is used to view the bronchial tree and to remove foreign obstructions, obtain tissues for biopsy, or for suctioning fluid.

HOW DOES THE TEST WORK?

The patient is anesthetized and a bronchoscope is inserted into the patient's mouth and down the trachea and bronchial tree. The bronchoscope contains a tiny video camera and probes that the physician manipulates to perform the procedure.

WHAT TO DO?

- Before the procedure:
  - The patient must sign an informed consent for an invasive procedure.
  - The patient is NPO for 8 hours except in an emergency, to reduce chances of vomiting when the bronchoscope is passed down the throat.
- During the procedure:
  - Monitor vital signs, respiratory effort, and skin color; cardiac monitor.
- After the procedure:
  - The patient remains nothing by mouth (NPO) until the gag reflex returns to avoid aspiration.
  - Verify the cough and gag reflex returns.
  - Monitor respirations for rate, effort, use of accessory muscles, and breath sounds.
  - Monitor heart rate and respiratory status for changes.
  - Monitor sputum for blood due to irritation within bronchi.

Chest X-ray

WHY IS IT DONE?

Used to detect the size and position of the heart and structural abnormalities of the lungs.

HOW DOES THE TEST WORK?

An x-ray machine directs x-rays through the chest and onto film positioned behind the patient. As x-rays are directed to the patient, some are absorbed by the body and others pass through to the film. Areas of the body that absorb x-rays appear light on the film. Dark areas on the film represent x-rays that passed through the body.

WHAT TO DO?

- Before the procedure:
  - Explain the test to the patient and that the patient will be asked to hold his or her breath while the x-ray is taken.
  - Before the test, remove all jewelry, zippers, hooks, and any metal on the part of the body being x-rayed.
- During the procedure:
  - Patient should hold his or her breath during the image to get a clear picture.

Pulmonary Angiography

WHY IS IT DONE?

Provides a view of the pulmonary circulatory system so that the physician can determine the condition of blood flow to the lungs.

HOW DOES THE TEST WORK?

Radiopaque dye is inserted into the patient's veins after a catheter has been passed through the heart into the pulmonary artery fluoroscopically. The image is watched on a screen as the dye flows through the pulmonary circulatory system.

WHAT TO DO?

- Before the procedure:
  - Verify that the patient is not allergic to contrast dye, iodine, or shellfish. If the patient is, then either another diagnostic study will be done, or the patient will be premedicated for this test if no other test is deemed appropriate. Diphenhydramine and prednisone may be given prior to the test to lessen or prevent an allergic reaction while closely monitoring the patient.
  - The patient must sign an informed consent based on institutional policy.
  - Instruct the patient that a flushed feeling is common when the dye is injected intravenously.
- During the procedure:
  - Monitor patient for tolerance of procedure and possible reaction to dye.
- After the procedure:
  - Monitor the insertion site for bleeding.

Sputum Culture and Sensitivity

WHY IS IT DONE?

Sputum from the patient is cultured to determine which, if any, bacteria is contained in the sputum and determine which antibiotic kills the bacteria.

HOW DOES THE TEST WORK?

Sputum is collected from the patient in a sterile container and sent to the lab where the sample is smeared in petri dishes and incubated to grow the bacteria. Samples of the bacteria are stained and examined under a microscope to identify the bacteria. The samples are checked periodically, but are usually given 72 hours to complete the testing process. Once identified, bacteria are exposed to known antibiotics to determine which antibiotic kills the bacteria.

WHAT TO DO?

- Before the test:
  - Use a sterile specimen container to determine that the bacteria that grow in the lab have come from the patient and not from contamination.

- Collect sputum only and not saliva—there are bacteria naturally found in the mouth, so saliva samples will grow bacteria in the lab even though it is not causing any infection.
- After the test:
  - Sample needs to go to the lab.
- Teach the patient:
  - How to properly obtain sputum sample.

Thoracentesis

WHY IS IT DONE?

Removal of fluid from the pleural sac to drain fluid or identify the contents of the fluid

HOW DOES THE TEST WORK?

The patient either sits at the edge of the bed or lies on the unaffected side. The affected site is anesthetized. A needle is inserted into the plural sac and fluid is drained using a syringe.

WHAT TO DO?

- Before the test:
  - The patient must sign an informed consent for an invasive procedure.
  - Position the patient at the edge of the bed or lying on the unaffected side with the head of the bed elevated 30 degrees.
- During the test:
  - Monitor the patient for tolerance of the procedure.
  - Monitor respiratory status for rate, effort, skin color, use of accessory muscles, and breath sounds.
- After the test:
  - Lay the patient on the affected side for 1 hour following the procedure. This applies direct pressure to the puncture site, reducing the chance of bleeding.
  - Monitor the injection site for leakage; reinforce dressing if drainage noted.
  - Monitor respiratory status for changes.

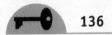

Pulmonary Function Test (PFT)

WHY IS IT DONE?

This test assesses the lungs' ability to move air. Monitor change from normal function; differentiate obstructive from restrictive disease.

HOW DOES THE TEST WORK?

The patient takes a deep breath. The spirometer is inserted into the patient's mouth and the patient breathes outward quickly at full force until all air is expelled. A deep breath is then taken in through the mouthpiece and this process is repeated three times. A computer then calculates the lungs' volume and vital capacity by measuring the amount of air moving in and out. The force of the air flow is measured. The duration of time of exhalation is measured.

WHAT TO DO?

- Before the test:
  - The patient should not smoke prior to the test. Smoking may have an effect on the outcome of the test.
- During the test:
  - Instruct the patient to take a deep breath and then exhale completely into the spirometer, followed by deep inhalation.
- After the test:
  - Administer bronchodilators after the initial testing is done and repeat the test if indicated. This will show the effect of bronchodilators on pulmonary function. Albuterol or levalbuterol are typically used.

Arterial Blood Gas (ABG)

WHY IS IT DONE?

This determines the patient's ventilation, tissue oxygenation, and acid-base status.

HOW DOES THE TEST WORK?

Three to five milliliters of blood is sampled from an artery in a heparinized syringe. If the sample cannot be analyzed right away, it should be placed on ice.

- The normal results are:
    - pH 7.35–7.45
    - PaO_2 80–100 mmHg
    - $PaCO_2$ 35–45 mmHg
    - HCO_3 22–26 mEq/L

WHAT TO DO?

- Before the test:
    - Provide the lab with information on whether or not the patient is receiving supplemental oxygen or mechanical ventilation as well as the amount of oxygen received or the setting of the ventilator. Oxygen supplementation at the time of testing will be reported with the results.
    - Note the patient's temperature. Alteration in temperature may alter the results of the test.
- After the test:
    - Apply mechanical pressure to puncture site for 5 minutes.
    - Apply pressure dressing to puncture site for 30 minutes once bleeding has stopped.
    - Monitor the puncture site for bleeding.

Ventilation-Perfusion Scan (V/Q scan)

WHY IS IT DONE?

Enables visualization of the flow of blood in the lungs to determine if lung tissue is adequately perfused.

HOW DOES THE TEST WORK?

The patient inhales radioactive gas mixed with oxygen for the ventilation phase. Radioisotopes are intravenously injected into the patient's veins using an IV access for the perfusion phase.

WHAT TO DO?

- Before the test:
  - Explain the procedure to the patient.
- During the test:
  - The patient must lie still for the testing, holding his or her breath as directed.

Mantoux Intradermal Skin Test (PPD)

WHY IS IT GIVEN?

This determines if the patient has antibodies to the *Mycobacterium tuberculosis* bacteria, which indicates that the patient has been exposed to the bacteria.

HOW DOES THE TEST WORK?

An injection of tuberculin is given intradermally. The test is positive if an indurated area appears around the injection site after 48 to 72 hours. A positive test indicates the presence of antibodies. Further testing is used to confirm that the patient has TB. Following a positive Mantoux test, the patient will typically be sent for a chest x-ray and may have a sputum culture for mycobacterium done.

WHAT TO DO?

- Before the test:
  - Explain to the patient why the test is being done, and that a positive result means that the patient has been exposed to TB. Further testing would need to be done to know if disease is currently present.

- During the test:
  - The injection needs to be given intradermally on the forearm. If it is given at the wrong depth, the reading will not be accurate and there may be irritation or damage to the tissue.
- After the test:
  - Patients need to return in 48 to 72 hours to have the injection area evaluated for induration.
- Teach the patient:
  - That a positive test result means they have been exposed to the disease.
  - Further testing may need to be done depending on the outcome of this test.
  - There may be slight redness at the injection site later on the day of injection. This does not mean that the test is positive or that the patient has TB. The result is read at 48 to 72 hours.

Lung Biopsy

WHY IS IT DONE?

Removal of a tissue sample to be examined by the histology lab for abnormalities.

HOW DOES THE TEST WORK?

A tissue sample can be extracted by inserting a needle through the chest and into the lung or by using a bronchoscope. A biopsy can also be performed as an open procedure through the chest wall, opening the lung to remove tissue samples.

WHAT TO DO?

- Before the test:
  - The patient must sign an informed consent. This is required for an invasive procedure which will remove something from the body.
  - NPO for 8 hours to decrease the chance of aspiration if done as an open procedure.
- During the test:
  - Monitor vital signs, skin color, and respiratory effort; cardiac monitor.

- After the test:
  - Examine the incision site for bleeding.
  - Monitor respiration for changes, potential for pneumothorax development after a piece of the lung has been removed.

Quiz

1. Following an asthmatic attack, a mother asks you how to prevent another asthmatic attack. You should:

   (a) Tell her that asthmatic attacks cannot be prevented.

   (b) Help the mother identify triggers that cause asthmatic attacks and show her how to avoid them.

   (c) Ask her physician to change her medication.

   (d) Immediately move her family to a dry climate.

2. The patient presents with difficulty breathing and a barrel chest. He is diagnosed with emphysema. The patient asks why increasing oxygen therapy doesn't relieve his difficulty breathing. The best response is:

   (a) Difficulty breathing is due to air trapped in your lungs, reducing the lungs' ability to exchange oxygen and carbon dioxide. Increasing oxygen does not resolve the trapped air.

   (b) You must lie on your right side for oxygen therapy to work properly.

   (c) Your barrel chest has decreased, causing your lungs to over-expand.

   (d) You must take deeper breaths when receiving oxygen therapy.

3. The physician has scheduled a thoracentesis. The patient asks why there is so much fluid in the pleural space. The best response is:

   (a) An error occurred and you were administered too much IV medication.

   (b) Your body is unable to remove fluid, resulting in a build-up of fluid in the pleural space around your lungs.

   (c) This is the result of oxygen therapy.

   (d) This is a normal side effect of bumetanide, which is the medication ordered by your physician.

4. Your patient is apprehensive about undergoing bronchoscopy. He cannot imagine having anything inserted into his throat. What is the best response?

(a) Your physician performs this procedure hundreds of times a week.

(b) I had it performed three years ago and I was fine.

(c) The thought of this procedure seems to be disturbing you. You will be asleep during this procedure. I will ask your physician to visit you again and answer any questions that you have regarding the procedure.

(d) You won't feel a thing. You'll be fine.

5. A 25-year-old nonsmoker who is normally in good health reports having a bad cough for the past three weeks. He has crackles and rhonchi and shows you a small clear plastic container that has discolored, blood-tinged sputum that he produced this morning. What would his physician want to rule out?

(a) Lung cancer.

(b) The flu.

(c) Pneumonia.

(d) Asthma.

6. Your patient returns from the operating room. Why would you monitor the patient for atelectasis?

(a) All postoperative patients are at risk for infection.

(b) Postoperative patients might have received too much oxygen during surgery.

(c) Immobility, anesthesia, and lack of deep breathing places the patient at risk for atelectasis.

(d) Postoperative patients do not receive enough oxygen during surgery.

7. A patient reports sudden difficulty breathing with tachypnea and tachycardia and localized chest pain. The physician suspects a pulmonary embolism. What test would you expect the physician to order?

(a) Helical CT scan.

(b) EKG.

(c) ECC.

(d) Vital capacity.

8. The patient hospitalized with bronchitis is concerned that she might have chronic bronchitis. She asks you to explain the difference between acute and chronic bronchitis. What is the best response?

    (a) Acute bronchitis lasts for three consecutive months and is reversible.

    (b) Acute bronchitis lasts seven to ten days.

    (c) Chronic bronchitis lasts three consecutive months in two consecutive years, resulting in blockage of the airways and cannot be reversed. Acute bronchitis is caused by a viral or bacterial infection and lasts about ten days. Blockage of the airways is reversible in acute bronchitis.

    (d) I will ask your physician to explain the differences during his rounds.

9. A patient who has successfully been treated for a pulmonary embolism is about to be discharged. How can he lower the risk of experiencing another pulmonary embolism?

    (a) Avoid sitting and standing for too long and do not cross legs.

    (b) Take vitamin K with heparin.

    (c) Avoid confined spaces.

    (d) Jog five miles each day.

10. The physician orders a pulmonary function test. The patient asks you how the test is performed. The best response is:

    (a) A tube is inserted into your lungs while you are asleep to expand your lungs to their full capacity.

    (b) You breathe through a mouthpiece into a spirometer until all air in your lungs is expelled. Then you will take a deep breath through the mouthpiece. This is done three times and a computer calculates the capacity of your lungs.

    (c) You breathe into a spirometer to measure your lung capacity.

    (d) A computer is used to measure your volume and vital capacity.

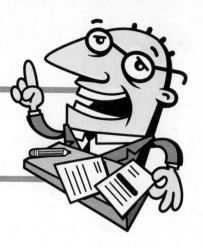

CHAPTER 3

Immune System

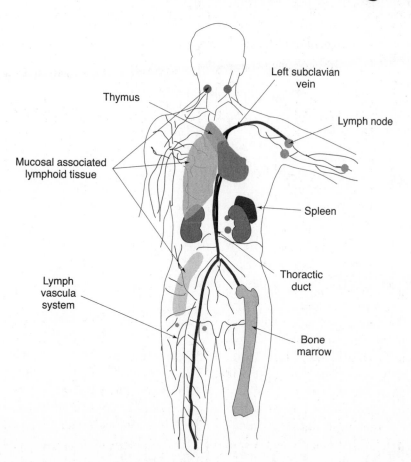

Learning Objectives

1 Acquired immunodeficiency
   syndrome (AIDS)

2 Anaphylaxis

3 Ankylosing spondylitis

4 Kaposi's sarcoma (KS)

5 Lymphoma

6 Rheumatoid arthritis

7 Scleroderma

8 Mononucleosis

9 Epstein-Barr virus/
   Chronic fatigue syndrome

10 Lyme disease

11 Septic shock

12 Systemic lupus erythematosus
    (SLE)

Key Terms

Allergies
Anaphylaxis
Antigen
Autoimmune disorders
B-cells
Exudation

Histamines
Human immunodeficiency virus
   (HIV)
Hypersensitivity reactions
Immunodeficiency disorders
Lymphocytes

Reed-Sternberg cells
T-cells
Tryptase
Urticaria
Western blot

How the Immune System Works

Normal functioning of the immune system protects the body against the invasion of outside organisms. A variety of organisms are capable of this; however, not all are harmful. The cells of the immune system recognize organisms that invade the body, then isolate and destroy them. At times, the immune system is not able to adequately function in this capacity. This results in infection, immunodeficiency disorders, autoimmune disorders, allergies, and hypersensitivity reactions.

Lymphocytes are the primary cells of the immune system. Lymphocytes are divided into B-cells and T-cells. B-cells provide a humoral immune response, since they produce an antigen-specific antibody. T-cells provide a cellular immune response. Mature T-cells are composed of CD4 and CD8 cells. CD8 cells are responsible for destroying foreign and viral inhabited cells, and suppress immunological functions. CD4 cells, also known as helper T-cells, stimulate immune functions, such as B-cells and macrophages. A macrophage is a cell whose functions include ingesting foreign or invading cells.

Just the Facts

1 Acquired Immunodeficiency Syndrome (AIDS)

WHAT WENT WRONG?

The human immunodeficiency virus (HIV) causes malfunction of T-cells which protect the body from invading microorganisms. When it enters a cell, HIV replicates, causing the cell to reproduce more infected cells. It also frequently causes cell death. The CD4 lymphocyte is most often affected, followed by B-lymphocytes and macrophages. Immunodeficiency results.

PROGNOSIS

Prognosis has improved since HIV was discovered in 1981. Fewer patients are progressing from HIV to AIDS, and both classes are living longer. New drugs and therapies are decreasing the number of deaths. Patients are living with fewer disabilities and comorbidities.

HALLMARK SIGNS AND SYMPTOMS

- Anorexia—secondary to GI manifestations, oral disease, and side effects of medications.
- Fatigue—cells dying at an abnormal rate; opportunistic infections due to a poorly functioning immune system.

- Night sweats—immune system triggered response.
- Fever—may be due to a concurrent infection related to a low WBC count.
- Malnutrition—due to poor appetite, poor nutrition, nausea and vomiting, and most often from a secondary infection; decreased protein synthesis.

INTERPRETING TEST RESULTS

- Less than 200 T-cells per microliter—the CD4 lymphocyte is the most commonly used count; <200 cells/μl signals the process from HIV to AIDS, and thus, increases the risk for malignancies and advancing infection.
- Positive HIV antibody titer—95 percent positive 6 weeks after contact. Often used with the Western blot to confirm diagnosis.
- Positive Western blot—confirms positive HIV test.

TREATMENT

- High-calorie and high-protein diet to combat wasting and weight loss.
- Administer antibiotics to combat opportunistic infections:
  - trimethoprim/sulfamethoxazole
- Administer antiviral medication to suppress HIV replication, causing support of the immune system and fewer opportunistic infections.
  - Nucleoside analogs (have antiviral activity):
    - didanosine
    - zidovudine
    - stavudine
    - zalcitabine
  - Nucleotide analog:
    - tenofovir
  - Protease inhibitors (suppress HIV replication):
    - fortovase
    - ritonavir
    - indinavir
    - nelfinavir
  - Nonnucleoside reverse transcriptase inhibitors (stop reverse transcriptase at a different site):

- nevirapine
- delavirdine
- efavirenz
- Administer antiemetic to combat nausea:
  - prochlorperazine
- Administer antifungal medication to combat fungal infections, which are often opportunistic:
  - fluconazole

NURSING DIAGNOSES

- Hopelessness
- Social isolation
- Ineffective protection

NURSING INTERVENTION

- Maintain activity as tolerated and schedule rest periods to maintain physical functioning.
- Avoid exposure to blood to prevent the spread of the virus.
- Explain to the patient:
  - Use of condoms to prevent the spread of the virus.

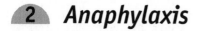 *Anaphylaxis*

WHAT WENT WRONG?

An allergen, usually food or medication, enters the body causing the release of histamines, which result in capillaries dilating and smooth muscle contracting. This results in edema, respiratory distress, hypotension, and skin changes, leading to an allergic reaction. Lesser degrees of extreme allergy are urticaria (hives) and angio-edema (swelling caused by exudation).

PROGNOSIS

Prognosis may be guarded, depending on how severe the reaction is and how quickly treatment is rendered. Patients need to be monitored for 1 to 2 days after treatment and cautioned about reexposure to the offending item.

HALLMARK SIGNS AND SYMPTOMS

- Shortness of breath due to swelling of the larynx
- Hypotension and shock due to generalized vasodilation
- Sneezing—a common occurrence to an allergan
- Anxiety secondary to difficulty in breathing
- Rales (crackles) heard in the lungs—due to fluid in the lungs
- Wheezing (rhonchi) due to bronchospasm

INTERPRETING TEST RESULTS

Tryptase levels are from mast cells which increase in anaphylaxis. After the acute episode is over, allergy skin testing is recommended.

TREATMENT

- Administer emergency medications:
  - epinephrine to open airways and to reduce bronchospasm
  - corticosteroids to reduce symptoms
  - antihistamines to mitigate symptoms
- Administer circulatory volume expanders to treat hypotension caused by vasodilation:
  - saline
  - plasma
  - IV fluids
- Administer vasopressors to counteract vasodilation and to increase blood pressure:
  - norepinephrine
  - dopamine

- Oxygen therapy to support breathing.
- Insert endotracheal tube to maintain airway.

NURSING DIAGNOSES

- Decrease cardiac output
- Risk for suffocation
- Anxiety

NURSING INTERVENTION

- Maintain airway to facilitate breathing.
- Monitor for hoarseness and difficulty breathing to check for symptoms of decreased respiration.
- Explain to the patient:
  - Avoid exposure to allergens to prevent future occurrences.
  - Seek medical help immediately if exposed to allergens to prevent anaphylaxis.

3 *Ankylosing Spondylitis*

WHAT WENT WRONG?

Ankylosing spondylitis (AS) is a progressive form of arthritis that affects <1 percent of the population. Joints between the spine and pelvis become inflamed, as do some of the ligaments, resulting in instability of the joints. Heredity factors play an important role in the development of AS. The disease is strongly associated with the presence of histocompatibility antigen HLA-B27 on the chromosomes of affected individuals. It begins in the sacroiliac joints and spreads up the spine.

PROGNOSIS

The course of the disease may vary in each case and from individual to individual. Some have episodes of transient back pain while others have more chronic severe back pain that leads to varying degrees of spinal stiffness over time. The disease is characterized by acute painful exacerbations and remissions.

HALLMARK SIGNS AND SYMPTOMS

- Severe lower back pain after a period of inactivity due to inflammation and stiffness
- Reduced motion of the lumbar area of the spine due to the pain of inflammation

INTERPRETING TEST RESULTS

- Spinal x-ray: joints show the characteristic Bamboo spine that is a late sign. Early x-rays may show arthritic erosion.
- Blood serum contains the HLA-B27 antigen, which is present in about 90 percent of those with AS.
- Elevated ESR.

TREATMENT

Nonpharmacologic measures include patient education, family education, genetic counseling, positioning, extension exercises, and physical therapy. The primary goals are to relieve pain, decrease inflammation, begin strengthening exercises, and maintain good posture and function. Medications take an empiric approach. If one NSAID is not effective for that particular patient, another is tried. Corticosteroids should not be utilized for long-term management due to the systemic effects.

- Stretching exercises—to maintain flexibility.
- Back brace—to maintain posture.
- Administer nonsteroidal anti-inflammatory agent—to decrease inflammation and for the analgesic effect.
  - aspirin
  - ibuprofen
  - indomethacin
  - sulfasalazine
  - sulindac
- Physical therapy.

NURSING DIAGNOSES

- Activity intolerance
- Impaired physical mobility
- Chronic pain

NURSING INTERVENTION

- Administer intermittent heat to the lumbar area of the spine for symptom relief.
- Massage the lumbar area of the spine for symptom relief.
- Provide comfort to the patient.
- Explain to patient:
  - It is best to sit in a high back chair for posture.
  - Repeated attempts to maintain erect posture.

4   *Kaposi's Sarcoma (KS)*
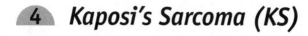

WHAT WENT WRONG?

Overgrowth of blood vessels that leads to malignant tumors and cancer of lymphatic tissue and skin commonly found in patients with AIDS. Usually seen in cases of advanced AIDS.

PROGNOSIS

Kaposi's sarcoma is often associated with AIDS. The treatment of AIDS with antiretrovirals usually helps the symptoms of KS.

HALLMARK SIGNS AND SYMPTOMS

- Red, brown, and purple lesions on the buccal mucosa, lips, gums, tongue, and palates because it is a malignancy affecting the skin and mucosa.
- Difficulty breathing (dyspnea) if the malignancy invades the pulmonary system.

INTERPRETING TEST RESULTS

- Biopsy to look for the HIV virus, and B-lymphocytes.
- CT scan to determine metastasis of the lesion to ascertain the severity of the disease.

TREATMENT

The treatment for KS is often specific for the individual lesion, using radiation. Treatment for AIDS will also ameliorate, to some degree, the effects of AIDS.

- Radiation in the affected tissue to shrink and treat tumors. Laser surgery may be utilized to remove some lesions.
- Administer antiemetic medication to counter effects of chemotherapy and radiation:
  - trimethobenzamide
- Administer chemotherapy medication to slow or halt the disease:
  - doxorubicin
  - etoposide
  - vinblastine
  - vincristine

NURSING DIAGNOSES

- Disturbed body image
- Ineffective protection
- Risk for infection

NURSING INTERVENTION

- Monitor skin for lesions to determine new lesions and/or metastasis.
- Daily weighing to determine changes in weight from baseline.
- Explain to the patient:
  - The need for dietary changes, such as a high-protein, high-calorie diet.
  - How to conserve energy.
  - Hospice care.

5 *Lymphoma*

WHAT WENT WRONG?

Functionless and damaged cells of the lymphatic system undergo overgrowth, decreasing the effectiveness of the lymphatic system. There are two main types of lymphoma, characterized by painless lymph node swelling:

- Hodgkin's disease is malignant lymphoma characterized by presence of Reed-Sternberg cells. There are four stages of Hodgkin's disease:
    - Stage I—Reed-Sternberg cells appear in one lymph node region.
    - Stage II—Reed-Sternberg cells appear in multiple lymph node regions on the same side of the diaphragm.
    - Stage III—Reed-Sternberg cells appear in multiple lymph node regions on both sides of the diaphragm.
    - Stage IV—Reed-Sternberg cells appear throughout the body.
- Non-Hodgkin's lymphoma (NHL) are cancers of the B-lymphocytes and are characterized by the absence of Reed-Sternberg cells.

The lymphomas are caused by a disruption of cells during differentiation. Diagnosis is made on lymph node biopsy.

PROGNOSIS

Prognosis depends on what stage the patient was in upon diagnosis, and on response to treatment. Survival is generally <10 years for non-Hodgkins; may be more for Hodgkins, with an optimistic staging.

HALLMARK SIGNS AND SYMPTOMS

- B symptoms (night sweats, fever, and weight loss)
- Enlarged, painless lymph nodes in cervical region, mesentery, abdomen, and pelvis.

INTERPRETING TEST RESULTS

- Lymph node biopsy contains Reed-Sternberg cells, which typify Hodgkin's disease.
- Bone marrow biopsy contains follicular type cells (Non-Hodgkin's lymphoma).

TREATMENT

Treatment depends on the staging, which is based on the number of involved lymph nodes, and the number of cavities, and bone marrow involvement.

- Radiation in the affected tissue to shrink the nodes.
- Administer Hodgkin's disease medication:
  - vincristine
  - doxorubicin
  - bleomycin
  - dacarbazine
- Administer non-Hodgkin's lymphoma medication:
  - cyclophosphamide
  - vincristine
  - doxorubicin
  - rituximab
  - prednisone
  - radiation

NURSING DIAGNOSES

- Impaired tissue integrity
- Risk for infection
- Ineffective protection

NURSING INTERVENTION

- Monitor vital signs to determine variations from baseline.
- Monitor for complications such as new palpable lymph nodes and fever.
- Increase fluid intake.
- Increase calories, protein, iron, calcium, and vitamins and minerals to counter-act weight loss.
- Administer prescribed antiemetic medication for nausea.
- Monitor laboratory results for blood counts in response to chemotherapy.

- Explain to the patient:
  - Consult with physician before using over-the-counter medication.

6 *Rheumatoid Arthritis*

WHAT WENT WRONG?

Antibodies from the bloodstream move into the synovial lining of joints, causing joints to swell. The swelling affects the functionality of tendons, bones, and ligaments that move the joint, resulting in pain with movement. Etiology is unknown, although genetics plays a part. The usual age of onset is 20 to 40 years, and it affects about 2 percent of the population. Inflammation and nodules around joints are common, usually involving the wrists, hands, knees, and feet.

PROGNOSIS

Prognosis is variable. Some patients go into remission and need only moderate treatment. Others progress with decreased functioning, with cardiac, renal, and respiratory disease. Life expectancy is greatly lessened for this group.

HALLMARK SIGNS AND SYMPTOMS

- Morning stiffness in joints due to the inflammation
- Enlarged joints from swelling
- Pain when moving due to the stiffness
- Limited range of motion because of the inflammation and pain
- Fever, malaise, and weight loss

INTERPRETING TEST RESULTS

- Rheumatoid factor is positive in blood test.
- Positive antinuclear antibody (ANA).

- Positive ESR.
- Gamma globulins.
- X-rays show changes in the affected joints.

TREATMENT

Reduction of pain and inflammation is the goal of treatment, along with preserving range of motion of the joint. Treatment is divided into nonpharmacological and pharmacological methods.

- Administer nonsteroidal anti-inflammatory (NSAID) medication to decrease inflammation and pain:
  - ibuprofen
  - indomethacin
  - flurbiprofen
  - naproxen
  - sulindac
  - diflunisal
- Administer disease-modifying antirheumatology agents (DMARDS):
  - methotrexate is an antimetabolite
  - TNF1—tumor necrosis factor increases lymphocytes and leukocytes found in the joint fluids
  - etenercept
  - infliximab
  - adalimumab
  - antimalarials
  - hydroxychloroquine
- Administer corticosteroids:
  - prednisone
- Administer antacids to coat the stomach:
  - magnesium hydroxide
  - aluminium hydroxide

- Physical therapy and occupational therapy to maintain ADL and independence.

- Cold and heat therapy for pain relief, anti-inflammatory effect, to help muscles and joints.

- Splints to maintain joints in positions that are most used.

- Exercises to maintain flexibility and ROM (range of motion).

NURSING DIAGNOSES

- Chronic pain
- Activity intolerance
- Disturbed body image

NURSING INTERVENTION

- Assist patient in placing a splint on affected joint.
- Weight loss to place less stress on joints.
- Explain to the patient:
- Get a full night's sleep.
- Avoid the cold.
- Reduce stress.

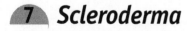 *Scleroderma*

WHAT WENT WRONG?

Antibodies attack connective tissues in an autoimmune response. This results in scar tissue (fibrosis) forming on skin, organs, GI tract, blood vessels, and muscles, causing systemic sclerosis.

It is a chronic disease of unknown etiology, usually seen in 30-to-50-year-olds.

PROGNOSIS

Scleroderma is a progressive disease causing early death, especially in those patients with diffuse disease. Organ damage indicates an earlier demise; those with limited organ involvement have longer life expectancies.

HALLMARK SIGNS AND SYMPTOMS

- Stiffness and pain due to the fibrosis
- Skin thickens
- Edema, malaise, and fever

INTERPRETING TEST RESULTS

- Positive antinuclear antibody.
- Dermis appears thickened in skin biopsy.

TREATMENT

Treatment is based on treating the patient's symptoms to ensure comfort. No known medications are able to stop the disease. Various medications may be used to treat the symptoms of the affected organs caused by scleroderma.

- Physical therapy to maintain joint mobility.

NURSING DIAGNOSES

- Impaired physical mobility
- Impaired skin integrity
- Pain

NURSING INTERVENTION

- Monitor for increasing blood pressure, which is the leading cause of death to scleroderma patients due to the renal effects of the disease.

- Explain to the patient:
  - That there is no cure for scleroderma, but it may go into remission and then relapse.
  - Schedule rest periods during activities.
  - Avoid the cold.

8 *Mononucleosis*

A viral syndrome consisting of sore throat, enlarged lymph glands, and fevers. Usually caused by the Epstein-Barr Virus, but sometimes other viruses are the cause. Occasionally, a rash may be seen. The spleen is sometimes enlarged due to sequestration of cells during the immune response.

WHAT WENT WRONG?

A virus was transmitted from contact to contact. Oftentimes, a secondary bacterial infection, streptococcus, is found.

PROGNOSIS

Prognosis is good. Since it is a disease of young people, recovery is generally uncomplicated.

HALLMARK SIGN AND SYMPTOMS

- General malaise
- Fever
- Myalgias
- Headache
- Sore throat

INTERPRETING TEST RESULTS

- Mono Spot or a positive heterophil antibody test is used to identify the Epstein-Barr Virus.
- CBC, chemistry.
- Throat culture for strep.

TREATMENT

Treatment is supportive with rest and over-the-counter medications for symptom resolution.

- Penicillin or erythromycin for the streptococcal throat.

NURSING DIAGNOSES

- Fatigue
- Activity intolerance
- Impaired physical mobility

NURSING INTERVENTIONS

- Encourage adequate rest.
- Assure fluids and nutritional intake.
- Monitor fever and vital signs.
- Throat culture, if indicated.
- Analgesics.

9 *Epstein-Barr Virus/ Chronic Fatigue Syndrome*

WHAT WENT WRONG?

Chronic Fatigue Syndrome (CFS) is a chronic, multisymptom, multisystem syndrome in a previously healthy adult. It results from any of five so far known viruses: Epstein-Barr, cytomegalovirus, coxsackievirus B, adenovirus type I, and human herpes virus 6. In an unknown way, the viruses disturb the immune system which is then unable to adequately fight off the virus.

PROGNOSIS

The prognosis varies as the disease waxes and wanes. Remissions and exacerbations may be frequent. By adulthood, most of the population in the United States will test positive for EB virus.

SIGNS AND SYMPTOMS

Persistent fatigue unrelieved by rest, impairment of memory and concentration, myalgias, arthralgias, headache, change in sleep, malaise, depression, and labile mood. Insomnia is a common occurrence.

INTERPRETING TEST RESULTS

Since CFS is a diagnosis of exclusion, testing is done to rule out other etiologies for the symptoms. These may include CBC, metabolic panel, thyroid studies, HIV, ESR, rheumatoid factor, Lyme, EBV, and CMV titers.

TREATMENT

Treatment is empirical and based on symptoms. Treating and eliminating other diagnoses is imperative. Allowing for frequent rest periods, and adequate nutrition are necessary. Pharmacological treatment may include NSAIDs and analgesics. As there is a higher prevalence of past and present psychiatric diagnoses in patients with CFS, an evaluation may be indicated. Psychotherapy may help. Physical therapy is often indicated and routine exercising has been found to be helpful.

NURSING DIAGNOSES

- Activity intolerance
- Fatigue
- Chronic pain

NURSING INTERVENTIONS

- Provide supportive care.
- Encourage fluids and adequate nutrition.
- Rest.
- Offer psychotherapy.
- Exercise regimen.

10 *Lyme Disease*

WHAT WENT WRONG?

A bite from a deer tick causes the bacteria (a spirochete) *Borrelia burgdorferi,* to be transmitted into the human blood stream. The patient presents with fever, myalgias and the classic bull's eye rash, erythema chronicum migrans up to three weeks following the bite.

PROGNOSIS

Early treatment generally leads to a better outcome. Lingering constitutional symptoms occasionally occur.

HALLMARK SIGNS AND SYMPTOMS

- Fever
- Generalized aches
- Headache
- Rash at site of the bite (patient may not recall bite)

INTERPRETING TEST RESULTS

- IgM antibody is elevated.
- Lyme titers may be drawn.

TREATMENT

- doxycycline, 100 mg bid (twice a day) × 14 to 21 days.
- aqueous penicillin G, 20 million units.
- ceftriaxone, 4 grams/day IM or IV.

NURSING DIAGNOSES

- Impaired skin integrity
- Impaired physical mobility

NURSING INTERVENTIONS

- Cover all exposed skin while outside.
- Use appropriate insect repellant.
- Inspect arms and legs for ticks when coming in from outside.
- Inspect pets.
- Educate on proper way to remove tick.

11 *Septic Shock*

WHAT WENT WRONG?

Septic shock starts with bacteremia, usually gram negative bacteria infecting the blood. The sources are usually genito-urinary system, gastrointestinal tract, and lungs. The infection may be underlying for some time before shock develops. Once the cascade from bacteremia to septic shock starts, it may be difficult to halt the process. Shock may occur more quickly in patients who are elderly, immune-compromised, or with other comorbidities. In response to a bacterial infection, TNF-alpha and other inflammatory chemicals are released into the blood, causing an increase in the blood leaking from vessels into both the infected and non-infected tissues (vascular permeability).

PROGNOSIS

Prognosis depends on the general state of the patient, on the type of bacteria, how quickly a definitive diagnosis is made, and the originating source(s) of the bacteremia. Mortality rates vary from 40 to 80 percent.

HALLMARK SIGNS AND SYMPTOMS

- Nausea and vomiting from the source of the infection
- Temperature over 101°F due to infection
- Hypotension due to fluid displacement, vasodilation
- Tachycardia from fever and infection
- Tachypnea from fever and infection
- Lactic acidosis results from poor oxygenation

INTERPRETING TEST RESULTS

- WBC 15,000 to 30,000—indicates infection.
- Decreased platelet count—blood coagulopathies are common in shock.
- Abnormal PT and PTT—blood coagulopathies.

TREATMENT

Treatment results depends on the individual. Varying responses are due to the variable immune and inflammatory responses of each patient and their comorbidities. Treatment depends on identifying the organism, the source of the bacteremia, the appropriate antibiotic, and maintaining normal vital signs.

- Antibiotic specific for the type of bacteria present.
- Fluid resuscitation.

NURSING DIAGNOSES

- Decreased cardiac output
- Deficient fluid volume
- Skin integrity

NURSING INTERVENTION

- Monitor vital signs, especially fever.
- Monitor fluid intake and output to assess for fluid overload and hydration status.
- Monitor coagulation factors.

12 *Systemic Lupus Erythematosus (SLE)*

WHAT WENT WRONG?

SLE is a chronic inflammatory immune disorder affecting the skin and other body organs. Antibodies to DNA and RNA cause an autoimmune inflammatory response, resulting in swelling and pain. It is most common in young women, and has a strong genetic factor. The etiology is not known.

PROGNOSIS

Prognosis is good but is consistent with many remissions and exacerbations. Most patients do quite well on a course of medications, but some progress rapidly with severe organ involvement and subsequently, death. Certain medications may produce lupus-like symptoms in patients. A review of medications is indicated before a diagnosis is made.

HALLMARK SIGNS AND SYMPTOMS

- Butterfly rash on face due to deposition of immunoglobulin and complement in the skin.
- Fatigue may be due to anemia
- Anemia due to inflammation
- Fever, malaise
- Joint pain

INTERPRETING TEST RESULTS

- Positive antinuclear antibody test—antibodies are present in the blood.
- Positive rheumatoid factor.

TREATMENT

Treatment of SLE is supportive. The drugs used should match the stage the patient is in at the time. Treatment of systemic signs is dependent on the organ system involved.

- Administer NSAIDs to decrease the inflammation and give analgesic effects:
  - ibuprofen
  - flurbiprofen
  - indomethacin
  - sulindac
  - naproxen
  - diclofenac
- Antimalarials—used to treat joint manifestations and skin rashes.
- Administer immunosuppressants in patients who are unresponsive to corticosteroids:
  - azathioprine
  - cyclophosphamide
- Administer analgesic:
  - NSAIDs
  - aspirin
  - acetaminophen
  - tramadol

NURSING DIAGNOSES

- Impaired mobility
- Disturbed body image

- Ineffective protection
- Chronic pain

NURSING INTERVENTION

- Avoid sunlight.
- Cover butterfly rash with cosmetics.
- Reduce stress.
- Monitor for infections.

Crucial Diagnostic Tests

Immunologic Blood Studies

WHY IS IT GIVEN?

These tests are used to identify immunological factors in the blood:

- *ANA.* The antinuclear antibodies test is a screening test for the detection of antibodies to nuclear antigens. Close to 100 percent of patients with SLE will show positive evidence.
- *ESR.* The erythrocyte sedimentation rate is useful in differentiating between inflammatory and neoplastic disease. Serial values are helpful to track disease severity.
- *SS-A* and *SS-B.* SS-A antibodies can be detected in about 30 percent of SLE patients. SS-B antibodies have a high specificity for the sicca complex, caused by diminished secretion from glands.
- *Rheumatoid factor.* Rheumatoid factor is an IgM antibody that is associated with rheumatoid arthritis. Blood is drawn from a vein and a study is conducted to determine if the blood contains this immunoglobulin antibody. 50 percent of the patients with rheumatoid arthritis have this antibody.
- *Scleroderma autoantibodies.* The sclerodema antibody is found in venous blood of patients who have scleroderma. The autoantibodies are positive in about 25 to 40 percent of scleroderma patients.

HOW DOES THE TEST WORK?

A small amount of blood is removed from the patient and is examined for immunoglobulins, and their antibodies, antinuclear antibodies, rheumatoid factor, and lupus erythematosus cell preparation. A positive finding indicates that the patient has the corresponding immunologic disease, or has had some exposure.

WHAT TO DO?

- After the procedure:
  - Make sure that the site of the venipuncture isn't bleeding to ensure that adequate clotting has occurred.
- Results should be available in several days.

Enzyme-Linked Immunosorbent Assay (ELISA)

WHY IS IT GIVEN?

This determines if the patient's blood contains antibodies for the human immuno-deficiency virus (HIV) to determine if the patient is HIV-positive.

HOW DOES THE TEST WORK?

A small sample of blood is taken and examined for the presence of the HIV antibody. This is generally used for screening and confirmation is necessary with a Western Blot test.

WHAT TO DO?

- Before the procedure:
  - Obtain written informed consent due to legal requirements.
  - Explain the purpose of the test and how the test results are interpreted.

- After the procedure:
  - Explain when the test results will be available to the patient.
  - Assess the site of the venipuncture to confirm adequate clotting.

Western Blot Tests

WHY IS IT GIVEN?

This test looks for the presence of HIV-related viral proteins in the patient's blood to confirm if the patient is HIV-positive.

HOW DOES THE TEST WORK?

A small amount of blood is taken and examined for the presence of HIV viral proteins.

WHAT TO DO?

- Before the procedure:
  - Obtain written informed consent due to legalities.
  - Explain the purpose of the test and how the test result is interpreted.
- After the procedure:
  - Explain when the test results will be available to the patient.
  - Make sure that the site of the venipuncture isn't bleeding to ensure adequate clotting.

Culture and Sensitivity of Sputum

WHY IS IT GIVEN?

Sputum from the patient is cultured to find which, if any, bacteria is contained in the sputum and determine which antibiotic will be effective.

HOW DOES THE TEST WORK?

Sputum is collected from the patient either from a deep cough or from suctioning and sent to the lab where samples are smeared on petri dishes and incubated for 48 to 72 hours to grow the bacteria. Samples of the bacteria are stained and examined under a microscope to identify the bacteria. Once identified, known antibiotics are administered to the bacteria in the petri dish to determine which antibiotic kills the bacteria.

WHAT TO DO?

- Before the test:
  - Determine which, if any, antibiotic the patient is taking.
  - Use a sterile specimen container to avoid contamination.
  - Collect sputum only and not saliva as the mouth contains many bacteria.
- During the test:
  - Deep coughs are necessary to generate sputum.
- After the test:
  - Continue taking the prescribed antibiotic.

Lymphangiography

WHY IS IT GIVEN?

This test produces a radiographic image of the lymphatic system to determine if there are any abnormalities, such as edema of the legs, Hodgkin's disease, lymphoma, lymphadenopathy, and lymphatic metastases. The results are useful in the staging of lymphoma and Hodgkin's disease and to determine the efficacy of treatment.

HOW DOES THE TEST WORK?

A radiopaque dye is injected via catheter into the lymphatic system and then the patient is x-rayed. The dye remains present for up to one year so repeat testing can be done.

WHAT TO DO?

- Before the test:
  - The patient must sign an informed consent due to the invasive nature of the test.
  - Make sure that the patient is not allergic to seafood, iodine, or contrast dye.
  - Check renal function (BUN, creatinine) as the kidneys are responsible for processing the dye.
- During the test:
  - Check for allergic reaction to the dye such as skin rash, itching, shortness of breath, and swelling.
- After the test:
  - Administer fluids to aid in elimination of the dye.
  - Monitor peripheral pulses to ensure adequate circulation in the feet.
  - Examine injection site for complications such as infection, bleeding, and edema.
  - Urine, stool, and skin might have a blue color from the dye.

Quiz

1. A cell whose functions include ingesting foreign or invading cells is a (an):
   (a) T-cell.
   (b) B-cell.
   (c) Macrophage.
   (d) Erythrocyte.

2. A confirmatory lab test for HIV includes:
   (a) Western Blot.
   (b) Low WBC.
   (c) Comprehensive metabolic panel.
   (d) Enzyme-linked immunosorbent assay (ELISA).

3. When assessing a patient for anaphylaxis, you would be alert for:

   (a) Chest pain and indigestion.

   (b) Hives and dyspnea.

   (c) Hypertension and blurred vision.

   (d) Headache and photophobia.

4. Patients with rheumatoid arthritis typically have pain:

   (a) With activity.

   (b) Upon awakening.

   (c) Late in the evening.

   (d) All day without remission.

5. The joints most commonly involved with rheumatoid arthritis include:

   (a) Symmetrical involvement of major joints.

   (b) Small joints of hands and feet.

   (c) Spine, from the sacrum upward to cervical.

   (d) Slightly movable joints of the axial skeleton.

6. The primary mode of treatment for ankylosing spondylitis is:

   (a) Relaxed posture for comfort.

   (b) Strict bedrest.

   (c) Physical therapy.

   (d) Respiratory therapy.

7. In your patient with a CD4 count <200, the most important nursing assessment would include:

   (a) Bowel movements.

   (b) Urinary output.

   (c) Fever.

   (d) Blood pressure.

8. The best treatment for mononucleosis is:

   (a) Antibiotics.

   (b) Physical therapy.

   (c) Nonsteroidal anti-inflammatories (NSAIDs).

   (d) Rest and fluids.

9. During exacerbations of Systemic Lupus Erythematosus, patients are often treated with:

   (a) Antiemetics.

   (b) Antineoplastics.

   (c) Corticosteroids.

   (d) Antibiotics.

10. Which of the following would have the highest priority in septic shock?

   (a) Monitoring temperature.

   (b) Monitoring ABC (airway, breathing, circulation).

   (c) Monitoring pupillary reaction.

   (d) Monitoring ANA and RF levels.

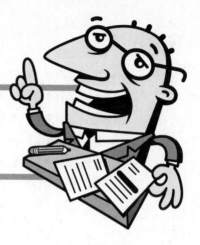

CHAPTER 4

Hematologic System

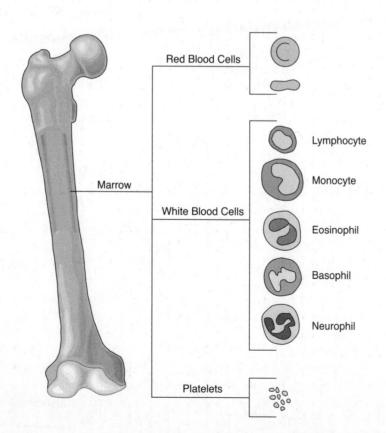

Red Blood Cells

Marrow

White Blood Cells

Lymphocyte

Monocyte

Eosinophil

Basophil

Neurophil

Platelets

Learning Objectives

1 Anemia

2 Aplastic anemia (Pancytopenia)

3 Iron deficiency anemia

4 Pernicious anemia

5 Disseminated intravascular coagulation (DIC)

6 Hemophilia

7 Leukemia

8 Multiple myeloma

9 Polycythemia vera

10 Sickle cell anemia

11 Deep vein thrombosis (DVT)

12 Idiopathic thrombocytopenic purpura (ITP)

 Key Terms

Clotting factors
Ecchymosis
Epistaxis
Hematocrit
Hemoglobin
Hemolysis

Leukopenia
Lymphocytes
Macrophages
Microemboli
Petechiae
Prothrombin

PT
PTT
Purpura
Stem cells
Thrombocytopenia

How the Hematologic System Works

The hematologic system refers to the blood and blood-forming organs. The formation of red blood cells, white blood cells, and platelets begins in the bone marrow. Stem cells are produced in the bone marrow. Initially, these cells are not differentiated and may become red blood cells (RBCs), white blood cells (WBCs), or platelets. In the next stage of development, the stem cell becomes committed to a particular precursor cell, to become either a myeloid or lymphoid type of cell and will differentiate into a particular cell type when in the presence of a specific growth factor.

The spleen is found in the left upper quadrant of the abdomen. The spleen filters whole blood. It removes old and imperfect white blood cells, lymphocytes and macrophages, and RBCs. The spleen also breaks down hemoglobin and stores of RBCs and platelets.

The liver is found in the right upper quadrant of the abdomen and is the main production site for many of the clotting factors, including prothrombin. Normal liver function is important for vitamin K production in the intestinal tract. Vitamin K is necessary for clotting factors VII, IX, X, and prothrombin.

Just the Facts

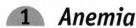

1 *Anemia*

WHAT WENT WRONG?

A low hemoglobin or red blood cell (RBC) count results in decreased oxygen-carrying capability of the blood. This may be due to blood loss, damage to the red blood cells due to altered hemoglobin or destruction (hemolysis), nutritional deficiency (iron, vitamin B_{12}, folic acid), lack of RBC production, or bone marrow failure. Some patients have a family history of anemia due to genetic transmission, such as thalassemia or sickle cell.

PROGNOSIS

Anemia is a symptom of something else happening. The cause of the anemia needs to be determined in order to correct the anemia and its symptoms.

HALLMARK SIGNS AND SYMPTOMS

- Fatigue due to hypoxia from less oxygen being available to the tissues of the body
- Weakness due to hypoxia
- Pallor due to less oxygen being available to the surface tissues
- Tachycardia as the body attempts to compensate for less available oxygen by beating more rapidly to increase blood supply
- Systolic murmur due to increased turbulence of blood flow
- Dyspnea or shortness of breath due to hypoxia as body attempts to get more oxygen
- Angina as the myocardium is not getting enough oxygen

pallor
hypoxia

- Headache due to hypoxia
- Lightheadedness due to hypoxia
- Bone pain due to increased erythropoiesis as body attempts to correct anemia
- Jaundice in hemolytic anemia due to increased levels of bilirubin as red blood cells break down

INTERPRETING TEST RESULTS

- Hemoglobin level low.
- Hematocrit level low.
- RBC count low.
- MCV (mean corpuscular volume) shows size of cell—normal (normocytic), microcytic (low), or macrocytic (high).
- MCH (mean corpuscular hemoglobin) shows color of cell—normal (normochromic), hypochromic (low).
- RDW (red cell distribution width) elevated—shows the variation of the cell sizes; there is greater variation in cell size when body is attempting to compensate for anemia.
- Reticulocyte count elevated when RBC cell production is increased to compensate for the anemia.

TREATMENT

Correction of the underlying cause is necessary. Treatment may include dietary modifications and supplementations. See specific anemias below.

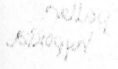

NURSING DIAGNOSIS

- Fatigue
- Activity intolerance

NURSING INTERVENTION

- Check vital signs for changes.
- Monitor CBC—hemoglobin, RBC, MCV, MCH, RDW.

- Plan nursing care based on patient tolerance of activity.
- Monitor for angina.

2　*Aplastic Anemia (Pancytopenia)*

WHAT WENT WRONG?

The bone marrow stops producing a sufficient amount of RBC, WBC, and platelets, thereby increasing the risk of infection and hemorrhage. The red cells remaining in circulation are normal in size and color. This may be due to chemical exposure, high-dose radiation exposure, or exposure to toxins. Cancer treatments such as radiation therapy and chemotherapeutic agents may suppress bone marrow function, which will result in anemia (low RBC), thrombocytopenia (low platelets), and leukopenia (low WBC). The cause may also be unknown or idiopathic.

PROGNOSIS

The bone marrow dysfunction may be slow-onset or sudden. The lifespan of the RBC is longer than the platelets and WBC, so the anemia may show up later than the effects of losing the other cells. Some exposures to toxic agents or medications are severe and potentially fatal in susceptible individuals.

HALLMARK SIGNS AND SYMPTOMS

- Fatigue due to hypoxemia
- Weakness due to tissue hypoxia
- Pallor due to lack of oxygen reaching superficial tissues due to anemia
- Infections due to low white blood cell production, causing decreased ability to fight infection
- Bruising (ecchymosis), and tiny subcutaneous (SC) hemorrhages (petechiae) due to decrease in platelets, altering clotting ability
- Bleeding from mucous membranes (GI tract, mouth, nose, vagina)

INTERPRETING TEST RESULTS

- Low hemoglobin.
- Low hematocrit.
- Low RBC count.
- Thrombocytopenia—low platelet count.
- Leukopenia—low WBC.
- Reticulocyte count low.
- Positive fecal occult blood test.
- Decreased cell counts in bone marrow biopsy as body stops producing.

TREATMENT

- Administer hematopoietic growth factor to correct anemia in patients with low erythropoietin levels:
  - erythropoietin, epoetin alfa (recombinant human erythropoietin) by SC injection or IV
- Administer human granulocyte colony-stimulating factor (G-CSF) to correct low WBC levels:
  - filgrastim by SC injection or IV
  - granulocyte-macrophage colony-stimulating factor (GM-CSF) sargram-ostim by IV infusion
- Packed RBC transfusions when anemia is symptomatic.
- Platelet transfusion for severe bleeding.
- Bone marrow transplant replaces functioning stem cells.
- Administer immunosuppressive drugs, antithymocyte globulin, and cortico-steroids.
- Splenectomy when spleen is enlarged and destroying RBCs.

NURSING DIAGNOSES

- Risk for infection
- Activity intolerance
- Risk for deficient fluid volume

NURSING INTERVENTION

- Monitor vital signs for changes.
- Record intake and output of fluids.
- Protect patient from falls.
- Avoid IM injections due to altered clotting ability.
- Explain to the patient:
  - No aspirin due to effect on platelet aggregation (clotting ability).
  - Plan to take rest periods during activities due to fatigue.
  - Only use an electric razor to decrease risk of bleeding due to decreased platelet count.
  - Call your physician, nurse practitioner, or physician assistant for signs of bleeding or bruising.

 Iron Deficiency Anemia

WHAT WENT WRONG?

A lower-than-normal amount of iron in blood serum results in decreased formation of hemoglobin and a decreased ability for the blood to carry oxygen. Iron stores are typically depleted first, followed by serum iron levels. Iron deficiency may be due to blood loss, dietary deficiency, or increased demand due to pregnancy or lactation. As red blood cells age, the body breaks them down and the iron is released. This iron is reused for the production of new blood cells. A small amount of iron is lost daily through the GI tract, necessitating dietary replacement. When RBCs are produced without a sufficient amount of iron, the cells are smaller and paler than usual.

PROGNOSIS

Iron deficiency anemia is a very common type of anemia. Typically patients respond to oral supplementation of iron. Occasionally a patient will have problems absorbing iron from the intestinal tract. These patients will need parenteral supplementation. Once iron stores are replaced, the anemia should correct and hemoglobin levels return to normal. Some patients may need lifelong supplementation, depending on the cause of the deficiency.

HALLMARK SIGNS AND SYMPTOMS

- Weakness due to anemia and tissue hypoxia
- Pallor due to decreased amount of oxygen getting to surface tissues
- Fatigue due to anemia and hypoxemia
- Koilonychia—thin, concave nails raised at edges, also called spoon nails
- Tachycardia and tachypnea on exertion due to increased demand for oxygen

INTERPRETING TEST RESULTS

- Decrease in serum hemoglobin as fewer RBCs are made.
- Serum ferritin is low.
- Mean corpuscular volume (MCV) initially normal, then low—microcytic anemia.
- Mean corpuscular hemoglobin (MCH) initially normal, then low—hypochromic anemia.
- Serum iron level is low.
- Serum iron-binding capacity is increased.
- Transferrin saturation decreases.
- Peripheral blood smear shows poikilocytosis (red blood cells of different shapes).
- Platelet count may increase.

TREATMENT

Iron replacement therapy is continued to correct the deficiency and replace the lost stores of iron in the body. The typical timeframe for oral therapy is to continue for 3 to 6 months after the anemia has been corrected. There have been documented incidents of anaphylactic reactions to iron dextran. Patients new to this treatment typically have a smaller test dose initially, prior to the initiation of treatments.

- Administer iron to replace what has been lost to return stores to normal levels:
  - Oral replacement in split doses (three times a day):
    - ferrous sulfate
    - ferrous gluconate
    - ferrous fumarate

- Parenteral iron replacement for those who cannot tolerate or do not respond to oral therapy, have gastrointestinal illness, or continued bleeding:
    - iron dextran given deep IM or IV
    - iron sodium gluconate given IV
    - iron sucrose complex given IV
  - IM injection of iron using Z-track method.
- Increase dietary intake of iron.

NURSING DIAGNOSES

- Imbalanced nutrition, less than what body requires
- Activity intolerance

NURSING INTERVENTION

- Monitor intake and output.
- Monitor vital signs for tachycardia or tachypnea.
- Monitor for reactions to parenteral iron therapy.
- Explain to the patient:
  - Check for bleeding.
  - Increase iron in diet.
  - Teach dietary sources of iron.

4   *Pernicious Anemia*

WHAT WENT WRONG?

The body is unable to absorb Vitamin B_{12}, which is needed to make RBC, resulting in a decreased RBC count. More common in people of northern European descent, the anemia typically develops in adulthood. The intrinsic factor is normally secreted by the parietal cells of the gastric mucosa and are necessary to allow intestinal absorption of vitamin B_{12}. Destruction of the gastric mucosa due to an autoimmune response results in loss of parietal cells within the stomach. The ability of vitamin B_{12} to bind with intrinsic factor is lost, decreasing the amount that is absorbed. Typical onset is between the ages of 40 and 60.

PROGNOSIS

Ongoing replacement of vitamin B_{12} is necessary to correct the deficit and alleviate symptoms that may have developed. Without treatment, the neurologic effects will continue, ultimately leading to dementia.

HALLMARK SIGNS AND SYMPTOMS

- Pallor due to anemia
- Weakness and fatigue due to anemia
- Tingling in hands and feet—"stocking-glove paresthesia"—due to bilateral demyelination of dorsal and lateral columns of spinal cord nerves
- Diminished vibratory and position sense
- Poor balance due to effect on cerebral function
- Dementia appears later in the disease
- Atrophic glossitis—beefy red tongue
- Nausea may lead to anorexia and weight loss
- Premature graying of hair

INTERPRETING TEST RESULTS

- Decreased hemoglobin due to decreased production of RBCs.
- Increased MCV—macrocytic anemia.
- Positive Schilling test due to decrease in intrinsic factor.
- Decreased amount of hydrochloric acid in the stomach (hypochlorhydria) due to changes within the parietal cells of the gastric mucosa.
- Postitive Romberg test due to ataxia and neurologic changes.
- Diminished sensation when testing for vibration, position sense, or propioception of extremities.

TREATMENT

Lifelong replacement with vitamin B_{12} will correct the anemia and improve the neurologic changes that have occurred. Initially the patient is given weekly injections of

B_{12} to combat the deficiency. The injections eventually become monthly for lifelong maintenance. Oral supplementation is not effective in these patients because they cannot adequately absorb vitamin B_{12} due to insufficient intrinsic factor.

- Administer vitamin B_{12} by IM injection.
- Transfusion of packed RBC if anemia is severe.

NURSING DIAGNOSES

- Impaired gas exchange
- Imbalanced nutrition, less than what body requires
- Risk for injury

NURSING INTERVENTION

- Prevent injuries.
- Explain to the patient:
  - Use soft toothbrush due to oral changes.
  - Avoid activities that could lead to injury due to paresthesias or changes in balance.
  - Inspect feet each day for injury due to paresthesia.

5 Disseminated Intravascular Coagulation (DIC)

WHAT WENT WRONG?

Blood coagulates through the entire body within the vascular compartment. This depletes platelets and the body's ability to coagulate, resulting in an increased risk of hemorrhage. It occurs as a complication of some other condition. The coagulation sequence is activated causing many microthrombi to develop throughout the body. The clots that form are the result of coagulation proteins and platelets, resulting in the risk of bleeding or severe hemorrhage. It is often due to obstetric complications, posttrauma, sepsis, cancer, or shock.

PROGNOSIS

The prognosis varies depending on the underlying disease process and the ability to reverse the coagulopathy.

HALLMARK SIGNS AND SYMPTOMS

- Unexpected bleeding—oozing from puncture sites (venipuncture, IVs, surgical wounds)
- Petechiae as clotting factors are lost
- Purpura as clotting factors are lost
- Severe hemorrhage as clotting factors are lost
- Uncontrolled postpartum bleeding
- Tissue hypoxia from microemboli
- Hemolytic anemia, as cells are destroyed trying to pass through partially blocked vessels

INTERPRETING TEST RESULTS

- PT prolonged.
- PTT normal or prolonged.
- Platelet count low—thrombocytopenia.
- Fibrin degradation products elevated:
  - D-dimer may be elevated.

TREATMENT

Treatment needs to decrease coagulation ability (to prevent further clot development) and replace clotting components (to prevent further bleeding). Other interventions may be necessary depending on the locations of clot development and any compromise of body system function due to clot formation.

- Transfusion:
  - Packed RBC to replace what has been lost due to bleeding.
  - Fresh frozen plasma—replaces coagulation factor deficiency.

- Platelets—replaces needed cells.
- Cryoprecipitate—replaces fibrinogen.
- Administer anticoagulant drugs to decrease coagulation; not done in all patients:
  - heparin
- Bed rest.

NURSING DIAGNOSES

- Ineffective tissue perfusion
- Risk for deficient fluid volume

NURSING INTERVENTION

- Monitor for bleeding from obvious sites (wounds, suture lines, venipuncture, etc.) and occult sites (GI, urine).
- Avoid cleaning clots from exposed areas—may start bleeding from the site and not have sufficient clotting factors to stop.
- Explain to the patient:
  - Avoid situations that might cause bleeding—use electric razor, soft toothbrush, don't floss between teeth.

6 *Hemophilia*

WHAT WENT WRONG?

The patient is missing a coagulation factor that is essential for normal blood clotting and as a result the blood does not clot when the patient bleeds. It is an X-linked recessive inherited disorder, passed on so that it presents symptoms in males, and rarely in females. Hemophilia A is the result of missing clotting factor VIII. Hemophilia B is the result of missing clotting factor IX and is also known as Christmas disease.

PROGNOSIS

The most common sites of bleeding are into the joints, muscles, or from the GI tract. Mild forms of the disease will only cause bleeding after surgery or trauma, whereas severe forms of the disease will cause bleeding without any prior cause.

HALLMARK SIGNS AND SYMPTOMS

- Tender joints due to bleeding
- Swelling of knees, ankles, hips, and elbows due to bleeding
- Blood in stool (tarry stool) due to GI blood loss
- Blood in the urine (hematuria)

INTERPRETING TEST RESULTS

- PTT prolonged.
- PT normal.
- Bleeding time normal.
- Fibrinogen level normal.
- Decrease in clotting factor VIII found in blood serum in Hemophilia A.
- Decrease in clotting factor IX found in blood serum in Hemophilia B.

TREATMENT

- Avoid aspirin.
- For hemophilia A administer factor VIII concentrates.
- Cryoprecipitate.
- DDAVP for patients with mild deficiency.
- For hemophilia B administer factor IX concentrates.

NURSING DIAGNOSES

- Acute pain
- Impaired gas exchange

NURSING INTERVENTION

- No IM injections.
- No aspirin.
- To stop bleeding:
  - Elevate site.
  - Apply direct pressure to the site.
- Explain to the patient:
  - Wear a medical alert identification.
  - Contact physician for any injury.
  - Avoid situations where injury might occur.

Leukemia

WHAT WENT WRONG?

Replacement of bone marrow by abnormal cells results in unregulated proliferation of immature white blood cells entering the circulatory system. These leukemic cells may also enter the liver, spleen, or lymph nodes, causing these areas to enlarge. Leukemia is classified according to the type of cell it is derived from, lymphocytic or myelocytic, and as either acute or chronic. Lymphocytic leukemias involve immature lymphocytes originating in the bone marrow and typically infiltrate the spleen, lymph nodes, or central nervous system. Myelogenous or myelocytic leukemia involves the myeloid stem cells in the bone marrow and interferes with the maturation of all blood cell types (granulocytes, erythrocytes, thrombocytes).

The exact cause of leukemia is unknown. There is a higher incidence in people who have been exposed to high levels of radiation, who have had exposure to benzene, or who have a history of aggressive chemotherapy for a different type of cancer. There may be a genetic predisposition to develop acute leukemia. Patients with Down's syndrome, Fanconi's anemia, or a family history of leukemia also have a higher-than-average incidence of this disease.

PROGNOSIS

Patients with acute leukemia typically have a more aggressive disease process, which may have a shorter course from the time of diagnosis. Patients with chronic leukemia are more likely to have a less aggressive disease process that runs over

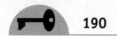

a longer course. The chronic patients typically have an insidious onset and a better prognosis.

HALLMARK SIGNS AND SYMPTOMS

- Acute patients:
  - Fatigue and weakness due to anemia
  - Fever due to increased susceptibility to infection
  - Bleeding, petechiae, ecchymosis (bruising), epistaxis (nosebleed), gingival (gum) bleeding—due to decreased platelet count
  - Bone pain due to bone infiltration and marrow expansion
  - Lymph nodes (lymphadenopathy) enlarged as leukemic cells invade nodes
  - Liver (hepatomegaly) and spleen (splenomegaly) enlarged as leukemic cells invade
  - Headache, nausea, vomiting, and weight loss
  - Papilledema, cranial nerve palsies, seizure if there is central nervous system involvement
- Chronic patients:
  - Fatigue due to anemia
  - Weight loss due to chronic disease process and loss of appetite
  - Poor appetite
  - Enlarged lymph nodes (lymphadenopathy) due to infiltration of lymph nodes
  - Enlarged spleen (splenomegaly) due to involvement of the spleen

INTERPRETING TEST RESULTS

- Low RBC count, low hemoglobin—anemia.
- Low platelet count—thrombocytopenia.
- Elevated WBC count—leukocytosis.
- Abnormal amount of immature WBC shown in bone marrow biopsy.

TREATMENT

- Acute myelogenous leukemia.
  - Administer an anthracycline (idarubicin or daunorubicin) plus cytarabine.

- Combination: Daunorubicin, vincristine, prednisone, asparaginase.
- Administer platelet transfusions.
- Administer Filgrastim for neutropenia.
- Administer antibiotics for infections.
- Bone marrow transplant.
  - Administer immunosuppressives to avoid transplant rejection.
- Chronic myelogenous leukemia.
  - Administer Signal transduction inhibitor:
    - Imatinib
    - Interferon-α
    - Busulfan
    - Hydroxyurea
- Chronic lymphocytic leukemia.
  - Administer alkylating agents:
    - cyclophosphamide
    - chlorambucil
  - Administer antienoplastics:
    - Vincristine
    - Prednisone
    - Doxorubicin
  - Monoclonal antibody targeted therapy:
    - alemtuzumab
    - Combination of fludarabine and rituxumab.
  - Transfusion if hemolytic anemia or bleeding:
    - Packed RBCs.
    - Whole blood.
    - Platelets.
  - Bone marrow transplant and immunosuppression.
  - High protein diet.

NURSING DIAGNOSES

- Risk for infection
- Chronic pain
- Imbalanced nutrition, less than what body requires

NURSING INTERVENTION

- Monitor for bleeding—platelet count may be decreased.
- Monitor for infection—patients have increased susceptibility to infection.
- Monitor pain control.
- Small, frequent meals.
- Teach patients about infection control:
  - Avoid others with infection.
  - Report signs of infection, sore throat, fevers, etc.
- Explain to the patient:
  - Use an electric razor.
  - Use soft toothbrush.
  - Watch for bleeding or bruising.

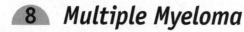 *Multiple Myeloma*

WHAT WENT WRONG?

A malignancy of the plasma cells causes an excessive amount of plasma cells in the bone marrow. Masses within the bone marrow cause destructive lesions in the bone. Normal bone marrow function is reduced as the abnormal plasma cells continue to grow. Immune function is diminished and the patient develops anemia. The disease typically affects older adults.

PROGNOSIS

Patients are susceptible to infection and often have significant pain from bone involvement of the disease. The survival time from diagnosis averages about 3 years.

HALLMARK SIGNS AND SYMPTOMS

- Severe bone pain due to involvement in back or ribs
- Anemia due to invasion of the bone marrow

- Skeletal fractures due to loss of normal bone structure (osteoporosis)
- Increased risk of infection due to bone marrow failure to produce white blood cells
- Spinal cord compression as mass enlarges
- Renal failure due to protein effect in renal tubules

INTERPRETING TEST RESULTS

- Presence of the Bence Jones protein in urine.
- Serum protein electrophoresis shows a monoclonal protein spike.
- CBC shows anemia.
- Rouleau formation on peripheral smear, a group of RBCs clump together in a stack (like a stack of coins).
- Abnormal plasma cells in bone marrow biopsy.
- X-rays of bone show lytic lesions.
- Elevated calcium in blood (hypercalcemia).
- Protein in urine (proteinuria).
- Elevated erythrocyte sedimentation rate.

TREATMENT

Treatment regimens undergo changes based on patient response and current research findings. Combination therapy is common in treatment of multiple myeloma.

- Pain management.
- Combination chemotherapy:
  - alkylating agent (melphalan) and prednisone
  - thalidomide and dexamethasone
  - nonalkylating combination (vincristine, doxorubicin, and dexamethasone)
  - proteosome inhibitor (borteozomib) and thalidomide derivative (lenalidomide)
- Diet high in protein, carbohydrates, vitamins, and minerals.
- Small frequent meals.
- Transfusion of packed RBCs if anemia is severe.
- Bone marrow transplantation.

NURSING DIAGNOSES

- Pain
- Impaired mobility
- Risk for injury

NURSING INTERVENTION

- Protect the patient from falling.
- Monitor input and output due to renal function changes.
- Perform muscle-strengthening exercises.
- Explain to the patient:
  - No lifting.
  - Be alert for fractures.

9 *Polycythemia Vera*

WHAT WENT WRONG?

A myeloproliferative disorder that results in an overproduction of blood cells and a thickening of blood. The hallmarks of polycythemia vera include excessive production of red blood cells, white blood cells, and platelets. The excess of cells present in the blood causes problems with the flow of blood through vessels, especially the smaller ones. There will be an increase in peripheral vascular resistance causing increased pressure, and vascular stasis in the smaller vessels, potentially causing thrombosis or tissue hypoxia. Organ damage may result because of these changes.

PROGNOSIS

After diagnosis of polycythemia vera, the average survival time is 10 to 15 years with appropriate treatment, less than 2 years without treatment. Some patients may go on to develop acute leukemia. Complications usually arise from thrombosis or tissue hypoxia.

HALLMARK SIGNS AND SYMPTOMS

- Facial skin and mucous membranes dark and flushed (plethora)
- Hypertension due to increased peripheral vascular resistance and thickening of the blood
- Itching worse after warm shower due to histamine release from increased basophils within dilated vessels
- Headache and difficulty concentrating
- Vision blurred, tinnitus (ringing in ears), and hearing changes
- Thrombosis due to vascular stasis
- Spleen enlargement (splenomegaly)
- Tissue hypoxia and possible infarction of heart, spleen, kidneys, and brain due to thrombosis

INTERPRETING TEST RESULTS

- Increased RBC count.
- Increased hemoglobin.
- Increased hematocrit level.
- Increased WBC count.
- Increased basophils.
- Increased eosinophils.
- Increased platelet count.
- Increased uric acid level.
- Increased potassium.
- Increased vitamin B_{12} level.
- Bone marrow panhyperplasia; iron stores absent.

TREATMENT

Treatment is aimed at maintaining bloodflow to the smaller vessels and diminishing the amount of excess blood cells being made by the bone marrow.

- Periodic scheduled phlebotomy—the removal of 500 ml of blood—to reduce the hematocrit level to below 45; may be done weekly.

- Adequate hydration.
- Anticoagulants such as aspirin.
- Administer myelosuppressive medication:
  - hydroxyurea
  - anagrelide
  - radioactive phosphorus 32
- Administer medication to lower uric acid level if necessary:
  - allopurinol
- Alkylating agents:
  - melphalan
  - busulfan
- Radiation therapy.
- Antihistamine for pruritis.

NURSING DIAGNOSES

- Ineffective tissue perfusion
- Disturbed sensory perception
- Risk for injury

NURSING INTERVENTION

- Monitor vital signs.
- Monitor for bleeding.
- Monitor for signs of infections.
- Keep the patient mobilized to decrease chance of clot formation.
- Increase fluid intake.
- Explain to the patient:
  - Maintain activity.
  - Use electric razor, use soft toothbrush, and avoid flossing to decrease chances of bleeding.
  - Avoid activities that could cause injury.

10 *Sickle Cell Anemia*

WHAT WENT WRONG?

This is an autosomal recessive disorder in which an abnormal gene causes damage to the RBC membrane. The abnormal hemoglobin within the red blood cell is called hemoglobin S. Dehydration or drying of the RBC makes it more vulnerable to sickling (forming a crescent-like shape), as do hypoxemia and acidosis. Hemolytic anemia results as RBCs are destroyed due to the damage to the outer membrane. The sickled cells can also clump together, causing difficulty getting through the smaller vessels.

PROGNOSIS

Sickle cell anemia will become a chronic multisystem disease. Causes of death in these patients are usually related to organ failure. Patients may also inherit a single gene for sickle cell. These patients may develop sickle cell trait, in which symptoms would only be present in the setting of extreme circumstances (vigorous exercise at high altitude, especially with rapid ascent).

HALLMARK SIGNS AND SYMPTOMS

- Acute pain (especially back, chest, and long bones) from vascular occlusion of the small vessels as the sickled cells clump
- Fever as body responds to acute sickling episode and accompanying provoking event
- Painful, swollen joints due to vaso-occlusive process
- Fatigue due to chronic anemia
- Stroke (cerebrovascular accident) due to vaso-occlusive process
- Enlarged liver (hepatomegaly)
- Enlarged heart and systolic murmur

INTERPRETING TEST RESULTS

- Low RBC count due to chronic hemolytic anemia; the RBCs have a shorter lifespan.

- Elevated WBCs.
- Increased reticulocytes.
- Presence of Howell-Jolly bodies and target cells.
- Sickle cells appear in blood smear.
- Indirect bilirubin level elevated.
- Hemoglobin electrophoresis shows majority hemoglobin S (80 to 98 percent).

TREATMENT

During acute episodes pain control, hydration, and oxygenation are the focus of treatment. The underlying cause that sent the patient into crisis will also need to be treated concurrently.

- Administer analgesics to alleviate the pain associated with the vaso-occlusive process:
  - narcotic pain control necessary when pain is severe
- Warm compresses on joint.
- Blood transfusion of packed RBC when anemia indicates.
- Supplemental oxygen if hypoxic.
- Adequate hydration, using IV fluids.
- Treat infections.

NURSING DIAGNOSES

- Fatigue
- Acute pain
- Impaired gas exchange

NURSING INTERVENTION

- Increase fluid intake.
- Monitor IV fluids.
- Monitor pain control.

- Record fluid intake and output to monitor renal function.
- Administer supplemental O_2 to increase available oxygen.
- Explain to the patient:
  - Avoid the cold.
  - No cold compresses.
  - Plan for rest periods during the day.

11 *Deep Vein Thrombosis (DVT)*

WHAT WENT WRONG?

Thrombophlebitis, or the formation of a clot within the vein, commonly occurs within the deep veins in the legs, and may also occur in the arms. Initially platelets and white cells clump together, sticking to the inside of the vessel wall. As blood flows over the area, other cells may deposit onto the area, making the thrombus larger. Compression of blood flow, which will increase the venous pressure or sluggishness of the blood flow, can increase the risk of clot formation. Immobility, obesity, or hormonal changes such as pregnancy can all contribute to increased risk.

PROGNOSIS

The clot may develop without any outward signs for some time. It may also be due to another disease process or medication which affects clotting abilities. A small piece of the clot may break free to become an embolus and travel elsewhere in the body. This embolus may lodge in a vessel in the lung (a pulmonary embolism), causing acute respiratory symptoms, possibly even death.

HALLMARK SIGNS AND SYMPTOMS

- Some patients will be asymptomatic
- Unilateral leg (or arm) pain or tenderness (calf, thigh, groin, upper or lower arm) depending on location of thrombosis
- Unilateral swelling of leg (or arm) due to vascular occlusion

- Positive Homan's sign (pain on dorsiflexion of foot) seen in minority of patients with DVT
- Warmth over the site

INTERPRETING TEST RESULTS

- Doppler flow studies.
- Venous duplex ultrasound.
- Impedence plethysmography looks at venous outflow; better at diagnosis in thigh than in calf.
- Venography uses contrast dye to visualize the thrombus; not commonly done due to need for dye and other available tests.
- MRI direct thrombus imaging useful for inferior vena cava and pelvic vein locations.
- PT, PTT, INR, and CBC with platelet count as baseline.
- D-dimer to test for hypercoagulable state.

TREATMENT

Most patients undergo medical management and rest. Preventive measures are instituted for future occurrences. Patients with repeat occurrences may have an umbrella filter implanted.

- Bedrest with elevation of extremity.
- Warm, moist soaks of the area.
- Monitor prothrombin time (PT), partial thromboplastin time (PTT), international normalized ratio (INR).
- Weight-dosed heparin IV.
- Low molecular weight heparin.
- Warfarin.
- Thrombolytic therapy to dissolve clot with drugs such as recombinant tissue plasminogen activator (t-PA).
- Umbrella filter is inserted into the inferior vena cava for patients with recurring DVT.
- Thrombectomy is the surgical removal of the thrombus.

NURSING DIAGNOSIS

- Impaired physical mobility
- Risk for acute pain

NURSING INTERVENTIONS

- Monitor vital signs for changes.
- Monitor for signs of pulmonary embolism, shortness of breath, chest pain, tachycardia (rapid heart rate), tachypnea (rapid respirations), and diaphoresis (sweating).
- Avoid massaging the area to lessen the possibility of dislodging the clot.
- Intermittent warm, moist soaks. Assess skin between changes.
- Follow weight-dosed heparin protocol.
- Monitor lab results: PT, PTT, INR, and CBC with platelets.
- Low molecular weight heparin (enoxaparin, dalteparin).
- Warfarin orally.
- Monitor for signs of bleeding or bruising.
- Instruct patient to:
  - Report signs of bleeding or bruising to physician, nurse practitioner, or physician assistant.
  - Avoid injury.
  - Use of electric razor and soft toothbrush; avoid flossing between teeth.
  - Diet restrictions, and to check with health care provider or pharmacist about interactions of any medications, if on warfarin as outpatient.

12 *Idiopathic Thrombocytopenic Purpura (ITP)*

WHAT WENT WRONG?

An autoimmune disorder in which antibodies are developed to the patient's own platelets. Antibodies attach to the platelets and macrophages within the spleen. The body destroys the platelets within the spleen. ITP is typically more common in women and becomes chronic in adults who are in early to mid-adulthood.

PROGNOSIS

Problems for the patient are most likely the result of bleeding due to inadequate platelets. Prednisone can control the majority of cases of ITP.

HALLMARK SIGNS AND SYMPTOMS

- Bleeding in mucous membranes or skin due to low platelet count:
  - epistaxis
  - oral bleeding
  - menorrhagia (heavy menstrual bleeding)
  - purpura
  - petechiae

INTERPRETING TEST RESULTS

- Thrombocytopenia—low platelet count.
- Mild anemia—usually secondary to bleeding.
- PT normal.
- PTT normal.

TREATMENT

The use of prednisone in patients with ITP is to decrease the body's action on the antibody-tagged platelets. Initially, the use of prednisone will also help to enhance vascular stability. High-dose therapy needs to be tapered down. Most patients will be on long-term maintenance doses of prednisone. Splenectomy provides complete or partial remission.

- Prednisone—bleeding will stop even before platelet count begins to rise.
- High-dose IV immunoglobulin.
- Danazol.

- Immunosuppressive therapy:
  - vincristine, azathioprine, cyclosporine, cyclophosphamide
  - rituximab
- Stem cell transplantation.

NURSING DIAGNOSIS

- Risk for infection
- Disturbed body image
- Risk for ineffective individual coping

NURSING INTERVENTIONS

- Monitor vital signs for changes.
- Monitor for signs of bleeding or bruising.
- Decrease chance of bleeding:
  - Use soft toothbrushes, no flossing, only electric razors.
- Protect from potential infection, sick visitors, etc.
- Encourage patient to discuss feelings about illness.

Crucial Diagnostic Tests

Bone Marrow Biopsy

WHY IS IT DONE?

The removal of bone marrow by needle aspiration to determine blood cell formation.

HOW DOES THE TEST WORK?

Local anesthetic used at the site: posterior iliac crest, sternum, and ribs. Skin cleansed per protocol for a sterile procedure. Specimen removed from within bone, properly labeled and delivered to lab.

WHAT TO DO?

- Before the test:
  - The patient must sign an informed consent for an invasive procedure per policy.
  - Position the patient lying appropriately for selected site and drape for privacy.
- After the test:
  - Place pressure on the site of the aspiration to reduce risk of bleeding.
  - Monitor the aspiration site for bleeding.

Fecal Occult Blood Test

WHY IS IT GIVEN?

To determine if blood is being passed in the stool, even though it can't be seen.

HOW DOES THE TEST WORK?

Stool sample is collected and applied to a card. A reagent is applied to the sample to test. If blood is present in the stool sample, a color change occurs.

WHAT TO DO?

- Before the test advise patient:
  - No eating red meats, beets, turnips, and horseradish 48 hours before the test; these may interfere with the test.
  - No aspirin, vitamin C, iron, or nonsteroidal anti-inflammatory medications 48 hours before the test; these may interfere with test results.

Coagulation Studies

WHY IS IT DONE?

This determines the effectiveness of the patient's ability to clot.

HOW DOES THE TEST WORK?

- PT—prothrombin time—checks for prothrombin deficiency, warfarin therapy 11 to 15 seconds.
- INR—monitors effectiveness of warfarin therapy.
- PTT—partial thromboplastin time—monitors effectiveness of therapeutic range for heparin, 25 to 38 seconds.
- Bleeding time—the amount of time necessary to stop bleeding from a small break made in the skin—3 to 7 minutes.

Complete Blood Count

- WBC—white blood cell count
- RBC—red blood cell count
- Hemoglobin
- Hematocrit
- MCV—mean corpuscular volume
- MCH—mean corpuscular hemoglobin
- MCHC—mean corpuscular hemoglobin concentration
- RDW—red cell distribution width
- Platelets
- Reticulocyte count
- Neutrophils
- Lymphocytes
- Monocytes
- Eosinophils

IRON STUDIES

- Serum iron
- TIBC—total iron binding capacity
- Percent iron saturation
- Ferritin transferrin
- Vitamin B_{12} levels
- Folate

Quiz

1. Your patient is diagnosed with anemia and is often fatigued. She asks you why she feels this way. You tell her that it is because of:

   (a) Destruction (hemolysis) of the red blood cells.

   (b) Decreased oxygen-carrying capability of the blood.

   (c) Paleness (pallor) of the skin.

   (d) Lack of nutritional intake of essential nutrients, such as iron or B_{12}.

2. Your patient is diagnosed with iron deficiency anemia. She asks you how this happened to her. The best response is:

   (a) Insomnia.

   (b) An increase in iron intake.

   (c) Low salt intake.

   (d) Heavy menses or an inadequate intake of iron.

3. Your patient is showing signs of clotting and bleeding concurrently. You recognize this as signs of:

   (a) Disseminated intravascular coagulation.

   (b) Hemophilia.

   (c) Multiple myeloma.

   (d) Polycythema vera.

4. Patients with idiopathic thrombocytopenic purpura (ITP) have an increased risk of bleeding. Therefore you must carefully monitor:

   (a) Platelet count and RBC.

   (b) WBC and bleeding time.

   (c) PT and PTT.

   (d) Iron and ferritin levels.

5. Your patient is diagnosed with deep vein thrombosis (DVT). A priority intervention is:

   (a) Daily monitoring of platelet counts.

   (b) Use of intermittent warm soaks of the affected area.

   (c) Application of ice packs to the affected area every 4 to 6 hours.

   (d) Increasing dietary intake of foods rich in vitamin K.

6. A patient is recently diagnosed with hemophilia. What signs and symptoms should you teach your patient to recognize?

    (a) Clot formation, especially in the veins of the lower extremities.

    (b) Excessive bleeding after minor trauma.

    (c) Low blood counts and fatigue due to lack of adequate red blood cell production.

    (d) Anemia, bone pain, and infection.

7. As part of a treatment plan for patients with leukemia, a bone marrow transplant may be performed. You know that as a result of the care needed after the bone marrow transplant, these patients will have an increased risk for:

    (a) Bleeding.

    (b) Clot formation.

    (c) Infection.

    (d) Nausea and vomiting.

8. While patients are on immunosuppressive therapy post–bone marrow transplant, it is important to teach the patient:

    (a) To avoid other people with signs of infection.

    (b) To report signs of infection, such as sore throat or fever.

    (c) To take the medications as directed.

    (d) All of the above.

9. You are caring for a patient with sickle cell anemia. The treatment plan for this patient will include:

    (a) IV fluids to adequately hydrate.

    (b) Narcotic pain management when pain is severe.

    (c) Transfusion of red blood cells to correct anemia.

    (d) All of the above.

10. Patients with pernicious anemia are treated with:

    (a) Oral iron.

    (b) Oral folic acid.

    (c) Parenteral vitamin B_{12}.

    (d) Oral prednisone.

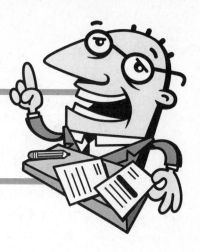

CHAPTER 5

Nervous System

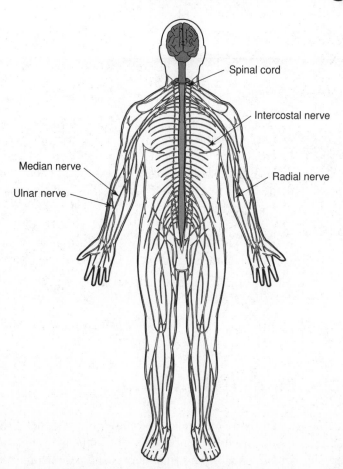

Spinal cord

Intercostal nerve

Median nerve

Ulnar nerve

Radial nerve

Learning Objectives

1. Head injury
2. Amyotrophic lateral sclerosis (ALS)
3. Bell's palsy
4. Brain abscess
5. Brain tumor
6. Cerebral aneurysm
7. Encephalitis
8. Guillain-Barré syndrome
9. Huntington's disease (Chorea)
10. Meningitis
11. Multiple sclerosis (MS)
12. Myasthenia gravis
13. Parkinson's disease
14. Spinal cord injury
15. Stroke
16. Seizure disorder

Key Terms

Arachnoid mater
Astrocytoma
Battle's sign
Broca's area
Cerebral edema
Closed head injuries
Concussion
Coutrecoup injury
Dura mater

Electromyogram
Epidural hematoma
Gliomas
Haemophilus influenzae
Idiopathic facial paralysis
Intracerebral bleed
Lou Gehrig's disease
Meningiomas
Neisseria meningitides

Occipital lobe
Oligodendroglioma
Open head injuries
Pia mater
Raccoon sign
Skull fractures
Streptococcus pneumoniae
Surgical debulking
Wernicke's area

How the Nervous System Works

The nervous system is divided into the central and peripheral nervous systems. The central nervous system is comprised of the brain and spinal cord. The peripheral nervous system contains the spinal nerves and peripheral nerves.

The basic component of the nervous system is the nerve cell or neuron. A neuron is composed of the nucleus (within the cell body), a dendrite, (which receives the signal), an axon (the extension of the cell that can pass on an impulse to the next nerve cell), and the axon terminals (which can transmit the signals to other cells). The messages are sent from one nerve cell to another, crossing a synapse (or gap) between cells. Neurotransmitters are chemicals released by the presynaptic neuron to enhance the communication between nerve cells. There are specific receptor sites for the different neurotransmitters on the postsynaptic neuron. Electrically charged ions transmit signals along the cell membranes of the nerve cells. A myelin coating on the outer surface of the nerve cells helps to speed the transmission along the nerve cells. This myelin coating also gives a white color to the nerve cells.

Some neurons are afferent neurons. They carry sensory information from the peripheral areas of the body to the central nervous system. These neurons do not have dendrites. Motor neurons that transmit information from the central nervous system to the muscles or glands are efferent neurons.

The brain is protected within the skull. The outermost layer of the brain is the cerebral cortex, made up primarily of neural cell bodies, giving a gray appearance. The cerebral cortex is divided into right and left hemispheres and into frontal, parietal, occipital, and temporal lobes. The frontal lobe has motor and pre-motor areas, as well as Broca's area, which controls speech articulation, behavior, moral decision-making, and emotional outburst. The parietal area interprets sensory stimuli, pain, and touch. The temporal lobe is involved in auditory processing, language interpretation (Wernicke's area), and memory formation, and storage. The occipital lobe houses the visual cortex. The diencephalon includes the thalamus, hypothalamus, and the basal ganglia. The thalamus relays the sensory information from the body to the appropriate part of the cerebral cortex. Descending messages from the cerebral cortex are passed through the thalamus to the body. The hypothalamus controls neuroendocrine function and maintains homeostasis, or constancy, within the body. The basal ganglia control highly skilled movements that require precision without intentional thought. The brainstem is comprised of the pons, medulla oblongata, and midbrain.

The spinal column is protected within the vertebral column. Both motor and sensory fibers are found within the spinal column. Motor nerves are located along the anterior horns and sensory nerves are located along the posterior horns of the spinal column. The motor nerve fibers are more protected from traumatic injury this way. If a patient sustains an external injury to the back that damages the spinal column, the first area to be impacted will be the sensory nerves, hopefully maintaining motor function. If enough damage has occurred, then both sensory and motor function will be lost. Peripheral nerve fibers leave the spinal column to travel to the rest of the body. Impulses travel from the central nervous system to muscle fibers to control voluntary motion and involuntary function of organs. Impulses are also sent from the body to the central nervous system for input.

Just the Facts

 Head Injury

WHAT WENT WRONG?

The patient experiences a trauma to the head. The resulting injury may be a minor scalp laceration or a major internal injury with or without a skull fracture. There may be internal hemorrhage or cerebral edema resulting in hypoxia and a decrease in cognitive and functional capabilities. There are a variety of injuries that may be sustained. Open head injuries are typical of projectile wounds from gunshots or knifes. Closed head injuries are typical of trauma from falls, motor vehicle accidents, sports, or fights.

Concussion involves a blow to the head where there is a bruising-type injury as the brain is thrust against the inside of skull. The point of injury where the brain makes impact against the skull is referred to as a coup injury. There is also a contrecoup injury as the head recoils away from the point of impact and the brain is thrust against the inside of the skull at the opposite point of the head, resulting in injury there as well. Patients with concussion may experience a transient loss of consciousness associated with bradycardia, or slowing of the heartrate; low blood pressure; slow, shallow breathing; amnesia of the injury and the events immediately following the injury; headache; and temporary loss of mental focus. Cerebral contusion is a more serious injury than concussion. Greater damage is done to the brain; cerebral edema or hemorrhage may occur and lead to necrosis. Patients typically have longer loss of consciousness with a cerebral contusion.

Hemorrhages can occur at a variety of levels, between the skull and the outer coverings (dura) of the brain, within the layers covering the brain, or within the brain tissue. The bleeding may occur acutely, at the time of injury, or hours to weeks later. An epidural hematoma happens at the time of injury from an arterial site. The blood accumulates between the skull and the dura mater, or the outermost layer covering the brain. The site is often in the temporal area. The patient is typically awake and talking immediately after the blow to the head. Within a short time, the patient becomes unstable and then unconscious. Emergency neurosurgery is necessary to relieve the pressure and stop the bleeding. Subdural hematoma is typically bleeding from a venous source into the area below the dura mater and above the arachnoid mater. This may occur acutely in some patients, but can also occur as a slow, chronic bleed, especially in the elderly patient. The elderly patient with a chronic bleed may have a significant amount of blood accumulate before symptoms occur due to age-related changes in volume of brain tissue. A subarachnoid hemorrhage causes blood to accumulate within the area below the arachnoid mater and above the pia mater. The cerebrospinal fluid is found in this area. An intracerebral bleed is an accumulation of blood within the tissues of the brain. This may be due to a shearing force on the brain tissue from a twisting motion between the upper part of the brain (cerebrum) and the brain stem or tearing of small vessels within the brain. There will be associated edema and elevation of intracranial pressure.

Simple skull fractures are displaced and do not require specific intervention. Depressed skull fractures have bone fragments that have been broken off from the skull and pressed down toward the brain tissue. These fractures need to be corrected surgically. A basilar skull fracture has classic signs that include periorbital bruising (raccoon sign), blood behind the ear drum (Battle's sign), and leaking of cerebrospinal fluid from the nose or ear (check for glucose content to distinguish from a runny nose).

PROGNOSIS

The prognosis following head injury varies greatly depending on the location of the injury, the severity of the damage that occurred, and the treatment that was received. Patients with loss of consciousness over 2 minutes have a more severe injury and therefore worse prognosis. Patients who have loss of memory, either about the incident or the events immediately following, also have a more severe injury and worse prognosis. Some patients develop hemorrhage as a late effect of head injury, occurring hours, or in some cases, days after the initial injury. Posttraumatic seizure disorder can also occur as a late effect of head injury.

HALLMARK SIGNS AND SYMPTOMS

- Headache due to direct trauma and/or increasing intracranial pressure
- Disorientation or cognitive changes
- Changes in speech
- Changes in motor movements
- Nausea and vomiting due to increased intracranial pressure
- Unequal pupil size—important to determine if due to neurologic change or if patient has always had unequal pupil size (small percentage of population has unequal pupil size)
- Diminished or absent pupil reaction due to neurologic compromise
- Decreased level of consciousness or loss of consciousness
- Amnesia

INTERPRETING TEST RESULTS

- Skull x-ray shows fractures.
- MRI shows edema and hemorrhage.
- CT scan shows hemorrhage, cerebral edema, displacement of midline structures.
- EEG indicates focal seizure activity.

TREATMENT

- Surgical interventions may be necessary (craniotomy):
  - Removal of hematoma
  - Ligation of bleeding vessel
  - Burr holes (drilling holes) for decompression
  - Debridement of foreign material and dead cells
- Administer antibiotics for open head injuries to prevent infection.
- Ventilatory assist if needed—intubation and mechanical ventilation.
- Administer low-dose opioids for restlessness, agitation, and pain in ventilator-dependent patients:
  - morphine sulfate or fentanyl citrate
- Administer osmotic diuretics to reduce cerebral edema:
  - mannitol
- Administer loop diuretics to decrease edema and circulating blood volume:
  - furosemide
- Administer analgesics:
  - acetaminophen (Tylenol)
- High-protein, high-calorie, high-vitamin diet.
- Platelet and packed RBC transfusions—if blood counts warrant transfusion.

NURSING DIAGNOSES

- Risk for injury
- Ineffective tissue perfusion
- Decreased intracranial adaptive capacity
- Risk for disturbed thought processes

NURSING INTERVENTION

- Avoid discussing the patient's condition in the presence of the patient—remember the patient can still hear you even though he or she is not conscious, and may recall the conversations after they regain consciousness.
- Monitor vital signs for stability—increased blood pressure with widening pulse pressure and slow pulse, suggestive of increased intracranial pressure.
- Monitor neurologic status for changes—typically use Glasgow Coma Scale or similar tool to grade response to stimuli (highest score 15):

  - Eye-opening response

spontaneous	4
to sound	3
to pain	2
none	1

  - Motor responses

obeys commands	6
localizes pain	5
withdrawal (normal)	4
abnormal flexion	3
extension	2
none	1

  - Verbal responses

oriented	5
confused conversation	4
inappropriate words	3
incomprehensible sounds	2
none	1

- Monitor for signs of intracranial pressure—report changes.
- Check for signs of infection at wound site in post-operative patients.
- Monitor signs for diabetes insipidus—increased risk due to injury to the pituitary gland.
- Monitor intake and output.
- Monitor urine specific gravity, serum, and urine osmolarity.
- Collaborate with dietician for appropriate diet, if any swallowing or oral sensory concerns.
- Seizure precautions per institution policy.
- Explain to the patient and family:
  - Any dietary restrictions.
  - Any activity restrictions.
  - Medication actions, side effects, interactions.

- What to do in case of a seizure, how to protect the patient from further injury, time the seizure, monitor for breathing, when to call the doctor or EMS.
- Call your physician at any signs of change in the level of consciousness—drowsiness, lethargy, change in personality.

2 *Amyotrophic Lateral Sclerosis (ALS)*

WHAT WENT WRONG?

ALS is commonly called Lou Gehrig's disease and is a progressive, degenerative disorder that involves both the upper and lower motor neurons. There is no change in mental status or sensory function with the disease. The disease does result in paralysis of the motor system, except the eyes. As the disease is more progressed, families often can communicate with the patient through eye movements. Males are affected more commonly than females. The disorder may present at any age, but the age at onset is usually between 40 and late 60s. There is a familial form of the disease that has been linked to an abnormality in chromosome 21.

PROGNOSIS

The disease is rapidly progressive and there is currently no known cure. As the muscles weaken and atrophy, paralysis develops. Over time, the respiratory muscles become involved. At first this results in poor air exchange, increasing the risk for respiratory infections, such as pneumonia. Eventually, the respiratory compromise leads to death from respiratory failure.

HALLMARK SIGNS AND SYMPTOMS

- Fatigue, especially with exertion
- Atrophy of muscles due to weakness
- Dysphagia (trouble swallowing) due to muscular weakness
- Weakness of muscles in the limbs
- Muscle twitching (fasciculation) due to changes within the muscles
- Slurred speech due to muscle weakness

INTERPRETING TEST RESULTS

- Electromyogram (EMG) shows fibrillation and fasciculation; motor conduction velocity normal or slightly slowed.
- Elevated creatinine kinase due to muscle changes.
- Muscle biopsy shows lower neuron degeneration.
- Pulmonary function testing shows decreased vital capacity.

TREATMENT

- Maintain adequate nutrition.
- Consult with speech pathologist for potential swallowing difficulties.
- Administer spasmolytic agent specific for amyotrophic lateral sclerosis, which reduces the transmission of glutamine across the neural synapse. Use of this drug appears to slow the progression of the disease:
  - riluzole
- Administer medications to control symptoms.
- BIPAP (bi-level positive airway pressure) to assist respiration either at nighttime, intermittently as needed, or all day.
- Refer to hospice for end-of-life care.

NURSING DIAGNOSES

- Impaired physical mobility
- Ineffective airway clearance

NURSING INTERVENTION

- Develop a method of communication within the patient's capabilities—verbal communication may not be possible; patient may not be able to use call bell system.
- Monitor vital signs—monitor respiratory function and cardiovascular status; as muscular function decreases the respiratory muscles may be affected.
- Monitor input and output.

- Assess gag reflex—as muscular changes occur, normal protective gag reflex will diminish.
- Explain to the patient:
  - How to suction oral pharynx to remove secretions or food particles. As muscle function decreases, the cough reflex will not be sufficient to remove these.
  - How to tuck chin while drinking and eating to decrease chance of aspiration.

3 *Bell's Palsy*

WHAT WENT WRONG?

This is an acute idiopathic facial paralysis of the seventh cranial nerve that affects one side of the face. Often due to inflammation, the disorder is more common in diabetic patients. One side of the face is paralyzed, making the patient unable to close the eyelid, raise the eyebrow, or smile on the affected side of the face. Some patients will experience pain around the ear on the affected side. The patient may have an associated change in taste.

PROGNOSIS

The more severe the symptoms at the time of presentation, the poorer the prognosis. Some patients will have long-term persistence of symptoms, like facial disfigurement. The majority of patients will have complete resolution of symptoms.

HALLMARK SIGNS AND SYMPTOMS

- Unilateral facial paralysis—inability to close eye, wrinkle forehead, puff out cheeks, or smile
- Pain near the ear and jaw
- Altered taste

INTERPRETING TEST RESULTS

- Electromyogram (EMG) used to indicate recovery time; can determine prognosis.

TREATMENT

- Administer corticosteroids to decrease inflammation (unclear if there is a definitive benefit):
  - prednisone in divided doses for first few days, then taper down
- Administer artificial tears to maintain moisture within eyes.

NURSING DIAGNOSES

- Disturbed sensory perception
- Disturbed body image

NURSING INTERVENTION

- Monitor for pain control.
- Monitor for visual changes—dryness of eye can lead to irritation of cornea.
- Monitor patient for reaction to medications.
- Provide meals in private—patient may have difficulty keeping food in mouth and may not feel food or liquid that is drooling out side of mouth.
- Explain to patient:
  - How to properly instill artificial tear drops.
  - How to use eye patch.

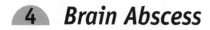

Brain Abscess

WHAT WENT WRONG?

Collection of pus creates a space-occupying area within the brain. Symptoms are similar to any other space-occupying lesion. The infection may be a primary site within the brain or may have traveled from nearby sites such as the ear or sinuses through bone erosion. It may also enter the brain via the systemic circulation from any infected site in the body, such as the lungs in bronchiectasis. The organism causes a local inflammatory reaction; there is pus and liquification of the affected tissue. Cerebral edema of the surrounding tissue occurs. The area becomes en-

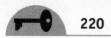

capsulated within 10 to 14 days from the onset of the infection. The infections are typically streptococci, staphylococci, anaerobes, or mixed-organism infections. Immunocompromised patients may have fungal or yeast present in the abscess. Up to 20 percent of the patients may have more than one abscess.

PROGNOSIS

Identification of the organism and appropriate treatment is imperative to resolution of the infection. There is a significant mortality rate in these patients.

HALLMARK SIGNS AND SYMPTOMS

- Drowsiness due to increased intracranial pressure
- Headache due to increased intracranial pressure
- Confusion or inattention
- Seizures due to irritation of brain tissue
- Increasing intracranial pressure
- Widened pulse pressure and bradycardia due to increased intracranial pressure
- Focal neurologic deficit, depending on location of abscess
- Nystagmus with cerebral abscess
- Aphasia with frontal lobe abscess
- Loss of coordination (ataxia) with a cerebellar abscess

INTERPRETING TEST RESULTS

- CBC elevated white blood cell count due to bacterial presence.
- CT scan shows area of abscess site differentiated from surrounding tissue.
- MRI shows area of abscess site possibly earlier than CT scan.
- Biopsy to positively identify organism.

TREATMENT

- Surgically drain (aspiration or open) the abscess to relieve intracranial pressure.

- Administer antibiotic intravenously, depending on organism:
  - nafcillin sodium (penicillinase-resistant penicillin)
  - penicillin G benzathine
  - chloramphenicol
  - metronidazole
  - vancomycin
- Administer corticosteroids in divided doses to decrease inflammation:
  - dexamethasone—taper dose down before stopping
- Administer anticonvulsants to reduce seizure risk; watch for drug interactions:
  - phenytoin
  - phenobarbital
- Administer osmotic diuretics to decrease cerebral edema:
  - mannitol

NURSING DIAGNOSES

- Risk for disturbed thought process
- Risk for falls

NURSING INTERVENTION

- Assess the patient's ability to think, reason, and remember.
- Assess the patient's speech capabilities.
- Assess the patient's movement and senses.
- Assess the patient's cranial nerve function.
- Monitor vital signs.
- Monitor fluid intake and output.
- Monitor for signs of infection in post-operative patients.
- Monitor for side effects of medications.
- Explain to the patient:
  - Need for continued antibiotic treatments.
  - How to administer IV antibiotics at home, how to monitor IV access, and when to call for problems.
  - Need for follow up CT scan or MRI imaging for monitoring.

5 *Brain Tumor*

WHAT WENT WRONG?

A brain tumor is a growth of abnormal cells within the brain tissue. The tumor may be a primary site that originated in the brain or a secondary site that has metastasized from a cancer site elsewhere in the body. Because the tumor is growing within the confined space of the skull, the patient will eventually develop signs of increased intracranial pressure. Some cell types grow faster than others; the patients with the more aggressive, fast-growing cancers will develop symptoms more quickly.

PROGNOSIS

Meningiomas are typically benign tumors that begin from the meninges (covering the brain). They are more common in women and in people as they age. Treatment is surgical removal, but the growth tends to recur.

Gliomas are malignant brain tumors of the neuroglial cells that tend to be fast-growing. Patients have nonspecific symptoms of increased intracranial pressure. Treatment typically includes surgical debulking of the tumor; complete removal is often not possible at the time of diagnosis. Surgery is followed by radiation and chemotherapy. Astrocytoma is the most common glioma and has a variable prognosis. Oligodendroglioma is more slow-growing and may be calcified. Glioblastoma is a poorly differentiated glioma with a poor prognosis.

HALLMARK SIGNS AND SYMPTOMS

- Cerebellum or brain stem:
  - Lack of coordination—cerebellum helps coordinate gross movements
  - Hypotonia of limbs
  - Ataxia
- Frontal lobe:
  - Inability to speak (expressive aphasia)
  - Slowing of mental activity
  - Personality changes
  - Anosmia (loss of sense of smell)

- Occipital lobe:
  - Impaired vision—defect in visual fields; patient may deny or be unaware of defect
  - Prosopagnosia (patient is unable to recognize familiar faces)
  - Change in color perception
- Parietal lobe:
  - Seizures
  - Sight disturbances result in visual field defect
  - Sensory loss—unable to identify object placed in hand without looking
- Temporal lobe:
  - Seizures
  - Taste or smell hallucinations
  - Auditory hallucinations
  - Depersonalization
  - Emotional changes
  - Visual field defects
  - Receptive aphasia
  - Altered perception of music

INTERPRETING TEST RESULTS

- MRI with gadolinium (contrast) defines tumor location, size.
- CT scan shows characteristic appearance of meningioma.
- Angiography will show blood flow to the area; some tumors will displace vessels as they grow.

TREATMENT

- Chemotherapeutic agents alone or in combination with radiation and surgery. May be given orally, intravenously or through an Ommaya reservoir. Drugs are chosen based on cell type:
  - carmustine, lomustine, procarbazine, vincristine, temozolomide, erlotinib, gefitinib

- Irradiation of the area to decrease tumor size.
- Craniotomy to remove the tumor if appropriate; this depends on location, size, primary site of cancer, and number of tumors. Some patients may have several small, scattered tumors, making surgery impractical.
- Administer glucocorticoid to reduce swelling or inflammatory response within confined space inside skull (no room to expand, bone does not give):
  - dexamethasone
- Administer osmotic diuretic to reduce cerebral edema:
  - mannitol
- Administer anticonvulsant to reduce chance of seizure activity:
  - phenytoin, phenobarbital, carbamazepine, divalproex sodium, valproic acid, levetiracetam, lamotrigine, clonazepam, topiramate, ethosuximide
- Administer mucosal barrier fortifier to reduce risk of gastric irritation:
  - sucralfate
- Administer H2 receptor antagonists to reduce risk of gastric irritation:
  - ranitidine, famotidine, nizatidine, cimetidine
- Administer proton pump inhibitors (PPIs) to reduce risk of gastric irritation:
  - lansoprazole, omeprazole, esomeprazole, rabeprazole, pantoprazole

NURSING DIAGNOSES

- Disturbed sensory perception
- Risk for injury

NURSING INTERVENTION

- Monitor neurologic function.
- Check for side effects to medications.
- Seizure precautions per institution protocol.
- Assess for pain control.
- Explain to the patient:
  - Home care needs.
  - Possible need for hospice.

6 *Cerebral Aneurysm*

WHAT WENT WRONG?

A cerebral aneurysm is a balloon-like out-pouching caused by a congenital or developed weakness in a cerebral artery. Trauma, infection, or vessel wall lesions due to atherosclerosis can all lead to the development of an aneurysm. Increased pressure within the vessel lumen may cause the aneurysm to rupture, causing significant intracranial bleeding.

PROGNOSIS

Patients are often asymptomatic with the aneurysm, until the time of the rupture. Some patients have the aneurysm identified on a radiological study as an incidental finding. The decision can then be made to monitor or treat the aneurysm. If an arterial aneurysm ruptures without warning, the patient will have significant bleeding—a hemorrhagic stroke. The blood may need to be evacuated from the intracranial area to relieve pressure. The rupture of the aneurysm may be fatal, or the patient may have long-term disability following the event.

HALLMARK SIGNS AND SYMPTOMS

- Asymptomatic until rupture
- Very bad headache due to hemorrhage and increased intracranial pressure
- Decreased level of consciousness due to increased intracranial pressure from blood accumulating within the brain

INTERPRETING TEST RESULTS

- Angiogram highlights the aneurysm due to structural abnormality.
- CT scan shows the aneurysm unless it is very small.
- Digital subtraction angiography shows the detail of the vasculature—abnormal structure.

- Diffusion/perfusion MRI or MRA (magnetic resonance angiography) shows vessel structure.
- Single photon emission computed tomography (SPECT) shows the perfusion of blood flow to a specific area of the brain.

TREATMENT

- Surgical repair of the aneurysm.
- Monitor level of consciousness and neurologic status.
- Administer corticosteroid drugs to reduce inflammation:
  - dexamethasone
- Administer anticonvulsant drugs to reduce seizure risk due to irritation of brain:
  - phenytoin, phenobarbital
- Administer stool-softener drugs to decrease need to strain (straining increases intracranial pressure):
  - docusate sodium
- Bed rest until otherwise ordered by physician, nurse practitioner, or physician assistant.
- Elevate head of bed 30 degrees.

NURSING DIAGNOSES

- Ineffective tissue perfusion
- Decreased intracranial adaptive capacity

NURSING INTERVENTION

- Monitor the patient's neurological function for changes—typically use Glasgow Coma Scale or similar tool to grade response to stimuli (highest score 15).
  - Eye-opening response

spontaneous	4
to sound	3
to pain	2
none	1

- Motor responses

obeys commands	6
localizes pain	5
withdrawal (normal)	4
abnormal flexion	3
extension	2
none	1

- Verbal responses

oriented	5
confused conversation	4
inappropriate words	3
incomprehensible sounds	2
none	1

- Monitor vital signs for changes—widened pulse pressure with bradycardia indicative of increased intracranial pressure.
- Explain to the patient:
  - Needs for homecare.
  - When to call healthcare provider.

7 *Encephalitis*

WHAT WENT WRONG?

Encephalitis is the inflammation of the brain tissue, most often caused by a virus, although it can also be due to bacteria, fungus, or protozoa. In the case of viral encephalitis, the patient typically will have had viral symptoms prior to the current illness. The virus enters the central nervous system via the bloodstream and begins to reproduce. Inflammation in the area follows, causing damage to the neurons. Demyelination of the nerve fibers in the affected area and hemorrhage, edema, and necrosis occur, which create small cavities within the brain tissue. Herpes simplex virus 1, cytomegalovirus, echovirus, Coxsackie virus, and herpes zoster can all cause encephalitis. Some forms of encephalitis can be transmitted by insects (such as mosquitoes or ticks) to humans, such as West Nile virus, St. Louis encephalitis, or equine encephalitis.

PROGNOSIS

Identification of the organism is important in order to individualize the treatment for the patient. The earlier that symptoms are recognized and the earlier the patient enters the healthcare system the better. Some patients will incur permanent disability from the irreversible damage that occurs to the brain. These patients may be in need of long-term custodial care.

HALLMARK SIGNS AND SYMPTOMS

- Fever due to infection
- Nausea and vomiting due to increased intracranial pressure
- Stiff neck due to meningeal irritation
- Drowsiness, lethargy, or stupor due to increased intracranial pressure
- Altered mental status—irritability, confusion, disorientation, personality change
- Headache due to increased intracranial pressure
- Seizure activity possible due to irritation of brain tissue

INTERPRETING TEST RESULTS

- Blood cultures used to help identify organism when patient is febrile.

TREATMENT

- Monitor respiratory status for compromise.
- Monitor vital signs for widened pulse pressure and bradycardia—signs of increased intracranial pressure.
- Monitor neurologic function for change.
- Administer corticosteroid to decrease inflammation:
  - dexamethasone
- Administer antipyretics to reduce fever:
  - acetaminophen
- Administer anticonvulsants to decrease chance of seizure activity:
  - phenytoin, phenobarbital
- Administer diuretics to decrease cerebral edema, if indicated:

- furosemide
- mannitol

NURSING DIAGNOSES

- Impaired physical mobility
- Disturbed thought processes

NURSING INTERVENTION

- Range of motion exercises—active or passive.
- Turn and position patient.
- Monitor neurologic status for changes—typically use Glasgow Coma Scale or similar tool to grade response to stimuli (highest score 15)
  - Eye-opening response
spontaneous	4
to sound	3
to pain	2
none	1
  - Motor responses
obeys commands	6
localizes pain	5
withdrawal (normal)	4
abnormal flexion	3
extension	2
none	1
  - Verbal responses
oriented	5
confused conversation	4
inappropriate words	3
incomprehensible sounds	2
none	1
- Provide a quiet environment to decrease unnecessary stimulation.
- Monitor fluid input and output.
- Explain to the patient and family:
  - Home care needs.
  - Necessity of turning and positioning.
  - Medication actions, side effects, and interactions.

8 Guillain-Barré Syndrome

WHAT WENT WRONG?

This is an acute, progressive autoimmune condition that affects the peripheral nerves. Symptoms occur as the myelin surrounding the axon on the peripheral nerves is damaged from the autoimmune effect. The disease typically follows a viral infection, surgery, other acute illness or immunization by a couple of weeks. Ascending Guillain-Barré exhibits muscle weakness and/or paralysis that begins in the distal lower extremities and travels upwards. The patient may also experience altered sensory perception in the same areas, such as the sensation of crawling, tingling, burning, or pain. The progression of symptoms may take hours or days. Descending Guillain-Barré begins with muscles in the face, jaw, or throat and travels downward. Respiratory compromise is a concern as the paralysis reaches the level of the intercostal muscles and diaphragm. Breathing can become compromised more quickly in patients with descending disease. Level of consciousness, mental status, personality, and pupil size are not affected.

PROGNOSIS

Patient support and monitoring are important during symptom progression. Involvement of respiratory muscles may result in respiratory compromise or failure. Involvement of ocular areas may cause blindness. If the nerve cell body is damaged during the acute phase, there may be permanent deficits for the patient in the involved area. Otherwise, the axons of the nerves may be able to repair the damage over several months.

HALLMARK SIGNS AND SYMPTOMS

- Burning or tickling feeling due to demyelination of the nerve axons
- Symmetrical weakness or flaccid paralysis, typically ascending in pattern
- Absence of deep tendon reflexes due to changes within the nerves—reflexes are a sensory-motor response that happens at the spinal level, not the brain
- Recent infection or other acute illness
- Facial weakness, dysphagia, visual changes in descending disease

- Labile blood pressure and cardiac dysrhythmias due to autonomic nervous system response

INTERPRETING TEST RESULTS

- Lumbar puncture will show cerebrospinal fluid (CSF) with increased protein; may not be present initially.
- Nerve conduction studies show slowed velocity.
- Pulmonary function tests show diminished tidal volume and vital capacity.

TREATMENT

- Monitor respirations and support ventilation if necessary.
- Plasmapheresis for plasma exchange to remove the antibodies in the circulation.
- Administer immunoglobulin intravenously after drawing labs for serum IgA.
- NG tube feeding if swallowing is a problem.

NURSING DIAGNOSES

- Ineffective breathing pattern
- Impaired gas exchange
- Impaired physical mobility
- Powerlessness

NURSING INTERVENTION

- Monitor for progression of change of sensation.
- Monitor respiratory status for change in effort or rate, use of accessory muscles, cyanosis, change in breath sounds, breathlessness when talking, irritability, and decreased cognitive awareness.
- Call physician if there are respiratory changes or decrease in pulse oximeter reading.

- Monitor gag reflex.
- Monitor for visual changes.
- Monitor for communication ability; the patient may need special method to communicate with staff if not able to use call bell system.
- Turn and reposition.
- Consult with social worker or chaplain for support services available to patient.
- Explain to the patient:
  - Importance of turning and positioning.
  - Care of the plasmapheresis access site.
  - Importance of planning for home care needs.

9 *Huntington's Disease (Chorea)*

WHAT WENT WRONG?

This is a degenerative disease that presents with a gradual onset of involuntary, jerking movements (chorea) and a progressive decline in mental ability, resulting in behavioral changes and dementia. The disease is transmitted genetically, as an autosomal dominant trait located on chromosome 4. Family members of patients can have genetic testing done to identify presence of the gene. The symptoms typically appear between the ages of 30 and 50 years.

PROGNOSIS

The patient may present with either abnormalities of movements or changes in intellectual function. In time, both will be present. The mental status changes will progress to dementia. The disease will prove to be fatal within 10 to 20 years from the time of onset.

HALLMARK SIGNS AND SYMPTOMS

- Personality changes
- Irritability or moodiness
- Psychiatric disturbance

- Progressive dementia as disease causes further neurologic degeneration
- Restlessness or fidgeting due to dyskinesia
- Abnormal, jerking movements (chorea)
- Depression

INTERPRETING TEST RESULTS

- Genetic testing can detect gene presence even prior to onset of symptoms.
- CT scan shows cerebral atrophy later in disease.
- MRI shows atrophy later in disease.
- Positron emission tomography (PET) shows decrease in glucose uptake in specific areas in a structurally normal brain.

TREATMENT

Huntington's disease is progressive and while there is no cure for it, medications can be used to control symptoms.

- Genetic counseling.
- Control dyskinesia and behavior with medication to block dopamine receptors:
  - phenothiazines
  - haloperidol
  - reserpine.

NURSING DIAGNOSES

- Risk for injury
- Impaired physical mobility
- Ineffective health maintenance

NURSING INTERVENTION

- Provide basic needs for the patient, assist with ADLs as needed.
- Protect the patient from suicide attempts due to depression.

- Assist the patient with positioning for safety and comfort.
- Explain to the patient:
  - Nature of disease.
  - Genetic counseling available for family members of patients.

10 *Meningitis*

WHAT WENT WRONG?

Meningitis is the inflammation of the meningeal coverings of the brain and spinal cord, most commonly due to bacteria or viral cause, although it can also be caused by fungus, protozoa, or toxic exposure. Bacterial meningitis is the most common and is typically due to *Streptococcus pneumoniae* (pneumococcal), *Neisseria meningitides* (meningococcal), or *Haemophilus influenzae*. The incidence of *H. influenzae* meningitis infections has decreased since the vaccine against *H. influenzae* began to be used routinely in infants in the early 1990s. Other organisms that can cause bacterial meningitis include *Staphylococcus aureus*, *Escherichia coli*, and *Pseudomonas*. Organisms typically travel either through the bloodstream to the central nervous system or enter by direct contamination (skull fracture or extension from sinus infections). Bacterial meningitis is more common in colder months when upper respiratory tract infections are more common. People in close living conditions, such as prisons, military barracks, or college dorms are at greater risk for outbreaks of bacterial meningitis due to likelihood of transmission.

Viral meningitis may follow other viral infections, such as mumps, herpes simplex or zoster, enterovirus, and measles. Viral meningitis is often a self-limiting illness.

Patients who are immunocompromised have an increased risk for contracting a fungal meningitis. This may travel from the bloodstream to the central nervous system or by direct contamination. *Cryptococcus neoformans* may be the causative organism in these patients.

PROGNOSIS

Identification of meningitis and the causative organism is important in order to adequately treat the patient. Bacterial meningitis still has a significant mortality rate and these patients need to be managed in the hospital. Some patients will have permanent neurologic effects following the acute episode. Viral meningitis is typically self-limiting. Fungal meningitis often occurs in patients who are immunocompromised. Patients who have comorbidities or are elderly have greater difficulty with the symptoms of meningitis.

HALLMARK SIGNS AND SYMPTOMS

- Stiff neck due to meningeal irritation and irritation of the spinal nerves
- Nuchal rigidity (pain when flexing chin toward chest) due to meningeal irritation and irritation of the spinal nerves
- Headache due to increased intracranial pressure
- Nausea and vomiting due to increased intracranial pressure
- Photophobia (sensitivity to light) due to irritation of the cranial nerves
- Fever due to infection
- Malaise and fatigue due to infection
- Myalgia (muscle aches) due to viral infection
- Petechial rash on skin and mucous membranes with meningococcal infection
- Seizures due to irritation of brain from increased intracranial pressure

INTERPRETING TEST RESULTS

- Lumbar puncture for cerebral spinal fluid analysis, glucose (bacterial low), protein (bacterial elevated), cell counts (bacterial elevated neutrophils), and culture.
- Increased cerebral spinal fluid pressure noted.
- Polymerase chain reaction (PCR) test of cerebrospinal fluid to test for organisms—results within a couple of hours.
- Culture and sensitivity—results may take up to 72 hours.
- Blood cultures.
- CT scan brain to rule out space-occupying lesion as cause of symptoms.

TREATMENT

- Administer antibiotics as soon as possible to improve outcome for bacterial meningitis:
  - penicillin G

- ceftriaxone
- cefotaxime
- vancomycin plus ceftriaxone or cefotaxime
- ceftazidime
- Fungal infections are typically treated with:
  - amphotericin B
  - fluconazole
  - flucytosine
- Administer corticosteroid to decrease inflammation in pneumococcal infection:
  - dexamethasone
- Administer osmotic diuretic for cerebral edema:
  - mannitol
- Administer analgesics for headache if needed:
  - acetaminophen
- Administer anticonvulsant if necessary:
  - phenytoin, phenobarbital
- Bed rest until neurologic irritation improves.

NURSING DIAGNOSES

- Risk for injury
- Powerlessness

NURSING INTERVENTION

- Monitor intake and output to check fluid balance.
- Keep room darkened due to photophobia.
- Monitor neurologic function at least every 2 to 4 hours, changes in mental status, level of consciousness, pupil reactions, speech, facial movement symmetry, and signs of increased intracranial pressure.
- Seizure precautions per institution policy.
- Isolation per policy depending on organism.

- Explain to the patient:
  - Why restrictions (bed rest) are necessary.
  - Vaccine available for meningococcal meningitis—the 2 different types are meningococcal polysaccharide vaccine (MPSV4) and conjugate vaccine (MCV4).

11 *Multiple Sclerosis (MS)*

WHAT WENT WRONG?

This is an autoimmune disease that results in demyelination of the white matter of the nervous system. Nerve impulses travel along the myelin coating on the outside of the nerve cells. With the disruption in the myelin on the outside of the nerve cells, the transmission of information from cell to cell within the nervous system is altered. The patient's sensations, movements, or mental function may be affected. A patient with relapsing-remitting disease will have episodes of exacerbation when symptoms occur and then months or years of symptom-free episodes. A portion of these patients will progress to enter a disease state that has a steady pattern of deterioration without relation to the periodic exacerbations; this is referred to as a secondary progressive disease. Other patients have a primary progressive disease and develop the steady deterioration from the onset of the disease.

PROGNOSIS

The actual cause of the disease is unknown, although it is thought to be autoimmune. The disease is progressive. Stress may be noted to aggravate symptoms. When damage is done to the nerve cells, it is not repairable, even when symptoms resolve in between periods of exacerbation. The pattern of symptoms will vary from one patient to the next. The time frame between exacerbations will also vary. As the disease progresses, the patient will lose more functional ability and will ultimately need assistance with basic self-care needs.

HALLMARK SIGNS AND SYMPTOMS

Symptoms have periods of exacerbation and remission. Symptoms typically resolve completely in between exacerbations early in the disease process.

- Double vision (diplopia)
- Blurred vision
- Fatigue
- Muscle weakness or unsteadiness
- Unsteady gait due to muscle weakness and general unsteadiness
- Intolerance of temperature changes
- Ataxia (decrease in motor coordination, gross motor movements)
- Increased deep tendon reflexes
- Slurred speech
- Burning tingling on the skin (paresthesia)
- Paralysis later in disease state
- Memory loss; loss of attention or mental focus
- Urinary urgency or hesitancy due to changes in sphincter control

INTERPRETING TEST RESULTS

- Increased immunoglobulin G (IgG) in cerebral spinal fluid.
- MRI shows demyelination and CNS plaques.
- CT scan shows increased density of white matter or plaque formation.

TREATMENT

- Use one of the following Biologic Response Modifiers on a continuous basis, not just during periods of exacerbation:
  - interferon beta-1a
  - interferon beta-1b
  - glatiramer acetate
- Administer immunosuppressants—may be helpful for secondary progressive MS:
  - cyclophosphamide
  - azathioprine
  - methotrexate
  - cladribine
  - mitoxantrone

- Administer corticosteroids:
  - methylprednisolone intravenously
  - prednisone 60 to 80 mg daily the first week, then tapered over the next couple of weeks
  - dexamethasone
- Administer one of the following for muscle relaxation:
  - dantrolene
  - baclofen
  - carisoprodol
  - metaxalone
  - tizanidine
  - diazepam
- Use of the following medications may help with fatigue symptoms:
  - modafinil
  - methylphenidate
- Administer antidepressants if indicated:
  - fluoxetine (selective serotonin reuptake inhibitor—SSRI)
  - sertraline (SSRI)
  - paroxetine (SSRI)
  - citalopram (SSRI)
  - escitalopram (SSRI)
  - venlafaxine (inhibits norepinephrine, serotonin, and dopamine reuptake)
  - bupropion (inhibits norepinephrine and dopamine reuptake)
  - duloxetine (inhibits norepinephrine and serotonin reuptake)
  - amitriptyline (tricyclic) may help with discomfort associated with paresthesia
- Administer medications to help with altered bladder function:
  - oxybutynin
  - hyoscyamine sulfate
  - darifenacin
  - solifenacin
  - tolterodine
- Remove antibodies by removing plasma (plasmapheresis).

NURSING DIAGNOSES

- Impaired physical mobility
- Fatigue
- Self-care deficit

NURSING INTERVENTION

- Monitor motor movements for interference with ADLs.
- Encourage activity balanced with rest periods.
- Assess cognitive function for changes, or deterioration.
- Explain to the patient:
  - Bladder training.
  - Teach self-catheterization if necessary (for patients with flexic bladder).
  - Increase fluid intake unless other medical problems contraindicate.
  - Importance of positioning.
  - Avoid temperature extremes.
  - Medication compliance.

12 *Myasthenia Gravis*

WHAT WENT WRONG?

This is a disorder of the peripheral nervous system involving antibodies that have been produced by the body; they bind to receptor sites that normally bind acetyl-choline. This prevents the acetylcholine from binding to the receptor sites on the skeletal muscle, inhibiting normal muscle contraction in the affected area. The areas of the body most commonly affected by the autoimmune disease include the muscles in the eyes, face, lips, tongue, throat, and neck, resulting in weakness and fatigue of these areas. The disease does not seem to be hereditary, but does have a family tendency toward autoimmune disorders. The majority of the patients have a hyperplasia (excessive growth of normal cells) of the thymus gland. Myasthenia gravis is more likely to develop in young adults and is more common in women.

PROGNOSIS

The disease can take a variety of forms from mild weakness and drooping of the eye muscles to generalized, progressive weakness that ultimately affects respiratory function. Progression of symptoms will vary from patient to patient. There are typically episodes of exacerbations and remissions. The more aggressive form of the disease progresses more rapidly, resulting in death from respiratory failure.

HALLMARK SIGNS AND SYMPTOMS

- Ptosis (drooping of the eyelid) due to muscular weakness
- Diplopia (double vision) due to inability to keep both eyes focused on the same object
- Trouble closing eyes completely; dry eyes due to muscle weakness
- Difficulty swallowing (dysphagia) due to muscle weakness
- Muscle weakness later in the day due to fatigue
- Proximal muscle weakness
- Fatigue
- In advanced disease—loss of bowel and bladder control; difficulty with respiratory function
- Myasthenic crisis is an exacerbation of symptoms due to insufficient medication:
  - Tachycardia
  - Tachypnea
  - Elevated blood pressure
  - Cyanosis
  - Decrease in urinary output
  - Incontinence of bowel and bladder
  - Loss of gag reflex
- Cholinergic crisis is an exacerbation of weakness due to too much cholinergic medication:
  - Blurred vision
  - Nausea, vomiting, diarrhea
  - Abdominal cramping
  - Paleness

- Twitching of facial muscles
- Small pupils (miosis)
- Low blood pressure

INTERPRETING TEST RESULTS

Symptoms are relieved temporarily after administering endrophonium (Tensilon) or neostigmine bromide (Prostigmin) because the drug will allow the acetylcholine to bind at the post-synaptic receptor site on the muscle at which it should normally bind.

- Acetylcholine receptor antibodies are present in greater than 80 percent of patients with myasthenia gravis.
- Electromyography (EMG) shows reduced muscle response to repeated stimulations.
- CT scan to rule out thymoma.

TREATMENT

- Administer immunosuppressants to induce remission and help control symptoms:
  - prednisone or dexamethasone initially to improve symptoms
  - azathioprine and cyclophosphamide in the long term to help control symptoms
- Administer cholinesterase inhibitors for long-term control of symptoms. These drugs have short duration of action, therefore have to be dosed several times during the day:
  - neostigmine
  - pyridostigmine
  - ambenonium
- Administer natural tears or other lubricant to keep eyes moist:
  - patch eyes if unable to close
- High-calorie diet of appropriate food type—patient may have difficulty swallowing.
- Removing antibodies from plasma (plasmapheresis) may be beneficial.
- BiPAP or CPAP for enhanced air movement and oxygenation.
- Thymectomy (surgical removal of thymus gland) for patients with thymoma.
- Avoid aminoglycoside antibiotics which may exacerbate symptoms.

NURSING DIAGNOSES

- Impaired physical mobility
- Impaired verbal communication
- Ineffective air exchange
- Self-care deficit

NURSING INTERVENTION

- Encourage frequent rest periods.
- Monitor vital signs.
- Monitor nutritional intake.
- Monitor weight.
- Monitor neurologic status for changes in pupil reaction, extraocular movements, eyelid movement, facial symmetry, hand grip strength, coordination, fine motor skills, and gait.
- Monitor respiratory status for changes in rate, effort, skin color, use of accessory muscles, or change in mental status.
- Monitor gag reflex.
- Arrange for appropriate communication with staff if patient is unable to use call bell system or unable to be heard over intercom from room.
- Explain to the patient:
  - Home care needs.
  - Medication use; need to maintain time schedule for medications.
  - Time meals one hour after medications to decrease chance of aspiration.
  - Teach use of oral-pharyngeal suctioning catheter to clear secretions.
  - Avoid heat extremes (hot tubs, saunas).
  - Alcohol may exacerbate symptoms.

13 *Parkinson's Disease*

WHAT WENT WRONG?

There is a gradual degeneration of the midbrain area known as the substantia nigra. The neurons use the neurotransmitter dopamine to send their signals from cell to cell. The loss of neurons within the substantia nigra continues and results in diminished voluntary fine motor skills due to dopamine loss. There is also development of sympathetic noradrenergic lesions, causing norepinephrine loss within the sympathetic nervous system. There is excess effect of the excitatory neurotransmitter acetylcholine on the neurons; this causes increased muscle tone, leading to rigidity and tremors. There seems to be a genetic tendency towards development of Parkinson's disease. Environmental factors such as exposure to airborne contaminants, occupational chemicals, toxins, or a virus have been implicated in the development of the disease. Typical age of onset is after the fifth decade of life.

PROGNOSIS

Parkinson's disease is a progressive disorder and does not have a cure. The symptoms can be managed with medications, but will return as the medications wear off. The dosages will need to be adjusted periodically, and additional medications may be needed to address the side effects of the medications used. Some patients develop mental status changes or dementia in conjunction with Parkinson's disease.

HALLMARK SIGNS AND SYMPTOMS

- Mask-like facial expressions
- Slow, shuffling gait
- Pill-rolling movements of hands
- Stooping posture
- Tremor at rest
- Change in handwriting—gets progressively smaller over time
- Bradykinesia (slow movement)
- Trouble chewing or swallowing
- Drooling
- Inability to control voluntary movement (dyskinesia) and fine-skilled movement, or to initiate movement—due to loss of dopamine which has an inhibitory effect and helps refine movements while acetylcholine retains the excitatory effect on the neurons
- Rigidity of limbs:
  - Cogwheeling—there is a rhythmic stopping or interruption of the movement of the extremity
  - Lead pipe—no bending; resists movement completely

- Orthostatic hypotension due to lack of norepinephrine within the sympathetic nervous system, affecting the cardiovascular system

INTERPRETING TEST RESULTS

- Cerebrospinal fluid levels may show low levels of dopamine.

TREATMENT

- Administer antiparkinsonian agents which are able to cross the blood-brain barrier. These drugs absorb better on an empty stomach:
  - levodopa
  - carbidopa-levodopa
- Administer dopamine receptor agonists to act directly on the dopamine receptor sites:
  - pergolide
  - bromocriptine
  - pramipexole
  - ropinirole
- Administer selegiline, a selective monoamine oxidase B inhibitor that slows the breakdown of dopamine and allows lower doses of levodopa to be used because it prolongs its effect.
- Administer catechol O-methyltransferase (COMT) inhibitors which help block the breakdown of levodopa:
  - entacapone
  - tolcapone
- Administer acetylcholine blocking drugs to decrease tremor and rigidity in patients:
  - biperiden
  - benztropine mesylate
  - procyclidine
  - orphenadrine
  - trihexyphenidyl
- Diet high in protein and calories.
- Soft food diet.
- Physical therapy.

NURSING DIAGNOSES

- Activity intolerance
- Impaired mobility
- Risk for injury

NURSING INTERVENTION

- Monitor neurological status for changes.
- Monitor respiratory status for changes.
- Encourage self-care, allow patient extra time.
- Encourage exercise; assist with passive ROM if necessary.
- Weigh patient.
- Record food intake.
- Explain to the patient:
  - Importance of following medication time schedule as well as effects of medication wearing off.
  - Reduce risk of falls at home.

14 *Spinal Cord Injury*

WHAT WENT WRONG?

Injury to the spinal cord results in compression, twisting, severing, or pulling on the spinal cord. The damage to the cord may involve the entire thickness of the cord (complete), or only a partial area of the spinal cord (incomplete). The most common cause of spinal cord injury is trauma. Any level of the spinal cord may have been affected by the injury. Loss of sensation, motor control, or reflexes may occur below the level of injury or within 1 to 2 vertebrae or spinal nerves above the level of injury. The loss may be unilateral or bilateral. Damage to the vertebrae may have occurred at the same time as the spinal cord injury. Swelling due to the initial trauma may make the injury seem more severe than it actually is. When the initial swelling resolves, the actual degree of permanent injury can be more accurately assessed.

PROGNOSIS

The level of injury will determine the degree of disability the patient is likely to sustain. A high-level injury, such as a cervical injury, will more likely result in quadraplegia (paralysis of all four extremities) and compromise of the respiratory drive. A complete spinal cord injury will result in greater disability than an incomplete injury. Spinal cord tissue does not regenerate after an injury. Swelling that occurs immediately following an injury may be controlled with medications and some clinical improvement may occur, but the damage to the cord cannot be undone.

HALLMARK SIGNS AND SYMPTOMS

- Loss of motor control due to damage to the anterior horn of the spinal cord
- Loss of reflexes due to damage of the spinal cord, the point of synaptic transmission of sensory impulse to motor response
- Flaccid paralysis
- Lack of bowel and bladder control
- Altered sensation (tingling—paresthesia; diminished—hypoesthesia; increased—hyperesthesia)
- Bradycardia, hypotension, hypothermia due to problems with the autonomic nervous system

INTERPRETING TEST RESULTS

- MRI shows vertebral or spinal cord injury and edema.
- CT scan shows vertebral or spinal cord injury and edema.

TREATMENT

- Immobilize the affected area of the spinal cord to decrease chance of further irritation.
- Place the patient in a flat position to avoid flexion or misalignment of the spine.
- Monitor traction or collar to prevent skin irritation.
- Administer corticosteroid to decrease inflammation at point of injury:
  - methylprednisolone

- prednisone
- dexamethasone
- Administer dextran, a plasma expander, which increases blood flow in the spinal cord, increasing oxygenation to the tissue.
- Assist respirations if indicated.
- Administer H2 receptor antagonists to protect stomach from stress ulcer formation:
  - cimetidine, ranitidine, famotidine, nizatidine
- Administer gastric mucosal protective agent to coat stomach lining:
  - sucralfate
- Place patient in a rotation bed for repositioning to prevent pressure on skin.
- Surgical repair of vertebral fracture or decompression may be necessary.

NURSING DIAGNOSES

- Impaired physical mobility
- Powerlessness

NURSING INTERVENTION

- Monitor respiratory status—assess for changes in rate, effort, use of accessory muscles, cyanosis, altered mental status, and pulse oximetry reading.
- Monitor neurologic status for changes—assess sensation, temperature, touch, position sense, comparing right to left.
- Monitor for spinal shock:
  - Flaccid paralysis, loss of reflexes below the level of injury, hypotension, bradycardia, possible paralytic ileus.
- Monitor pulse and blood pressure for changes—change in heart rate, hypotension, or hypertension.
- Assess skin for signs of pressure (redness) or breakdown.
- Assess abdomen and listen for bowel sounds.
- Explain to the patient:
  - Importance of regular bowel and bladder function to avoid autonomic dysreflexia due to distension: severe headache, hypertension, bradycardia, flushing, nasal congestion, sweating, nausea.
  - Use of incentive spirometer.

- Need for turning and positioning or special rotating bed to decrease pressure.
- Monitor intake and output.
- Home care needs—accessibility, equipment needs.
- Proper way to transfer from bed to wheelchair.
- Care of pin sites for cervical traction devices (e.g. halo traction).

15 *Stroke*

WHAT WENT WRONG?

A stroke is also known as a cerebrovascular accident (CVA) or a brain attack. Blood supply is interrupted to part of the brain, causing brain cells to die; this results in the patient losing brain function in the affected area. Interruption is usually caused by an obstruction of arterial blood flow (ischemic stroke), such as formation of a blood clot, but can also be caused by a leaking or ruptured blood vessel (hemorrhagic stroke). A blood clot may develop from a piece of unstable plaque lining a vessel wall that breaks free, or an embolus that travels from elsewhere in the body and lodges within the vessel. The bleeding may occur as a result of trauma or spontaneously, as in the setting of uncontrolled hypertension. Ischemia occurs when insufficient blood is getting to the brain tissue. This leads to lack of available oxygen (hypoxia) and glucose (hypoglycemia) for the brain. When these nutrients are not available for a sustained period, the brain cells die, causing an area of infarction. Permanent deficits result from infarction. There is increased risk for stroke in patients with a history of hypertension, diabetes mellitus, high cholesterol, atrial fibrillation, obesity, smoking, or oral contraceptive use.

Patients may also experience a transient ischemic attack (TIA) in which the symptoms result from a temporary problem with blood flow to a specific area of the brain. The symptoms have a duration between a few minutes and 24 hours.

PROGNOSIS

The degree of damage and location of the stroke will determine the outcome for the patient. Strokes occur suddenly and patients should seek immediate treatment for the best possible outcome. The majority of strokes are ischemic. Rapid entry into the healthcare system and treatment with thrombolytic agents (unless there are contraindications to this treatment) to break up a clot that has caused the ischemia gives the patient the best chance for recovery without permanent disability. Patients with hemorrhagic stroke may need surgery to relieve intracranial pressure or stop the bleeding. A large area of damage may lead to significant permanent disability or death.

HALLMARK SIGNS AND SYMPTOMS

- Mental impairment
- Disorientation, confusion
- Emotional changes, personality changes
- Aphasia (difficulty with speech; may be receptive, expressive)
- Slurring of words
- Sensory changes (paresthesia, visual changes, hearing changes)
- Unilateral numbness or weakness in face or limbs
- Seizure
- Severe headache due to increased intracranial pressure from hemorrhage
- TIA symptoms are similar but have a shorter duration and resolve

INTERPRETING TEST RESULTS

- CT scan identifies area of bleeding (usually for emergency use).
- MRI (magnetic resonance imaging) identifies location of ischemic areas (slower than CT scan).
- MRA (magnetic resonance angiography) can identify abnormal vasculature or vasospasm.
- Diffusion/perfusion MRI or MRA will show areas that are not getting adequate blood supply, but have not yet suffered an infarction.
- SPECT (single photon emission computed tomography) will show an area that is not perfusing adequately

TREATMENT

It is most important to determine whether the patient has suffered an ischemic or hemorrhagic stroke as the treatment is different. Giving a thrombolytic agent to the patient who has had a hemorrhagic stroke will only cause further bleeding into the brain. Caution is also recommended in patients with head trauma, uncontrolled hypertension, hemorrhagic retinopathy, gastrointestinal bleeding, recent surgery, recent MI, or pregnancy.

- Administer TPA (thromoblytic agent) within 3 hours of onset of symptoms, unless contraindicated.
- Administer anticoagulants for patients with ischemic stroke after use of TPA:
  - heparin, warfarin, low-molecular weight heparin, aspirin
- Administer antiplatelet medications to decrease platelet adhesiveness; used to prevent recurrent stroke:
  - clopidogrel, ticlopidine hydrochloride, dipyridamole
- Administer corticosteroid to decrease swelling:
  - dexamethasone (Decadron)
- Physical therapy to help maintain muscle tone or return function.
- Speech therapy to help with speech and swallowing.
- Occupational therapy to help regain function.
- Bed rest to reduce chance of injury.
- Adequate nutrition in appropriate food type for patient.
- Carotid artery endarterectomy to remove plaque from within the carotid artery if stenosis is present.
- Stenting of carotid artery to maintain bloodflow.
- Surgical correction of arteriovenous malformation, aneurysm, intracranial bleeding.

NURSING DIAGNOSES

- Risk for injury
- Ineffective tissue perfusion

NURSING INTERVENTION

- Monitor vital signs for changes.
- Assess neurological status for signs of deterioration—perform neurological checks at least every 4 hours—typically use Glasgow Coma Scale or similar tool to grade response to stimuli (highest score 15):
  - Eye-opening response   spontaneous   4
                                      to sound   3

	to pain	2
	none	1
• Motor responses	obeys commands	6
	localizes pain	5
	withdrawal (normal)	4
	abnormal flexion	3
	extension	2
	none	1
• Verbal responses	oriented	5
	confused conversation	4
	inappropriate words	3
	incomprehensible sounds	2
	none	1

- Monitor for signs of increased intracranial pressure—diminished level of consciousness, headaches, restlessness, confusion, nausea and vomiting, speech changes, or seizures.
- Notify healthcare provider of changes in neurologic status.
- Develop a means of communication with the patient—aphasia may compromise use of call bell system or intercom.
- Assess for neglect syndrome—patient may act as if unaware of the side affected by paralysis due to the stroke.
- Need for rehabilitation to return to prior functional ability.
- Explain to the patient:
  - Home care needs.
  - Proper technique to transfer from bed to chair.
  - Use of ambulatory assist devices: cane, crutch, walker.
  - Special dietary needs; use of Thick-it® for liquids.
  - Medication schedule, use, side effects, and interactions.

16 *Seizure Disorder*

WHAT WENT WRONG?

This is a disorder that involves a sudden episode of abnormal, uncontrolled discharge of the electrical activity of the neurons within the brain. The patient may experience a variety of symptoms depending on the type of seizure and the cause.

Generalized seizures	
Tonic clonic	Begins with tonic (stiffening/rigidity of muscles of limbs), loss of consciousness, then clonic (rhythmic jerking)
Tonic	Stiffening or rigidity of muscles; loss of consciousness
Clonic	Rhythmic jerking of muscle contraction and relaxation
Absence	Brief loss of conscious awareness and staring into space; appears to be daydreaming
Myoclonic	Brief stiffening or jerking of extremity, either single or in groups
Atonic	Loss of muscle tone
Partial seizures	
Simple partial	Begins with aura; may have unilateral unusual sensation or movement of extremity, autonomic (heart rate, flushing), or psychic changes; no loss of consciousness
Complex partial	Loss of consciousness; automatisms (lip smacking, picking, patting)

Seizures may be a symptom of another condition—such as a tumor or stroke which has increased the intracranial pressure, a metabolic disorder, withdrawal from alcohol or drugs—or may be due to a chronic seizure disorder such as epilepsy. Prior to the seizure, the patient may experience an aura, a sensory alteration involving sight, sound, or smell. After the seizure, the patient enters a post-ictal stage where there may be confusion and the patient is often fatigued. The patient may not recall any of the seizure or the time immediately surrounding the seizure.

INTERPRETING TEST RESULTS

- EEG (electroencephalogram) to identify areas of abnormal electrical activity within the brain.
- CT scan of the brain to identify causes of increased intracranial pressure (rule out tumor or bleed).
- MRI to identify causes of increased intracranial pressure (rule out tumor or bleed).
- PET (positron emission tomography) or SPECT (single photon emission computed tomography) to determine areas in the brain that are not adequately perfused.

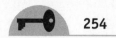

TREATMENT

If there is an underlying condition causing the disorder, removal of this condition will often result in resolution of the disorder. The patient with a primary seizure disorder will typically be managed with anticonvulsant medications. Some patients will need multi-drug regimens to adequately control the seizure disorder. Patients who do not respond to multiple antiepileptic drugs may be candidates for surgical intervention.

- Administer antiepileptic medications:
  - carbamazepine
  - phenytoin
  - phenobarbital
  - clonazepam
  - valproic acid
  - lamotrigine
  - gabapentin
  - levetiracetam
  - oxcarbazepine
  - primidone
  - tiagabine
  - topiramate
- Seizure precautions per institution.
- Maintain IV access with saline lock if no intravenous fluids needed for hospitalized patients.
- Surgery to remove seizure focal area or sever the connection between the cerebral hemispheres (corpus callostomy) to limit the amount of seizure activity for patients who do not have adequate control of seizures with medications.
- Vagal nerve stimulation where there is implantation of an electrical device that provides a predetermined pattern of vagal stimulation. This is used to decrease the frequency of seizures.

NURSING DIAGNOSES

- Risk for ineffective breathing pattern or airway clearance

- Risk for fall
- Anxiety

NURSING INTERVENTION

- Monitor patient during the seizure for breathing, skin color (cyanosis)—patient may have diminished oxygenation during seizure.
- May need supplemental oxygen post-seizure.
- Keep oxygen equipment and suction equipment and emergency airway management equipment at bedside (intubation may be performed by anesthesiologist, nurse anesthetist, or respiratory therapist).
- Monitor duration of seizure and progression of symptoms.
- Monitor for incontinence of bladder or bowel.
- Monitor for status epilepticus—prolonged seizures or repeated seizures, considered a medical emergency.
- Position patient to decrease risk of injury:
  - remove objects that may injure patient.
  - turn patient on side to reduce risk of aspiration.
  - do not insert anything in patient's mouth during seizure.
- Assess the patient post-seizure.
- Explain to the patient:
  - Medication use, side effects, and interactions.
  - Importance of taking medications on time, not skipping doses.
  - Importance of checking with prescriber before taking any new medications or over-the-counter (OTC) medications or supplements.
  - Have lab tests for drug level of antiepileptic drugs checked as directed.

Crucial Diagnostic Tests

X-ray

An x-ray of the skull or spine is done to determine the presence of fracture, dislocation, calcification into soft tissue areas, degree of curvature (normal anteroposterior curve of areas of the spine, versus lateral curvature of scoliosis).

CT scan with or without Contrast

Practitioner may do an initial test without contrast for first images and then give contrast and repeat images to compare. Done to check for bleeding, tumor, abscess, infarction, and hydrocephalus.

CT Angiography

This creates a three-dimensional reconstruction of the vasculature within the area imaged.

Cerebral Angiography

Contrast is injected to visualize the cerebral circulation, carotid, and vertebral arteries. This test is done to identify aneurysms, arteriovenous malformations, traumatic injuries, strictures, occlusions, and tumors.

The head is immobilized during the test. Wire is inserted via the femoral arterial site and passed to the carotid or vertebral vessel under fluoroscopic guidance. Contrast dye is injected so three-dimensional images can be obtained.

After the test, you need to monitor vital signs and perform neurologic checks and neurovascular checks of the extremity (capillary refill, peripheral pulses, skin color, and temperature). Check for bleeding at the site.

EEG

This test records the electrical activity from the cerebral hemispheres of the brain and creates a graphic recording. It determines general brain activity as well as the site of origin of seizure activity. It is also used to diagnose sleep disorders and determine brain death.

Lumbar Puncture

A spinal needle is inserted into subarachnoid space at level of L3–L4 or L4–L5 with patient lying on side with knees drawn up to chest. This test is performed under local anesthesia.

It is done to obtain pressure readings, obtain cerebrospinal fluid for analysis, inject contrast medium or air for diagnostic tests, inject medications, or reduce increased intracranial pressure.

The patient must lie flat for several hours after the procedure to reduce the risk of spinal headache due to leakage of spinal fluid. Encourage oral fluid intake.

MRI with Gadolinium

This test is done to detect differences in tissue integrity, tumors, and disc disease. Due to the use of a magnetic field to create images, an MRI is not for patients with implanted hardware (pacemakers, etc.) or for pregnant women.

MRA (Magnetic Resonance Angiography)

This is done to detect arterial blockages, aneurysm, and arteriovenous malformations.

PET (Positron Emission Tomography)

PET tells about the function of the brain involving glucose and oxygen metabolism. The test is done to detect areas of altered metabolism such as dementia, epilepsy, neoplasm, or degenerative disorders.

The patient is given a tagged isotope on deoxyglucose. There will be increased glucose uptake by areas with increased metabolic activity.

Single Photon Emission Computed Tomography (SPECT)

SPECT involves an intravenous injection of a radiopharmaceutical to enhance the image. It is done to detect cerebral blood flow, stroke, dementia, amnesia, neoplasm, head trauma, seizures, persistent vegetative state, brain death, and psychiatric disorders. This test is not for pregnant women.

Quiz

1. A patient arrived in the ER with a head injury. She is unconscious. You and a fellow nurse are the only staff members near the patient. He begins to criticize the attending physician and suggest that a different physician should care for this patient. What is the best response?

   (a) Report the nurse to the attending physician.

   (b) Call the nurse away from the patient and remind him that the patient can still hear even if unconscious.

   (c) Ask the nurse why he has such feelings.

   (d) Simply nod your head in agreement.

2. Your patient has unilateral facial paralysis and is unable to close his right eye. He is diagnosed with Bell's palsy. He asks you if there is any special care required for his eye. What is the best response?

   (a) No, since the symptoms will go away in a few weeks.

   (b) Wear sunglasses.

   (c) Increase fluid intake to prevent dryness of the eye.

   (d) Yes, you'll need to instill artificial teardrops and use an eye patch.

3. A new patient arrived in your unit. He has been diagnosed with a brain tumor. You are told that the patient is unable to speak. Based on this sign, where do you expect the tumor is located?

   (a) Frontal lobe.

   (b) Occipital lobe.

   (c) Cerebellum.

   (d) Parietal lobe.

4. The wife of a patient who has a ruptured aneurysm asks how this could have happened considering that he passed a physical three months ago. What is the best response?

   (a) Aneurysms are often asymptomatic.

   (b) The physician must have misread the x-ray.

   (c) The aneurysm must have developed since his physical.

   (d) Don't be too concerned because this happens all the time.

5. A 49-year-old patient is diagnosed with Huntington's disease. He thought he saw symptoms of the disease in his 15-year-old son. What is the best response?

   (a) Your son probably has the early symptoms of the disease.

   (b) Huntington's disease is genetically transmitted.

   (c) Symptoms usually appear between the ages of 30 and 50 years; however, you may want to ask your physician about genetic testing that can detect if your son has the gene that is associated with Huntington's disease.

   (d) Symptoms usually appear before the age of 30 years; however, you may want to ask your physician about genetic testing that can detect if your son has the gene that is associated with Huntington's disease.

6. A patient arrives in the ER with blurred and double vision, muscle weakness, and intolerance of temperature changes. The physician suspects multiple sclerosis. What test would you expect the physician to order to confirm her suspicions?

   (a) CBC with a very low WBC count.

   (b) CT scan showing plaque formation.

   (c) Endocrine function study with a low growth hormone and high T3 and T4.

   (d) Fasting glucose test with a result over 300 mg/dl.

7. A patient who was in an automobile accident 30 minutes ago reports that she is unable to move her legs. What is the best response?

   (a) Swelling due to the initial trauma may make the injury seem move severe than it actually is. A more accurate assessment will be made once the swelling goes down.

   (b) Swelling due to the initial trauma prevents you from moving your legs.

   (c) There are good rehabilitation centers that will help restore sensation to your legs.

   (d) You should have been wearing your seatbelt.

8. A husband visiting his wife in the hospital suddenly becomes confused and has difficulty with speech and starts slurring his words. The physician caring for his wife recognizes this as a cerebrovascular accident. What would you expect the physician to do?

    (a) Administer TPA since this is within 3 hours of the CVS.

    (b) Assess if the husband had an ischemic or hemorrhagic CVS.

    (c) Tell the husband to go home, get rest and to call the physician in the morning if the symptoms continue.

    (d) Admit the husband and place him on bed rest.

9. A patient is admitted to your unit diagnosed with advanced ALS. Which is the priority intervention?

    (a) Provide six small meals high in protein and assist with feeding.

    (b) Don't involve the patient in decisions about his health care because he does not have the mental status to respond.

    (c) Develop a method of communication.

    (d) Provide six normal meals high in protein and assist with feeding.

10. Your patient diagnosed with Guillain-Barré syndrome has a burning, tickling feeling and asks what causes that feeling. What is the best response?

    (a) The myelin cover of the nerve endings is absent.

    (b) You are lying too long on the affected side.

    (c) This is in response to your medication.

    (d) This is secondary to dysphagia.

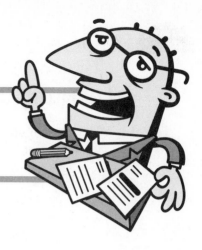

CHAPTER 6

Musculoskeletal System

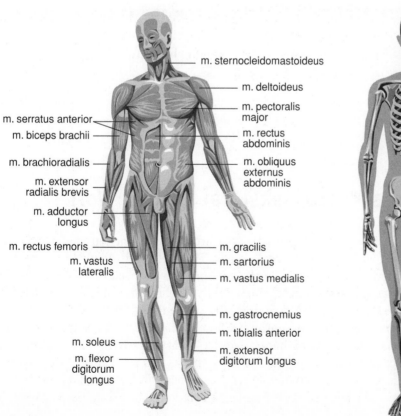

m. sternocleidomastoideus

m. deltoideus

m. pectoralis major

m. serratus anterior

m. biceps brachii

m. rectus abdominis

m. brachioradialis

m. obliquus externus abdominis

m. extensor radialis brevis

m. adductor longus

m. rectus femoris

m. gracilis

m. vastus lateralis

m. sartorius

m. vastus medialis

m. gastrocnemius

m. tibialis anterior

m. soleus

m. flexor digitorum longus

m. extensor digitorum longus

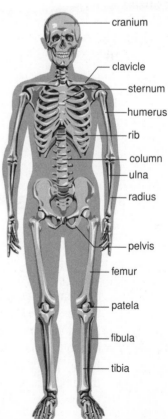

cranium

clavicle

sternum

humerus

rib

column

ulna

radius

pelvis

femur

patela

fibula

tibia

Learning Objectives

1. Carpal Tunnel Syndrome
2. Fractures
3. Gout
4. Osteoarthritis
5. Osteomyelitis
6. Osteoporosis

 Key Terms

Abduction	Eversion	Pronation
Adduction	Extension	Rotation
Bursa	Flexion	Supination
Cartilage	Inversion	Synovial joints
Circumduction	Osteoblasts	Synovium
Connective tissues	Osteoclasts	Tendons

How the Musculoskeletal System Works

The musculoskeletal system provides both structure and function for the body. The bones protect and support the vital organs. The skeleton is divided into the axial and appendicular areas. The axial skeleton protects the vital organs, surrounding the central nervous system and thoracic cavity. The appendicular skeleton attaches to the axial skeleton and consists primarily of the limbs. Bones are classified by both their shape and their composition. Short bones (like the phalanges) are found in the fingers and toes. Long bones (like the humerus or femur) are found in the limbs. Irregular bones are named for their shapes and are found in the joints of the ankle or wrist and in the middle ear. Flat bones (ribs or scapula) protect inner organs. The outer layer of bone tissue is a dense compact bone tissue called the cortex. Blood supply for the bone travels through small blood vessels within haversian canals located longitudinally within the cortical bone area. The inner layer is more spongy, cancellous tissue which has spaces filled with marrow. Production of blood cells occurs within the red bone marrow. Yellow bone marrow is composed primarily of fat cells. Osteoblasts (bone-building cells) and osteoclasts (bone-resorbing cells) are found in the outer layer of the bone.

Joints are the areas where two or more bones come together. Joints are described as being freely movable (synovial joints like the hip), partially movable (pelvic bones), or immovable (suture lines in the skull). Synovial joints are lined with synovium. This membrane secretes synovial fluid to lubricate the joint and act as a shock absorber during motion or weight bearing. Synovial joints have a variety of range of motion including flexion, extension, rotation, circumduction, supination, pronation, abduction, adduction, inversion, and eversion. Partially movable joints have specific small amounts of motion that are typical of the joint space. Pelvic bones and individual joints between the vertebral bones are partially movable. Immovable joints are areas where bones come together, but no movement is allowed.

Muscles work in groups, with one set of muscles relaxing as another set contracts to create motion. A small amount of muscle contraction is typical to maintain muscle tone within the muscles. Skeletal muscle is striated and voluntary. Connective tissues are the pieces that hold other parts together. Tendons attach muscles to bones; ligaments attach bones to bones. Cartilage provides a smooth surface within joints to ease movement and provide cushioning to weight-bearing joints. Bursa are small fluid-filled sacs, within joint areas or adjacent to bone which provide cushioning at points of friction.

Just the Facts

 Carpal Tunnel Syndrome

WHAT WENT WRONG?

The median nerve that passes through the carpal tunnel in the anterior wrist is compressed, resulting in pain and a numb sensation in the thumb, index finger, middle finger, and lateral aspect of the fourth finger in the hand. This is often the result of repetitive hand motions and may be work- or hobby-related. Carpal tunnel syndrome tends to be more common in women.

PROGNOSIS

Some patients respond to conservative treatments including nonsteroidal anti-inflammatory medications and rest of the affected area. A wrist brace may help to keep the wrist in a neutral position during this time. If this conservative treatment fails, the patient may need surgery to decompress the carpal tunnel area to relieve pressure on the nerve as it passes through the wrist into the hand. Long-term presence of carpal tunnel syndrome can lead to atrophy of muscles in the palm of the hand. Hand grip strength may be affected. After treatment, carpal tunnel syndrome may recur in the future.

HALLMARK SIGNS AND SYMPTOMS

- Tingling, numbness, or burning sensation (paresthesia) in the hand due to nerve compression
- Weakness in the hand due to nerve compression and, eventually, muscle wasting
- Pain in the hand due to nerve compression
- Tapping over the carpal tunnel area will cause tingling, numbness, or pain through the palm and affected fingers (Tinnel's sign)
- Pain, tingling, and burning sensation in the wrist and hand as a result of the blood pressure cuff being inflated on the upper arm to the level of the patient's systolic blood pressure

INTERPRETING TEST RESULTS

- Electromyography (EMG) or nerve conduction studies will show nerve dysfunction.
- Magnetic resonance imaging (MRI) will show swelling of the median nerve within the carpal tunnel.

TREATMENT

- Splint the wrist for 2 weeks to keep the wrist in a neutral position or slightly extended and decrease compression on the carpal tunnel area.
- Administer NSAID (nonsteroidal anti-inflammatory drugs) to decrease inflammation:

- diclofenac, diflunisal, etodolac, fenoprofen, flurbiprofen, ibuprofen, indomethacin, ketoprofen, ketorolac, meloxicam, nabumetone, naproxen, oxaprozin, piroxicam, salsalate, sulindac, tolmetin
- Administer corticosteroids to decrease inflammation:
  - hydrocortisone, dexamethasone, methylprednisolone, prednisolone, prednisone
  - Some are given orally.
  - Some may be injected into the carpal tunnel area.
- Surgery when decompression of the carpal tunnel is necessary to relieve pressure on the median nerve.

NURSING DIAGNOSES

- Pain
- Impaired mobility
- Disturbed sensory perception: tactile

NURSING INTERVENTION

- Assist the patient with hygiene if necessary before surgical correction and with postoperative dressings after surgery.
- Patients wearing wrist splints may need assistance with certain activities of daily living (ADLs).
- Assist the patient in exercising the hand; encourage performance of activities through physical therapy.
- Monitor the motion and sensation in the hand following surgery—check capillary refill, color, and sensation of fingers.
- Encourage movement of fingers after surgery.
- Monitor postoperative dressing for drainage.
- Explain to the patient:
  - Use, interactions, and side effects of anti-inflammatory medications.
  - Proper use of wrist splints.
  - Encourage appropriate exercises.
  - Use of ergonomic devices, such as wrist rests or keyboard trays for computer work.

2 *Fractures*

WHAT WENT WRONG?

Excess stress or direct trauma is placed on a bone, causing a break. This results in damage to surrounding muscles and tissue, leading to hemorrhage, edema, and local tissue damage. Initially after the fracture, bleeding in the area leads to hematoma formation at the site. Inflammatory cells enter the area. Granulation tissue replaces the hematoma. Cellular changes continue and a non-bony union known as a callus develops. Osteoblasts continue to enter the area. Fibrous tissue in the fractured area changes to bone.

The fracture site may be just a crack in the bone, without displacing any of the bone itself. A fracture that does not go all the way through the bone is considered an incomplete fracture. The fracture may also go all the way through a bone, breaking it into two (or more) pieces, which is referred to as a complete fracture. The surrounding muscle tissue that attaches above and below the fracture area in a limb will continue to create tension on their attachment points to the bone and pull the pieces further out of alignment. Some fractured bone pieces may penetrate through the skin; this is known as an open or compound fracture. Those that do not penetrate the skin are considered closed or simple fractures.

PROGNOSIS

The area of fracture needs to be identified (via an x-ray) and properly treated in order to heal. The fractured area typically needs to be realigned and then immobilized to allow for proper healing. During this time of immobilization, the bone cells come into the area to rebuild new bone to repair the damaged area. The period of immobilization typically lasts for 6 to 8 weeks, depending on the site and degree of damage. The full structural strength is not typically restored until months after the break, depending on the size and location of the fracture. Time for full healing varies from 6 weeks in young healthy adults with simple fractures to a couple of months in older patients with other health problems. Older patients have a significant increase in both morbidity and mortality following a hip fracture.

Complications following fractures include compartment syndrome, fat embolism, deep vein thrombosis (DVT), delayed union, nonunion, or misalignment. Compartment syndrome occurs when excess pressure builds up within a muscle compartment sheath. The pressure may be coming from internal or external sources of pressure. This is most common with fractures involving the lower leg or lower arm. Fat globules may be released from the yellow bone marrow into the bloodstream and embolize to other areas of the body. The risk for this is highest in the elderly and in men between 18 and 40. Decrease in mobility following fracture will increase the risk for DVT. Smoking, obesity, heart disease, and lower extremity surgery all increase this risk. Delayed union is when a fracture has not joined within 6 months, despite appropriate treatments. Nonunion is a fracture site that fails to completely heal. Misalignment is when the fracture site heals, but the anatomic alignment is not as it should be.

Muscle wasting may occur in the area that has been immobilized. Physical therapy can be very helpful for the patient to regain full functional strength of the area.

HALLMARK SIGNS AND SYMPTOMS

- Local bleeding—may or may not see skin level discoloration; it depends on amount of blood loss and distance between fracture and skin
- Edema at site due to inflammatory reaction to tissue damage
- Abnormal range of motion—need intact bone in order for muscle to pull and create movement; if fracture occurs near joint, swelling may limit ROM
- Shortening of the leg and external rotation is common following hip fracture

INTERPRETING TEST RESULTS

- X-ray shows fracture—may be displaced or not.
- CT scan shows fracture—useful when patient's body part cannot be turned or positioned for imaging (e.g. the neck).
- Bone scan will show increased cellular activity in area of fracture—useful for sites where fracture not easily seen or for hairline fractures not previously diagnosed.

TREATMENT

- Immobilize broken bone—to stabilize area, initially may be done with splint until fracture reduced (replaced into proper position) and cast applied or fixation device applied surgically.
- Open reduction is the surgical repair and direct visual realignment of fracture.
- Pain management as needed.

NURSING DIAGNOSES

- Risk for impaired skin integrity
- Risk for activity intolerance
- Impaired physical mobility

NURSING INTERVENTION

- Monitor circulation: check peripheral pulses, capillary refill, and skin temperature distal to the break. Compromise of blood flow will diminish pulses, slow capillary refill and cause cool skin temperature. Compare bilateral areas for symmetry.
- Monitor vital signs: check for elevated pulse, low BP, and elevated respiratory rate. The broken bone ends can lacerate a vessel causing internal bleeding; monitor for signs of shock. May see elevated temperature with infection from open fracture.
- Explain to the patient:
  - How to provide self-care—depending on the fracture area, the patient's ability to care for himself or herself may be compromised.
  - The importance of performing range-of-motion exercise to maintain muscle tone in the areas not immobilized.
  - Not to insert anything into the cast. The padding may become dislodged, causing pressure points under the hard cast which would lead to skin breakdown. The skin integrity may also be broken when scratching under the cast, leading to an infection.

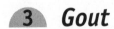 *Gout*

WHAT WENT WRONG?

This is a metabolic disorder in which the body does not properly metabolize purine-based proteins. As a result, there is an increase in the amount of uric acid, which is the end product of purine metabolism. As a result of hyperuricemia, uric acid crystals accumulate in joints, most commonly the big toe (podagra), causing pain when the joint moves. Uric acid is cleared from the body through the kidneys. These patients may also develop kidney stones as the uric acid crystallizes in the kidney.

A person may also develop secondary gout. This is due to another disease process or use of medication, such as thiazide diuretics or some chemotherapeutic agents.

PROGNOSIS

Gout is typically a chronic disorder. Patients need to understand the disease and its treatment so that medications can be initiated at the earliest point during a painful flare. Repeated flares in the same joint will ultimately cause joint damage. Chronic elevation of serum uric acid is associated with progression of atherosclerosis.

HALLMARK SIGNS AND SYMPTOMS

- Acute onset of excruciating pain in joint due to accumulation of uric acid within the joint
- Redness due to inflammation around the joint
- Nephrolithiasis (kidney stones) due to uric acid deposits in the kidney

INTERPRETING TEST RESULTS

- Elevated erythrocyte sedimentation rate (ESR).
- Elevated serum uric acid level—not seen in all patients with gout. Typical of primary gout patients prior to episode of acute joint pain.
- Elevated urinary uric acid levels.
- Arthrocentesis shows uric acid crystals within the joint fluid.

TREATMENT

Acute treatment is managed with colchicine and nonsteroidal anti-inflammatory medications. These medications are continued until the pain is controlled. Chronic gout is treated with allopurinol or an uricosuric agent to reduce the amount of uric acid in the system. These medications are used in the long term to reduce the amount of painful flares that occur.

- Administer colchicine during an acute episode to decrease the inflammatory response resulting from uric acid deposits. This will help reduce pain.
- Administer NSAID to decrease inflammation to aid in pain relief
  - indomethacin, ibuprofen, naproxen
  - Not aspirin; regular dosing causes retention of uric acid.
- Administer xanthine oxidase inhibitor medication to reduce total body uric acid. Given as long-term treatment to patients with recurrent episodes of gout:
  - allopurinol
- Administer uricosuric medications when the total body amount of urate needs to be decreased. Not used in patients who are already excreting a large amount of uric acid. Given to patients with chronic gout or recurrent episodes:
  - probenecid, sulfinpyrazone
- Low-fat, low-cholesterol diet—elevated uric acid levels accelerate athero-sclerosis.
- Immobilize the joint for comfort.

NURSING DIAGNOSES

- Impaired mobility
- Acute pain

NURSING INTERVENTION

- Have the patient drink 3 liters of fluid per day to avoid crystallization of uric acid in the kidneys. Increased fluids help flush the uric acid through the kidneys.
- Monitor uric acid levels in serum.
- Assist with positioning for comfort.
- Avoid touching inflamed joint unnecessarily. May need to keep clothing or bed linen away from area.
- Explain to patient:
  - Which foods are high-purine proteins—turkey, organ meats, sardines, smelts, mackerel, anchovies, herring, bacon.
  - Avoid alcohol, which inhibits renal excretion of uric acid.

Osteoarthritis

WHAT WENT WRONG?

A degenerative joint disease caused by the wear and tear of the articular cartilage. As the protective joint cartilage is worn away, the underlying bone becomes exposed, causing the exposed bones to rub. Degenerative changes within the bone tissue produce small areas of re-growth, causing jagged joint spaces and bone spurs. These rough areas project out into soft tissue or joint spaces, causing pain.

PROGNOSIS

Pain associated with osteoarthritis typically is related to activity and is relieved with rest. The major weight-bearing joints are more affected in overweight patients due to the excess wear and tear on the joints, especially affecting hips and knees. Initially patients respond well to rest periods and over-the-counter medications for pain control. As joints become more damaged over time, a joint replacement may be necessary to correct pain and to improve quality of life and mobility.

HALLMARK SIGNS AND SYMPTOMS

- Stiff joints for short time in morning, usually 15 minutes or less due to changes within joints
- Joint pain with movement or weight bearing due to joint remodeling
- Crepitus (grating feeling on palpation over joint during range of motion) due to loss of articular cartilage and bony overgrowth in joint
- Pain relief when joints are rested because lack of movements will relieve irritation in joint space
- Enlargement of joint due to bony overgrowth or remodeling
- Heberden's nodes—swelling of the distal interphalangeal joints

INTERPRETING TEST RESULTS

- X-ray shows narrowed joint spaces, bone spurs, or osteophytes around joints.
- Tests for inflammation will be normal—erythrocyte sedimentation rate, C-reactive protein.

TREATMENT

Initial treatment is usually with over-the-counter medications. The patients respond well to these medications. There is no underlying inflammatory disorder, so the medications can be used on an as-needed basis. Many of the patients are older and will be on other medications, so it is important that you check for medication interactions.

- Administer NSAID (nonsteroidal anti-inflammatory drug)—for any local inflammation from irritation at the joint area due to osteophytes or bone spur formation:
  - ibuprofen, naproxen
  - diclofenac, diflunisal, etodolac, fenoprofen, flurbiprofen, indomethacin, ketoprofen, ketorolac, meloxicam, nabumetone, oxaprozin, piroxicam, salsalate, sulindac, tolmetin
- Administer acetaminophen for pain relief.
- Glucosamine and chondroitin sulfate for relief of pain and stiffness.
- Capsaicin cream topically.
- Intra-articular injections of corticosteroid up to 3 or 4 times in a year.
- Intra-articular injections of:
  - hyaluronate sodium; series of 3 to 5 injections
  - hyaluron; series of 3 injections
  - hylan GF 20; series of 3 injections
- Exercise to maintain joint mobility and muscle tone.
- Walking aid for stability.

NURSING DIAGNOSES

- Pain
- Activity intolerance
- Impaired mobility

NURSING INTERVENTION

- Monitor pain to adequately treat pain, as needs may change.
- Diet modification for weight loss for overweight patients to decrease excess stress on weight-bearing joints.

- Explain to the patient:
  - When and how to take medications.
  - Importance of maintaining activity.
  - Disease process.

5 *Osteomyelitis*

WHAT WENT WRONG?

Osteomyelitis is an infection of the bone. In an adult, it is most commonly due to direct contamination of the site during trauma, such as an open fracture. Bacteria that cause infections elsewhere in the body may also enter the bloodstream and become deposited into the bone, starting a secondary infection site there. This is more common in children and adolescents. Some of the patients have been treated with antibiotics previously for the initial infection.

The causative organism is not always identified. More than three-quarters of the identified organisms are *Staphylococcus aureus*. Acute infection is associated with inflammatory changes in the bone and may lead to necrosis. Some patients will develop chronic osteomyelitis.

PROGNOSIS

The sooner the infected area can be made infection-free, the better the prognosis for the patient. There is a risk for developing chronic osteomyelitis. This risk is greater in patients with a compromised immune system or poor blood supply to the area (such as diabetics).

HALLMARK SIGNS AND SYMPTOMS

- Pain
- Fever, chills
- Malaise

INTERPRETING TEST RESULTS

- Elevated white blood count (WBC).
- X-ray osteolytic lesions (localized loss of bone density).

- Bone scan shows area of increased cellular activity—detects site of infection.
- Culture and sensitivity tests to determine the infecting organism and antibiotic—may be difficult to determine infecting organism.
- Bone biopsy to identify organism.

TREATMENT

Removal of necrotic bone tissue and local pus or drainage is often necessary to speed healing. Typically, patients need antibiotics for several weeks to properly treat the infection.

- Debridement of the area to remove necrotic tissue.
- Drain the infected site.
- Immobilize or stabilize the bone if necessary.
- Administer antibiotics parenterally for 4 to 6 weeks or orally for 6 to 8 weeks:
  - nafcillin, vancomycin, penicillin G, piperacillin, ticarcillin/clavulanate, ampicillin/sulbactam, pipercillin/tazobactam, clindamycin, cefazolin, linezolid, ceftazidime, ciprofloxacin
- Administer analgesic to relieve discomfort as needed:
  - ibuprofen, naproxen, acetaminophen
  - oxycodone, hydrocodone
- If there is vascular insufficiency or gangrene, amputation may be needed.

NURSING DIAGNOSES

- Impaired mobility
- Activity intolerance

NURSING INTERVENTION

- Monitor vital signs, changes in blood pressure, elevated pulse, elevated temperature and respiratory rate.
- Monitor wound site for redness, drainage, and odor.
- Monitor IV access site for patency.

- Explain to the patient:
  - When and how to take medications.
  - Importance of completing antibiotic medication.
  - How to flush venous access device.
  - Signs of infiltration, clotting of venous access device.
  - When to call for assistance with venous access.

6   *Osteoporosis*

WHAT WENT WRONG?

This is a decrease in bone density, making bones more brittle and increasing the risk of fracture. The body continuously replaces older bone with new bone through a balance between the osteoblastic and osteoclastic activity. When bone-building activity does not keep up with bone-resorption activity, the structural integrity of the bone is compromised.

Increased age, lack of physical activity, poor nutrition, having a small frame, being Caucasian, Asian, or female all increase the risk of osteoporosis. Osteoporosis can also occur as a secondary disease, due to another condition. These causes include use of medications such as corticosteroids or some anticonvulsants, hormonal disorders (Cushing's or thyroid), and prolonged immobilization.

PROGNOSIS

The risk of fracture is significantly increased in patients with osteoporosis. The most common fracture sites in patients with osteoporosis are hip, vertebrae, pelvis, and distal radius. Some fractures such as vertebral compression fractures affect quality of life. There is increased morbidity and mortality in patients who sustain a hip fracture. The cost of healthcare for these patients is significant, and includes the immediate care of the fracture as well as the necessary rehabilitation.

HALLMARK SIGNS AND SYMPTOMS

- Asymptomatic
- Back pain due to compression fractures in vertebral bodies

- Loss of height
- Excessive forward curvature of the thoracic spine (kyphosis) due to pathologic vertebral fractures; collapsing of the anterior portion of the vertebral bodies in the thoracic area
- Fracture with minor trauma

INTERPRETING TEST RESULTS

- X-ray shows demineralization of the bone—not an early sign.
- Dual energy x-ray absorptiometry (DEXA) shows decrease in bone mineral density in the hip and spine compared to young normal patients, and compared to age-matched, race-matched, sex-matched patients.

TREATMENT

It is much more cost-effective to focus on prevention of osteoporosis. Encourage adequate exercise and nutrition. Calcium supplementation may be necessary for patients who are not getting the recommended daily requirement of calcium in the diet. The body stores calcium in the bones. If there is insufficient dietary intake, the body will remove the calcium from the bone, further weakening the structural integrity. Once osteoporosis occurs, proper medical management is important to prevent fractures and increase bone density.

- Administer bisphosphonate drugs to inhibit osteoclastic bone resorption and increase bone density:
  - alendronate, risedronate, ibandronate sodium orally
  - parenteral preparations zoledronic acid, pamidronate
- Administer calcitonin nasal spray to increase bone density, also has analgesic effect on bone pain after 2 to 4 weeks.
- Administer selective estrogen receptor modulator for postmenopausal women for prevention of osteoporosis:
  - raloxifene
- Administer teriparatide to stimulate the production of collagenous bone to increase bone density.
- Administer vitamin D, which enhances the absorption of calcium; many patients with osteoporosis are also deficient in vitamin D.

- Administer calcium, 1000 to 1500 mg per day in divided doses to enhance absorption.
- Encourage weight-bearing activity.
- Perform range-of-motion activities.
- Increase vitamins and calcium in diet.

NURSING DIAGNOSES

- Impaired mobility
- Pain
- Risk for injury

NURSING INTERVENTION

- Pain control if fracture occurs.
- Explain to the patient:
  - How to properly take medications.
  - Bisphosphonates must be taken first thing in the morning on an empty stomach, with a full glass of water. The patient can't lie down for 30 to 60 minutes after taking the medication; this is to reduce risk of esophageal irritation.
  - Monitor for side effects of medications—GI effects with bisphosphonates.
  - Encourage weight-bearing activity.
  - Encourage appropriate nutrition.

Crucial Diagnostic Tests

X-ray

Body part to be imaged needs to be positioned properly to see underlying bone structure, identify fractures, and detect foreign bodies. The patient may need to lie, sit, or stand, depending on the body part to be imaged. Typically, two different views are taken of the same body part to allow better diagnostics.

Arthrogram

An x-ray of a joint area is taken after the injection of a contrast medium has been injected into the joint space to enhance its visibility. In a double-contrast study, a solution is injected, followed by air. This may be done to better assess the possibility of bone chips or torn ligaments within the joint space.

Determine if the patient has a history of allergy to contrast prior to the test.

Arthroscopy

- Fiberoptic scope used to visually examine the joint, performed under some type of anesthesia (local, epidural, conscious sedation, or general).
- This is done to perform surgery concurrently, diagnose injuries to joint spaces, and assess response to prior treatments.
- Postprocedure, check neurovascular status of the extremity—color, pulses, sensation, motion, and temperature.
- Teach patient to monitor for signs of infection—redness, swelling, fever, and increased pain.

Biopsy

A tissue sample is taken from a body part (muscle or bone) to determine disease state of tissue. The sample may be taken through closed (needle) biopsy or open (incisional) biopsy.

It is done to determine the presence of infection, cancer, muscular atrophy or inflammation, or presence of mitochondrial disorders.

Bone Scan

This is a peripheral intravenous injection of bone-seeking radiopharmaceutical followed by 2- to 3-hour delayed imaging. Patient must lie still for the duration of the scanning, about 30 to 60 minutes.

It is done to diagnose osteomyelitis, bone tumors, metastatic disease, fractures, and unexplained skeletal pain.

Encourage fluids after the injection to flush the radiopharmaceutical. Monitor for reaction to the radiopharmaceutical: rash, itching, hives, and so on.

Computed Tomography (CT) Scan

Computerized axial tomography—computer-manipulated pictures of radiologic images that are not obstructed by overlying anatomy. The patient needs to lie still during the exam for clear images.

This is done to detect fractures and bone metastasis.

Electromyography (EMG)

Multiple small needle–type electrodes are inserted into muscle areas to test muscle potential. The patient may be asked to move the area to allow for measurement during minimal and maximal contraction of the muscle. The amount of muscle and nerve activity is recorded graphically.

Explain to the patient that there may be some discomfort during the testing. Certain medications may need to be stopped prior to testing: muscle relaxants, stimulants, caffeine.

After the testing, the patient may complain of pain or anxiety.

The test is done to detect neuromuscular, peripheral nerve disorders, or lower motor neuron disorders, and may be done in conjunction with nerve conduction studies.

Magnetic Resonance Imaging (MRI)

Use of a super-conducting magnet and radio frequency signals cause hydrogen nuclei to send out an individual signal. As the radio waves bounce off the tissues in the body, different signals are sent based on the density of the tissues. The computer will create detailed images based on the information it receives. Contrast may be injected intravenously.

The MRI diagnoses problems within joints, soft tissue (tendons, ligaments), spine, intervertebral discs, and spinal cord.

Prior to the test, ask the patient about possible metallic objects (surgical clips, implants), pacemakers or implanted infusion pumps (may cause dysfunction of devices), or pregnancy.

Ask the patient about history of claustrophobia: closed machines are somewhat restrictive, while open machines are less claustrophobic. Tests typically last 60 minutes or longer.

Myelography

This is an injection of contrast medium into the subarachnoid space of the spine to allow for better visualization of the vertebral column, intervertebral discs, and spinal nerves. This is done when the patient is not a candidate for MRI or CT scan.

Posttesting, the patient typically is sitting to keep the contrast medium low in the spinal column, away from the brain.

Ultrasound

Sound waves are used to generate an image. This is done to determine the presence and location of mass, fluid, or surgical hardware.

Quiz

1. Patients who work in settings that require repetition of the same hand movements over a long period of time have an increased risk for which of the following disorders?

   (a) osteomyelitis.

   (b) osteoporosis.

   (c) carpal tunnel syndrome.

   (d) facture of the overused area.

2. You are caring for a patient who has just had open carpal tunnel release surgery. The surgeon has requested that the patient's hand and arm remain elevated above the level of the heart after the surgery. This is to:

   (a) reduce lymphatic drainage.

   (b) reduce postoperative swelling.

   (c) restrict hand movements.

   (d) decrease possibility of nosocomial infection.

3. In obtaining the patient history for your patient with carpal tunnel syndrome, you would expect to note a history of:

   (a) pain and numbness or tingling sensation in the hand (over the palmar surface of the thumb, index finger, middle finger, and lateral aspect of the ring finger) that is worse at night.

   (b) crepitus (grating feeling on palpation over joint during range of motion) due to loss of articular cartilage and bony overgrowth in joint.

   (c) excessive forward curvature of the thoracic spine (kyphosis) due to pathologic vertebral fractures, and collapsing of the anterior portion of the vertebral bodies in the thoracic area.

   (d) acute onset of excruciating pain in joint due to accumulation of uric acid within the joint.

4. Initial treatment of the patient with a fracture should include:

   (a) surgical reduction of the fracture.

   (b) insertion of internal fixation device.

   (c) reduction of the fracture.

   (d) immobilization of the area.

5. The first priority of care of the patient with a new fracture includes assessing:

   (a) respiratory rate and effort, pulse.

   (b) the fracture site for bleeding.

   (c) for signs of infection at the wound site of an open fracture.

   (d) for circulation and sensation distal to the fracture site.

6. Patients with a history of osteoporosis have an increased risk for:

   (a) infection in the bone.

   (b) peripheral blood clot formation.

   (c) painful joint inflammation.

   (d) fracture formation.

7. Teaching patients about proper use of bisphosphonate medications for treatment of osteoporosis should include taking medication:

   (a) on a full stomach.

   (b) first thing in the morning on an empty stomach with a full glass of water, 30 to 60 minutes before eating, without lying down.

   (c) just before getting into bed.

   (d) with an acidic liquid, like orange juice.

8. In order to allow for proper healing, patients with osteomyelitis may need to have:

    (a) debridement and drainage of the area.

    (b) immobilization of the area.

    (c) ice packs alternating with moist heat applied externally.

    (d) internal fixation device inserted.

9. You have been caring for a patient with osteomyelitis. In preparing the patient for discharge, you include teaching about:

    (a) the importance of multiple-week treatment with antibiotics.

    (b) the side effects and interactions of the medications.

    (c) symptoms that necessitate a call to the physician, nurse practitioner, or physician assistant.

    (d) all of the above.

10. The patient with gout will have periodic exacerbations of painful joint inflammation. Acute episodes are treated with:

    (a) nonsteroidal anti-inflammatory medications and colchicine.

    (b) allopurinol and aspirin.

    (c) antibiotics and acetaminophen.

    (d) bisphosphonates and calcium.

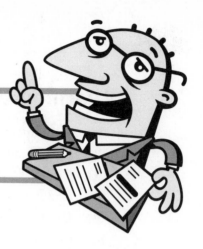

CHAPTER 7

Gastrointestinal System

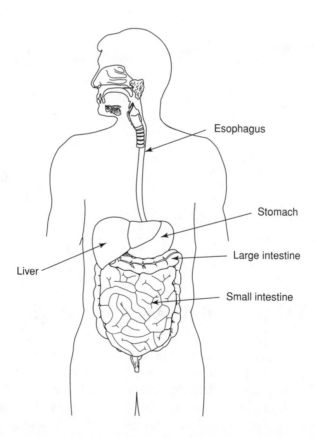

Esophagus

Stomach

Large intestine

Liver

Small intestine

Learning Objectives

1. Appendicitis
2. Cholecystitis
3. Cirrhosis
4. Crohn's disease
5. Diverticulitis disease
6. Gastroenteritis
7. Gastroesophageal reflux disease (GERD)
8. Gastrointestinal bleed
9. Gastritis
10. Hepatitis
11. Hiatal hernia
12. Intestinal obstruction and paralytic ileus
13. Pancreatitis
14. Peritonitis
15. Peptic ulcer disease (PUD)
16. Ulcerative colitis

 Key Terms

Accessory organs
Alimentary canal
Cholecystokinin
Fatty acids
Gastrin
Gastrointestinal tract
Glucagon
Hydrochloric acid
Ileocecal valve

Insulin
Islets of Langerhans
Lipase
Lower esophageal sphincter (LES)
Oropharynx
Pepsin
Pepsinogen
Plasma

Proteins
Secretin
Sphincter of Oddi
Triglycerides
Trypsin
Upper esophageal sphincter (UES)

How the Gastrointestinal System Works

The gastrointestinal system includes the alimentary canal (mouth, esophagus, stomach, small intestine, large intestine, rectum) and accessory organs (salivary glands, liver, pancreas, gallbladder) and ducts. The alimentary canal is a hollow tube lined with mucous membrane. The gastrointestinal tract functions to digest food, absorb nutrients, propel the contents through the lumen, and eliminate the waste products.

Digestion of food has both mechanical and chemical components. Both processes begin in the mouth. Chewing, movement through the gastrointestinal tract, and churning within the stomach are parts of the mechanical process. Saliva, hydrochloric acid, bile, and other digestive enzymes all contribute to the chemical process of digestion.

The esophagus extends from the oropharynx to the stomach. At the top of the esophagus is the upper esophageal sphincter (UES) to prevent the influx of air into the esophagus during respiration. At the bottom of the esophagus is the lower esophageal sphincter (LES) to prevent the reflux of acid from the stomach into the esophagus.

The contents of the esophagus empty into the stomach through the cardiac sphincter. The stomach secretes gastrin, which promotes secretion of pepsinogen and hydrochloric acid, pepsin, and lipase, all of which aid digestion and mucous which helps protect the stomach lining.

The liver is a very vascular organ located in the right upper quadrant of the abdomen under the diaphragm. It has two main lobes that are comprised of smaller lobules. The liver stores a variety of vitamins and minerals. It metabolizes proteins; synthesizes plasma proteins, fatty acids, and triglycerides; and stores and releases glycogen. The liver detoxifies foreign substances such as alcohol, drugs, or chemicals. The liver forms and secretes bile to aid in digestion of fat. Bile will release into the gall bladder for storage or into the duodenum if needed for digestion if the sphincter of Oddi is open due to secretion of the digestive enzymes secretin, cholecystokinin, and gastrin. The gall bladder is a small receptacle that holds bile until it is needed. It is located on the inferior aspect of the liver.

The pancreas is located retroperitoneally in the upper abdomen near the stomach and extends from just right of midline to the left toward the spleen. The pancreas has both endocrine and exocrine functions. The endocrine functions include secretion of insulin in response to elevations in blood glucose from the beta cells of the islets of Langerhans and glucagon in response to decrease in blood glucose from the alpha cells. The exocrine function includes secretion of trypsin, lipase, amylase, and chymotrypsin to aid in digestion.

The small intestine is comprised of the duodenum, jejunum, and the ileum. The duodenum attaches to the stomach, is about one foot long and C-shaped, and curves to the left around the pancreas. The common bile duct and pancreatic duct enter here. The jejunum is between the duodenum and ileum and is about eight feet long. The last portion of the small intestine is the ileum which is up to twelve feet long, depending on the size of the patient. The ileocecal valve separates the ileum from the large intestine. The appendix is found at this juncture. The large intestine can be broken down into the ascending colon, transverse colon, descending colon, and sigmoid colon. The sigmoid colon joins the rectum and ultimately the anal canal.

Just the Facts

 Appendicitis

WHAT WENT WRONG?

Inflammation of the vermiform appendix (a blind pouch located near the ileocecal valve in the right lower quadrant of the abdomen) is known as appendicitis. It may be due to obstruction from stool. The mucosal lining of the appendix continues to secrete fluid, which will increase the pressure within the lumen of appendix, causing a restriction of the blood supply to the appendix. This decrease in blood supply may result in gangrene or perforation as the pressure continues to build. Pain localizes at McBurney's point, located midway between the umbilicus and right anterior iliac crest. Appendicitis may occur at any age, but the peak occurrence is from the teenage years to 30.

PROGNOSIS

Rupture of the appendix is more likely to occur in acute appendicitis within the first 36 to 48 hours. Symptoms of peritonitis (inflammation of the peritoneum—the membrane lining the abdominal cavity) may occur as a complication of appendicitis. Rapid diagnosis and surgical intervention are necessary to avoid rupture of the appendix.

HALLMARK SIGNS AND SYMPTOMS

- Abdominal pain begins periumbical and travels to right lower quadrant
- Rebound pain (pain when pressure on the abdomen is quickly removed) occurs with peritoneal inflammation
- Guarding (protecting the abdomen from painful exam)
- Rigidity of the abdomen (abdomen feels more firm when palpating)
- Fever due to infection
- Nausea, vomiting, loss of appetite
- Right lower quadrant pain that improves with flexing the right hip suggests perforation

INTERPRETING TEST RESULTS

- Elevated white blood cell count (WBC).
- CT scan shows enlarged appendix or fecalith.
- Ultrasound may show enlarged appendix.

TREATMENT

- Surgical removal of the appendix—appendectomy (may be done via laparoscopy or open laparotomy).
- NPO—nothing by mouth to avoid further irritation of the intestinal area, and prep for surgery.
- Intravenous fluids until diet resumed.
- Pain medications after surgery as needed; pain medication is used cautiously preoperatively to maintain awareness of increase in pain due to possible rupture of appendix.
- Antibiotics postoperatively if needed.

NURSING DIAGNOSES

- Acute pain
- Hyperthermia
- Nausea

NURSING INTERVENTION

- Monitor vital signs for fever, increased heart rate, respiratory rate, and decrease in blood pressure.
- Assess pain level for changes.
- Monitor surgical site for appearance of wound, drainage.
- Monitor abdomen for distention, presence of bowel sounds.
- Monitor intake and output.
- Monitor bowel function.

2 *Cholecystitis*

WHAT WENT WRONG?

An inflammation of the gallbladder, often accompanied by the formation of gall-stones (cholelithiasis), is cholecystitis. The inflammation may be either acute or chronic in nature. In an acute cholecystitis, the blood flow to the gallbladder may become compromised which in turn will cause problems with the normal filling and emptying of the gallbladder. A stone may block the cystic duct which will result in bile becoming trapped within the gallbladder due to inflammation around the stone within the duct. Blood flow to the inflamed area will be minimized, localized edema develops, the gallbladder distends due to retained bile, and ischemic changes will occur within the wall of the gallbladder. Chronic cholecystitis occurs when there have been recurrent episodes of blockage of the cystic duct, usually due to stones. There is chronic inflammation. The gallbladder is often contracted, which leads to problems with storing and moving the bile. Patients may develop jaundice due to back-up of bile or obstructive jaundice. They will exhibit a yellowish tone to skin and mucous membranes. If patients have a naturally dark pigmentation to their skin, check palms and soles. Icterus is the yellow color change seen in the sclera (white) of the eye.

There is increased risk for gallbladder inflammation and development of gall-stones with increasing age, being female or overweight, having a family history of gallbladder disease, people on rapid weight loss diets, and during pregnancy.

PROGNOSIS

The ischemic changes of the gallbladder wall increase the risk of perforation of the organ or development of gangrene. Peritonitis is a potential risk in patients if a significant area of gallbladder perforates or there is associated infection or abscess that spreads. A small percentage of patients will develop cancer of the gallbladder. There is increased surgical risk for older patients or patients with comorbidities.

HALLMARK SIGNS AND SYMPTOMS

- Upper abdominal, epigastric, or right upper quadrant abdominal pain which may radiate to right shoulder
- Right upper quadrant (RUQ) pain increases with palpation of right upper abdomen during inspiration (Murphy's sign) causing the patient to stop taking deep breaths

- Nausea and vomiting, especially following fatty foods
- Loss of appetite
- Fever
- Increased air in intestinal tract (eructation, flatulence)
- Pruritis (itching) of skin due to build-up of bile salts
- Clay-colored stools due to lack of urobilinogen in gut (normally converted from bilirubin which was blocked with bile flow)
- Jaundice—yellowish skin and mucous membrane discoloration
- Icterus—yellowish discoloration of sclera (white of eye)
- Dark, foamy urine as kidneys attempt to clear out bilirubin

INTERPRETING TEST RESULTS

- Ultrasound of gallbladder shows cholelithiasis, inflammation.
- HIDA scan (hepatic iminodiacetic acid) may be more sensitive than ultrasound in showing obstructed duct.
- CT scan shows inflammation or cholelithiasis.
- MRCP (magnetic resonance cholangiopancreatography).
- ERCP (endoscopic retrograde cholangiopancreatography).
- Bilirubin direct (conjugated) and indirect (unconjugated) will be elevated if there is obstruction.
- White blood cell (WBC) count elevation with inflammation.
- Alkaline phosphatase, aspartate aminotransferase (AST), and lactate dehydrogenase (LDH) will be elevated with abnormal liver function.

TREATMENT

- Low-fat diet.
- Intravenous fluid replacement for vomiting.
- Administer antiemetics for control of nausea and vomiting:
  - prochlorperazine
  - trimethobenzamide
- Replace fat-soluble vitamins (A, D, E, K) as needed.
- Administer analgesics for adequate pain control:
  - meperidine

- avoid morphine (may cause spasm of sphincter of Oddi, increasing pain).
- Administer antibiotics for acute symptoms.
- Placement of stent into gallbladder if the patient is not a candidate for surgery.
- Ultrasound-guided aspiration of gallbladder.
- Surgical removal of gallbladder:
  - Laparoscopic cholecystectomy
  - Open cholecystectomy

NURSING DIAGNOSES

- Acute pain
- Chronic pain
- Risk for imbalanced nutrition: less than what body requires
- Nausea

NURSING INTERVENTION

- Monitor vital signs for changes in temperature, pulse rate, respiratory rate, and blood pressure.
- Assess abdomen for bowel sounds, distention, and tenderness.
- Assess pain level for adequate pain control.
- Assess postoperative wound for drainage, signs of infection.
- Monitor T-tube drainage in postoperative open cholecystectomy patients; empty and record at least every 8 hours.
- Advance diet to low-fat diet postoperatively as tolerated.

3 *Cirrhosis*

WHAT WENT WRONG?

Injury to the cellular structure of the liver causes fibrosis due to chronic inflammation and necrotic changes, resulting in cirrhosis. There are nodular changes to the liver. The bile ducts and blood vessels through the liver may become blocked due to both the nodular changes and fibrosis. These changes to the liver cause enlargement of the organ and change in texture. There is increased pressure within the portal vein. This causes resistance to blood flow throughout the venous system in the liver and also backs up venous blood to the spleen, causing enlargement of this organ also. Damage to the liver may be reversible if the cause if identified early and removed. The most common causes of cirrhosis include chronic alcohol use, liver damage secondary to exposure to drugs or toxins, viral hepatitis (especially hepatitis B, hepatitis C, and hepatitis D in those already infected with hepatitis B), fatty liver (steatohepatitis), autoimmune hepatitis, cystic fibrosis, metabolic disorders (excess iron storage—hemachromatosis), or genetic causes.

PROGNOSIS

As cirrhosis progresses, the patient may develop encephalopathy and coma. Early signs and symptoms of encephalopathy include altered level of consciousness, neuromuscular changes, and elevated serum ammonia levels.

HALLMARK SIGNS AND SYMPTOMS

- Initially asymptomatic
- Weakness, fatigue due to chronic disease
- Muscle cramps
- Weight loss
- Anorexia
- Nausea with possible vomiting
- Ascites—the accumulation of fluid within the abdominal cavity due to portal hypertension
- Abdominal pain
- Portal hypertension
- Pruritus (itching)
- Ecchymosis (bruises) or petechiae (small, pinpoint, round, reddish purple marks)
- Coagulation defects due to problems with vitamin K absorption, causing problems with production of clotting factors
- Amenorrhea
- Impotence due to inactivity of hormones
- Gynecomastia
- Jaundice due to problems with excretion of bilirubin
- Hepatomegaly (enlarged liver) in over one-half of the patients

- Spider veins—spider angiomas or telangiectasias on cheeks, nose, shoulders or upper chest
- Redness of palms—palmar erythema
- Glossitis due to vitamin deficiency
- Peripheral edema
- Dyspnea due to pressure on diaphragm from ascites
- Encephalopathy (asterixis, tremors, delirium, drowsiness, dysarthria, coma)

INTERPRETING TEST RESULTS

- Aspartate aminotransferase (AST) elevated.
- Alanine aminotransferase (ALT) elevated.
- Lactate dehydrogenase (LDH) elevated.
- Bilirubin direct (conjugated) and indirect (unconjugated) elevated.
- Urinary bilirubin elevated.
- Fecal urobilinogen decreased with biliary tract obstruction.
- Serum protein decreased.
- Serum albumin decreased.
- Anemia with elevated MCV, MCH.
- White blood cell (WBC) count low.
- Prothrombin time is prolonged due to changes in hepatic production of clotting factors.
- Platelet count low (thrombocytopenia).
- Ammonia level elevated as the disease advances.
- Abdominal x-rays show hepatomegaly.
- Abdominal CT scan shows hepatomegaly, ascites.
- Ultrasound shows hepatomegaly, ascites, portal vein blood flow.
- Liver biopsy shows fibrosis and regenerative nodules.
- Esophagogastroduodenoscopy (EGD) to detect esophageal varices.

TREATMENT

- Low-sodium diet; adequate calorie intake.
- Restrict fluid intake if hyponatremic (low serum sodium) or fluid overloaded.

- Restrict alcohol intake to prevent further damage.
- Administer vitamin supplements—folate, thiamine, multivitamin.
- Administer diuretics to reduce excess fluids:
  - furosemide
  - spironolactone
- Paracentesis to remove ascitic fluid.
- Monitor electrolytes for imbalance.
- Monitor coagulation profile (PT, PTT, INR).
- Administer lactulose to promote removal of ammonia in the gut.
- Administer antibiotics to destroy the normal GI flora which decreases protein breakdown and the rate of ammonia production:
  - neomycin sulfate
  - metronidazole
- Shunt placement:
  - Peritoneovenous—moves ascitic fluid from abdomen to superior vena cava.
  - Portocaval—diverts venous blood flow from liver to decrease portal and esophageal pressures.
  - Transjugular intrahepatic portal systemic—nonsurgical procedure performed in interventional radiology—sheath placed into jugular and hepatic vein; needle threaded through sheath and pushed into portal vein through the liver; balloon enlarges the tract and stent maintains.
- Gastric lavage.
- Esophagogastgric balloon tamponade for control of bleeding from esophageal varices.
- Administer blood products as needed for patients with bleeding esophageal varices.
- Sclerotherapy for esophageal variceal bleeding.

NURSING DIAGNOSES

- Ineffective breathing pattern
- Excess fluid volume
- Risk for infection

NURSING INTERVENTION

- Monitor intake and output.
- Monitor vital signs.
- Weigh patient daily.
- Measure abdominal girth—making sure to measure at level of umbilicus for consistency; marks are typically made at sides of abdomen to align tape measure on subsequent days.
- Assess peripheral edema.
- Assess heart and lung sounds for excess fluid.
- Elevate head of bed 30 degrees or greater to ease breathing.
- Elevate feet to decrease peripheral edema.
- Monitor for signs of bleeding or bruising.
- Monitor level of consciousness, orientation, recent and remote memory, behavior, mood, and affect.

Crohn's Disease

WHAT WENT WRONG?

A noncontinuous inflammatory disease that can affect any point from the mouth to the anus. The majority of cases involve the small and large intestine, often in the right lower quadrant at the point where the terminal ileum and the ascending colon meet. Patients typically have an insidious onset of intermittent symptoms. The disease causes transmural inflammation, going deeper than the superficial mucosal layer of the tissue to affect all layers. Over time the inflammatory changes within the gastrointestinal tract can lead to strictures or the formation of fistulas. The affected tissue develops granulomas and takes on a mottled appearance interspersed with normal tissue. There is a genetic predisposition and a bimodal peak of onset at 16 to 21 years old.

PROGNOSIS

Crohn's disease is a chronic disorder with periods of exacerbation and remission. Many patients will ultimately need surgery to deal with bowel obstruction, development of strictures, or fistula formation.

HALLMARK SIGNS AND SYMPTOMS

- Fever
- Right lower quadrant pain
- Diarrhea (non-bloody)
- Abdominal mass
- Weight loss (unintentional)
- Fatigue
- Bloating after meals (postprandial)
- Abdominal cramping due to spasm
- Borborygmi (loud, frequent bowel sounds)
- Fistula formation (bowel-bowel, bowel-stomach, bowel-bladder, bowel-skin, bowel-vagina)
- Aphthous ulcers (oral ulcerations)
- Nephrolithiasis

INTERPRETING TEST RESULTS

- Erythrocyte sedimentation rate will be elevated during exacerbations.
- Anemia—due to both vitamin B_{12} and folic acid deficiency.
- Albumin level will be low.
- Electrolytes may be abnormal due to loss from diarrhea and malabsorption.
- Barium studies will show "apple core" in area of stricture formation, narrowing due to inflammation, and fistula formation. Not performed if bowel perforation is a concern.
- CT scan shows abscess formation and thickening of bowel wall due to inflammation.
- Sigmoidoscopy or colonoscopy for direct visualization of lower GI tract or for biopsy.

TREATMENT

- Dietary restriction.
- Nutritional supplementation.

- Administer vitamin B_{12} and folic acid.
- Administer aminosalicylates to induce or maintain remission:
  - mesalamine
  - sulfasalazine
  - olsalazine
  - balsalazide
- Administer glucocorticoids to reduce inflammation:
  - hydrocortisone
  - budesonide
- Administer purine analogs to induce or maintain remission:
  - azathioprine
  - 6-mercaptopurine
- Administer methotrexate to induce or maintain remission.
- Administer antidiarrheal medications to decrease fluid loss; use with caution:
  - diphenoxylate hydrochloride and atropine sulfate
- Intravenous fluids to maintain hydration.
- Surgical correction of intestinal obstruction, fistula, perforation.

NURSING DIAGNOSES

- Acute pain
- Risk for imbalanced nutrition: less than what body requires
- Altered bowel elimination

NURSING INTERVENTION

- Monitor vital signs for temperature increase, pulse increase, and change in blood pressure.
- Monitor intake and output.
- Assess abdomen for bowel sounds, tenderness, masses.
- Assess postoperative wound for signs of infection, drainage.
- Wound care postoperatively.
- Proper skin care if bowel-skin fistula:
  - use of drainable pouch with skin wafer.

- cleaning skin promptly if drainage comes in contact with skin.
- Nutritional supplementation with Ensure®, Sustacal, Vivonex.
- Teach patient about home care needs.

5 *Diverticulitis Disease*

WHAT WENT WRONG?

Small out-pouchings called diverticula develop along the intestinal tract. Diverticulosis is the condition of having these diverticula. Any part of the large or small intestine may be involved. The area of the intestinal tract that most commonly develops diverticula is the lower portion of the large intestine. Certain types of undigested foods can become trapped in the pouches of the intestine. Bacteria multiply in the area, causing further inflammation. Diverticulitis is an inflammation of at least one of the diverticula. Diets that have a low fiber content, seeds, or nuts have been implicated in the development of diverticulitis. Perforation of the diverticula is possible when they are inflamed.

PROGNOSIS

Inflammation in diverticulitis increases the risk of perforation of the intestine. Peritonitis will develop from bacterial contamination after perforation of a diverticula. Bleeding from the intestinal mucosa in the area of inflammation can also occur. The presence of diverticula and repeated periods of inflammation may allow development of fistula formation from the diverticula to other areas within the abdomen, such as the intestine or bladder. Patients needing surgery may have a colostomy postoperatively. Depending on the location of the diverticulitis and the reason for the surgery, the colostomy may be reversible after healing has occurred.

HALLMARK SIGNS AND SYMPTOMS

- Asymptomatic in diverticulosis
- Change in bowel habits
- Bloating, increased gas
- Abdominal pain most often in the left lower quadrant with diverticulitis
- Rectal bleeding due to inflammation with diverticulitis

- Fever with diverticulitis
- Nausea, vomiting
- Tachycardia due to fever
- Peritonitis if diverticula ruptures

INTERPRETING TEST RESULTS

- Barium enema will show diverticula—not done if there is increased risk of perforation.
- Colonoscopy will show diverticula—not done during acute inflammation.
- CT scan will show thickening of bowel wall due to inflammation or abscess in diverticulitis.
- Elevated white blood count (WBC) during diverticulitis.

TREATMENT

- Administer antibiotics:
  - ciprofloxacin
  - metronidazole
  - trimethoprim-sulfamethoxazole
- Administer adequate intravenous hydration.
- Manage pain as needed.
- NPO or clear liquids (depending on order) during acute inflammation to rest intestinal tract.
- Surgical intervention to correct perforation of diverticula, abscess formaltion, bowel obstruction, fistula formation.
- NG tube postoperatively.

NURSING DIAGNOSES

- Acute pain
- Altered bowel elimination
- Disturbed body image

NURSING INTERVENTION

- Monitor vital signs for fever, increased heart rate, and decreased blood pressure.
- Assess abdomen for distention, presence of bowel sounds.
- Monitor intake and output.
- Postoperatively check:
  - Stoma at colostomy site
  - Wound site for drainage or signs of infection
  - Peripheral circulation, swelling due to increased risk of clot formation
- Teach patients:
  - Eat low-residue foods during flare-ups.
  - Eat high-fiber diet when asymptomatic, fresh fruits and vegetables, whole wheat breads, bran cereals.
  - Avoid laxatives and enemas due to increased irritation and intra-abdominal pressure.
  - Avoid lifting during exacerbation.
  - Avoid eating nuts and seeds.

 # Gastroenteritis

WHAT WENT WRONG?

An acute inflammation of the gastric and intestinal mucosa which is most commonly due to bacterial, viral, protozoal, or parasitic infection. It may also be caused by irritation due to chemical or toxin exposure or allergic response. Viral exposure is more likely in winter; bacterial exposure is more common in summer when food-borne illness exposure is likely.

PROGNOSIS

Symptoms may be self-limiting or may need prescription medication to resolve the illness. Older or debilitated patients may have more severe symptoms or require hospitalization due to dehydration.

HALLMARK SIGNS AND SYMPTOMS

- Nausea and vomiting due to gastric irritation
- Diarrhea—watery, soft, may be mixed with mucous or blood
- Abdominal pain due to intestinal irritation
- Abdominal distention
- Fever due to infection
- Anorexia due to gastric irritation
- Malaise due to infection
- Headache due to viral illness
- Signs of dehydration—dry, flushed skin and mucous membranes, decreased urine output, tachycardia, poor skin turgor, orthostatic blood pressure changes

INTERPRETING TEST RESULTS

- CBC may show leukocytosis or eosinophilia (parasites).
- Electrolytes show imbalance due to GI loss.
- BUN and creatinine elevated due to dehydration.
- Stool for ova and parasites show positive with parasitic infection.

TREATMENT

- Monitor intake and output.
- Replace fluids lost.
- Administer antiemetic medication for symptom relief:
  - prochlorperazine
  - trimethobenzamide
- Administer antidiarrheal medications for symptom relief:
  - loperamide
  - diphenoxylate
  - kaolin-pectin
  - bismuth subsalicylate
- Need to allow organism one way out of gastrointestinal system (either antiemetic or antidiarrheal, not both).

- Administer antimicrobials for infectious cause:
  - ciprofloxacin
  - metronidazole
- Intravenous fluids to correct dehydration.

NURSING DIAGNOSES

- Risk for imbalanced nutrition: less than what body requires
- Deficient fluid volume
- Altered bowel elimination
- Diarrhea
- Fatigue

NURSING INTERVENTION

- Monitor vital signs for changes.
- Monitor intake and output.
- Replace fluids lost.
- Assess skin and mucous membranes for signs of dehydration.
- Assess abdomen for bowel sounds, tenderness

7 Gastroesophageal Reflux Disease (GERD)

WHAT WENT WRONG?

The reflux of stomach acid and contents into the esophagus. This typically causes symptoms because the lining of the esophagus is not protected against the acid that is normally found only in the stomach. The pain that is produced is often referred to as heartburn, or may be mistaken for cardiac pain. The pain may also be referred to the back. The pain occurs more frequently in men, people who are obese, smokers, and those who use alcohol or medications that lower the muscle tone of the lower esophageal sphincter. The pain due to acid refluxing into the esophagus is worse after eating or when lying down. Patients with a hiatal hernia may also experience reflux due to the increased pressure that exists from a portion of the stomach protruding upward through the diaphragm.

PROGNOSIS

Control of symptoms is possible through lifestyle modification and use of medications to reduce acid production within the stomach. There has been no correlation shown between the severity of patient symptoms and the degree of damage being done to the tissue of the esophagus. Patients with ongoing symptoms should have an upper endoscopy to allow for visualization and biopsy of the area to monitor for the possibility of cancer of the esophagus developing due to long-term reflux. Barrett's esophagus is a premalignant condition of the esophagus that occurs due to reflux, where cellular changes have occurred and the patient needs to be monitored for progression to a malignant cell type. Some patients may develop trouble with swallowing due to the development of scarring from long-term exposure to acid. These patients may develop strictures over time. Procedures can be performed to help stretch the lumen of the esophagus to aid in swallowing.

HALLMARK SIGNS AND SYMPTOMS

- Epigastric burning, worse after eating
- Heartburn
- Burping (eructation) or flatulence
- Sour taste in mouth, often worse in the morning
- Nausea
- Bloating
- Cough due to reflux high in the esophagus
- Hoarseness or change in voice

INTERPRETING TEST RESULTS

- 24-hour pH monitoring of lower esophageal area will show elevations.
- Barium swallow or upper GI study may show reflux.

- Endoscopy or esophagogastroduodenoscopy shows irritation from cellular changes of chronic reflux is also used to monitor patients with Barrett's esophagus.
- Esophageal manometry to measure lower esophageal sphincter tone.

TREATMENT

- Administer antacids to neutralize acid; these medications act quickly:
  - Maalox, Mylanta, Tums, Gaviscon
- Administer H2 (histamine type 2) blockers to decrease the production of acid:
  - ranitidine, famotidine, nizatidine, cimetidine
- Administer proton pump inhibitors to reduce the production of acid:
  - omeprazole, esomeprazole, pantoprazole, rabeprazole, lansoprazole
- Have patient eat six small meals rather than three large ones to reduce intra-abdominal pressure.
- Surgery or endoscopic procedures may be performed to prevent the reflux from occurring.

NURSING DIAGNOSES

- Risk for imbalanced nutrition: less than what body requires
- Risk for imbalanced nutrition: more than what body requires
- Acute pain
- Chronic pain

NURSING INTERVENTION

- Monitor vital signs.
- Assess abdomen for distention, bowel sounds.
- Teach about medication management.
- Teach patient about lifestyle modifications:
  - Not to lie down after eating.
  - Elevate head of bed.

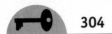

- Avoid wearing clothing that is tight at waist.
- Avoid acidic foods (citrus, vinegar, tomato), peppermint, caffeine, alcohol.
- Stop smoking.
- Lose weight if overweight

8 Gastrointestinal Bleed

WHAT WENT WRONG?

Bleeding from the gastrointestinal tract may cause significant blood loss. The bleeding may be from either the upper or lower gastrointestinal tract. Upper gastrointestinal bleeds are commonly from ulcers, esophageal varices, neoplasms, arteriovenous malformations, Mallory-Weiss tears secondary to vomiting, or anticoagulant use. Lower gastrointestinal bleeds are commonly due to fissure formation, rectal trauma, colitis, polyps, colon cancer, diverticulitis, vasculitis, or ulcerations.

PROGNOSIS

The amount and speed of blood loss coupled with the patient's age and co-morbidities account for the prognosis. The greater the loss of blood, the harder it is for the system to overcome the stress. Multiple transfusions to replace the lost blood increase the patient's risk for a reaction. Patients with blood-clotting disorders have a greater risk of a significant bleed. Patients may go into shock if the amount of blood loss is great, as they become hemodynamically unstable.

HALLMARK SIGNS AND SYMPTOMS

- Hematemesis—vomiting of blood (red, maroon, coffee ground)
- Melena—black, tarry stool
- Hematochezia—red or maroon blood rectally
- Orthostatic changes—drop in BP of at least 10 mmHg with position changes
- Tachycardia as body attempts to circulate lesser blood volume
- Pallor due to decrease in circulating blood volume
- Lightheadedness

- Diaphoresis (sweating)
- Nausea

INTERPRETING TEST RESULTS

- Positive fecal occult blood.
- Hemoglobin drops.
- Hematocrit drops.
- Anemia (iron deficiency) with chronic slow bleed.
- Nasogastric aspirate positive with upper GI bleed.
- Anoscopy, sigmoidoscopy, or colonoscopy may show site of lower GI bleed.
- Arteriography may show site of bleed.
- Bleeding scan may show site of bleed with radioisotope-tagged RBCs.

TREATMENT

- Maintain IV access.
- Administer isotonic fluids like normal saline.
- Monitor serial hemoglobin and hematocrit levels.
- Type and cross match for 3 to 6 units depending on amount of blood loss.
- Transfuse packed RBCs, type-specific when possible (type O negative when type-specific unavailable—no time to get results back from lab yet).
- May need to administer albumin or fresh frozen plasma, depending on amount of units transfused and comorbidities such as cirrhosis or clotting disorders.
- Endoscopic procedures to treat ulcer topically, with injectable or laser treatment.
- Esophageal varices may be treated by tamponade with Blakemore-Sengstaken tube.
- Surgery indicated when bleeding uncontrolled.

NURSING DIAGNOSES

- Deficient fluid volume
- Decreased cardiac output
- Anxiety

NURSING INTERVENTION

- Monitor vital signs for changes—drop in BP, increase in pulse or respiration.
- Monitor intake and output.
- Replace volume lost.
- Monitor abdomen for bowel sounds, tenderness, distention.
- Maintain large bore IV (14- to 18-gauge) access.
- Assess IV site for signs of redness or swelling.
- Monitor lab results—drop in lab values may lag behind blood loss.
- Monitor during blood transfusion as per institution protocol for checking blood unit, patient identity, frequency of vital signs, and documentation.

9 *Gastritis*

WHAT WENT WRONG?

Gastritis is an inflammation of the stomach lining due to either erosion or atrophy. Erosive causes include stresses such as physical illness or medications such as nonsteroidal anti-inflammatory drugs (NSAIDs). Atrophic causes include a history of prior surgery (such as gastrectomy), pernicious anemia, alcohol use, or *Helicobacter pylori* infection.

PROGNOSIS

Gastritis may cause changes within the cells of the stomach lining leading to malnutrition, lymphoma, or gastric cancer. Hospitalized patients, especially in critical care settings, should have preventive medications to avoid the development of gastritis.

HALLMARK SIGNS AND SYMPTOMS

- Nausea and vomiting
- Anorexia

- Epigastric area discomfort
- Epigastric tenderness on palpation due to gastric irritation
- Bleeding from irritation of the gastric mucosa
- Hematemesis—possible coffee ground emesis due to partial digestion of blood
- Melena—black, tarry stool

INTERPRETING TEST RESULTS

- Hemoglobin and hematocrit decrease.
- Anemia (iron deficiency) due to chronic, slow blood loss.
- Fecal occult blood positive.
- *Helicobacter pylori* may be positive.
- Upper endoscopy shows inflammation, allows biopsy.

TREATMENT

- Administer antacids:
  - Maalox, Mylanta, Tums, Gaviscon
- Administer sucralfate to protect gastric lining.
- Administer histamine 2 blockers:
  - ranitidine, famotidine, nizatidine, cimetidine
- Administer proton pump inhibitors:
  - omeprazole, esomeprazole, pantoprazole, rabeprazole, lansoprazole
- Eradicate *Helicobacter pylori* infection if present.
- Diet modification.
- Monitor hemoglobin and hematocrit.

NURSING DIAGNOSES

- Risk for imbalanced nutrition: less than what body requires
- Risk for imbalanced fluid volume
- Nausea

NURSING INTERVENTION

- Monitor vital signs.
- Monitor intake and output.
- Monitor stool for occult blood.
- Assess abdomen for bowel sounds, tenderness.
- Teach patient about:
  - Diet restrictions: avoid alcohol, caffeine, acidic foods.
  - Medications.
  - The need to avoid smoking.
  - The need to avoid NSAIDs.

10 *Hepatitis*

WHAT WENT WRONG?

Hepatitis is an inflammation of the liver cells. This is most commonly due to a viral cause which may be either an acute illness or become chronic. The disease may also be due to exposure to drugs or toxins.

Hepatitis A is transmitted via an oral route, often due to contaminated water or poor sanitation when traveling; it is also transmitted in daycare settings and residential institutions. It can be prevented by vaccine.

Hepatitis B is transmitted via a percutaneous route, often due to sexual contact, IV drug use, mother-to-neonate transmission or possibly blood transfusion. It can be prevented by vaccine.

Hepatitis C is transmitted via a percutaneous route, often due to IV drug use or, less commonly, sexual contact. There is currently no vaccine available.

Hepatitis D is transmitted via a percutaneous route and needs hepatitis B to spread cell to cell. There is no vaccine available for hepatitis D.

Hepatitis E is transmitted via an oral route and is associated with water contamination. There is no known chronic state of hepatitis E and no current vaccine available.

Hepatitis G is transmitted via a percutaneous route and is associated with chronic infection but not significant liver disease.

Exposure to medications (even at therapeutic doses), drugs, or chemicals can also cause hepatitis. Onset is usually within the first couple of days of use, and may be within the first couple of doses. Hepatotoxic substances include acetaminophen, carbon tetrachloride, benzenes, and valproic acid.

PROGNOSIS

Hepatitis may occur as an acute infection (viral type A, E) or become a chronic state. The patient with chronic disease may be unaware of the illness until testing of liver function shows abnormalities and further testing reveals presence of hepatitis. The chronic (viral type B, C) disease state creates the potential development of progressive liver disease. Some patients with chronic disease will need liver transplant. Recurrence rate post-transplant is high. Liver cancer may develop in those with chronic disease states.

HALLMARK SIGNS AND SYMPTOMS

- Acute hepatitis:
  - Malaise
  - Nausea and vomiting
  - Diarrhea or constipation
  - Low-grade fever
  - Dark urine due to change in liver function
  - Jaundice due to liver compromise
  - Tenderness in right upper quadrant of abdomen
  - Hepatomegaly
  - Arthritis, glomerulonephritis, polyarteritis nodosa in hepatitis B
- Chronic hepatitis:
  - Asymptomatic with elevated liver enzymes
  - Symptoms as acute hepatitis
  - Cirrhosis due to altered liver function
  - Ascites due to decrease in liver function, increased portal hypertension
  - Bleeding from esophageal varices
  - Encephalopathy due to diminished liver function
  - Bleeding due to clotting disorders
  - Enlargement of spleen

INTERPRETING TEST RESULTS

- AST elevated.
- ALT elevated.

- IgM anti-HAV in acute or early convalescent stage of hepatitis A.
- IgG anti-HAV in later convalescent stage of hepatitis A.
- HBeAg indicates current viral replication of hepatitis B and infectivity.
- HBsAg shows presence of the hepatitis B surface antigen which is indicative of either current or past infection with hepatitis B.
- IgM anti-HBc shows acute or recent infection with hepatitis B.
- IgG anti-HBc shows convalescent or past infection with hepatitis B.
- HBV DNA shows presence of hepatitis B DNA, most sensitive.
- Anti-HCV present with hepatitis C infection.
- HCV RNA present with hepatitis C infection.
- Anti-HDV present with hepatitis D infection.
- WBC count normal to low.
- Liver biopsy shows hepatocellular necrosis.
- Urinalysis shows protein and bilirubin.

TREATMENT

- Avoid medications metabolized in the liver.
- Avoid alcohol.
- Remove or discontinue causative agent if drug-induced or toxic hepatitis.
- Intravenous hydration if vomiting during acute hepatitis.
- Activity as tolerated.
- High-calorie diet; breakfast is usually the best tolerated meal.
- Administer interferon or lamivudine for chronic hepatitis B.
- Administer interferon and ribavirin for hepatitis C.
- Administer prednisone in autoimmune hepatitis.
- Liver transplantation.

NURSING DIAGNOSES

- Fatigue
- Risk for injury
- Impaired tissue integrity

NURSING INTERVENTION

- Monitor vital signs.
- Assess abdomen for bowel sounds, tenderness, ascites.
- Plan appropriate rest for patient in acute phase.
- Monitor intake and output.
- Assess mental status for changes due to encephalopathy.
- Assist patient to:
    - Plan palatable meals; remember that breakfast is generally the best tolerated meal.
    - Avoid smoking areas—intolerance to smoking.

11 *Hiatal Hernia*

WHAT WENT WRONG?

This is also known as a diaphragmatic hernia. A part of the stomach protrudes up through the diaphragm near the esophagus into the chest. Patients may be asymptomatic or have daily symptoms of gastroesophageal reflux disease (GERD). The hernia may be a sliding hiatal hernia which allows movement of the upper portion of the stomach including the lower esophageal sphincter up and down through the diaphragm. These patients typically have symptoms of GERD. Another type of hiatal hernia is a rolling hernia in which a portion of the stomach protrudes up through the diaphragm, but the lower esophageal sphincter area remains below the level of the diaphragm. These patients do not generally suffer from reflux.

PROGNOSIS

Lifestyle modifications may help control the symptoms of hiatal hernia. Some patients who do not get adequate control of symptoms or are refractory to treatment may need surgery to correct the movement through the diaphragm.

HALLMARK SIGNS AND SYMPTOMS

- Sliding hernia:
    - Heartburn
    - Difficulty swallowing (dysphagia)

- Burping (eructation)
- Chest pain
- Rolling hernia:
  - Chest pain
  - Shortness of breath after eating
  - Feeling of fullness after eating

INTERPRETING TEST RESULTS

- Barium swallow or upper GI study shows hiatal hernia.

TREATMENT

- Administer antacids for patients with reflux symptoms:
  - Maalox, Mylanta, Tums, Gaviscon
- Administer histamine type 2 (H2) blockers to reduce stomach acid:
  - ranitidine, nizatidine, famotidine, cimetidine
- Administer proton pump inhibitors to reduce the production of acid:
  - omeprazole, esomeprazole, pantoprazole, rabeprazole, lansoprazole
- Avoid lying down after eating.
- Modify eating schedule; small, frequent meals.
- Elevate head of bed.
- Avoid clothing that is tight around the waist.

NURSING DIAGNOSES

- Acute pain
- Chronic pain

NURSING INTERVENTION

- Monitor vital signs.
- Assess abdomen for distention, bowel sounds.
- Teach patient about lifestyle modifications:
  - Medication management.

- Not to lie down after eating.
- Elevate head of bed.
- Avoid wearing clothing that is tight at waist.
- Avoid acidic foods (citrus, vinegar, tomato), peppermint, caffeine, alcohol.
- Stop smoking.
- Lose weight if overweight.

12 *Intestinal Obstruction and Paralytic Ileus*

WHAT WENT WRONG?

An intestinal obstruction occurs when motility through the intestine is blocked. This may be caused by a mechanical obstruction due to the presence of a tumor, presence of adhesions from prior surgery, infection or fecal impaction. A paralytic ileus results when motility through the intestine is blocked without any obstructing mass. This may occur during the postoperative period following intra-abdominal surgery, during a severe systemic illness (sepsis), electrolyte imbalance, or because of a metabolic disorder (diabetic ketoacidosis).

PROGNOSIS

Disruption of intestinal function needs to be reestablished for return to homeostasis. In most cases the underlying cause must also be corrected in order for the intestinal function to be restored. Nutritional needs must be met during the treatment period.

HALLMARK SIGNS AND SYMPTOMS

- Obstruction:
  - Abdominal pain (cramping, intermittent or constant)
  - Abdominal distention
  - Vomiting of gastrointestinal contents (may eventually include stool as GI tract backs up)
  - Bowel sounds high-pitched
  - Constipation
  - Abdominal tenderness on palpation

- Paralytic ileus:
  - Abdominal pain (constant)
  - Abdominal distention
  - Vomiting of gastrointestinal contents
  - Bowel sounds diminished or absent

INTERPRETING TEST RESULTS

- Abdominal x-ray shows dilation of small bowel with air-fluid levels in obstruction; diffuse distention in ileus.

TREATMENT

- NPO to rest intestinal tract.
- Nasogastric tube attached to suction the contents from stomach.
- Intravenous fluid replacement with isotonic solution.
- Correction of electrolyte imbalances.
- Parenteral nutrition replacement and vitamin supplementation.
- Administer antiemetics if nausea continues after NG tube in place.
- Monitor electrolytes.

NURSING DIAGNOSES

- Risk for imbalanced nutrition: less than what body requires
- Risk for imbalanced fluid volume
- Altered bowel elimination

NURSING INTERVENTION

- Monitor vital signs for changes.
- Assess abdomen for bowel sounds, tenderness.
- Monitor intravenous access site for irritation, redness, swelling.
- Keep patient NPO.
- Monitor intake and output.
- Replace fluids lost from all sources

13 *Pancreatitis*

WHAT WENT WRONG?

Pancreatitis is an inflammation of the pancreas which causes destructive cellular changes. It may be an acute or a chronic process. Acute pancreatitis involves auto-digestion of the pancreas by pancreatic enzymes and development of fibrosis. Blood glucose control may be affected by the changes to the pancreas. Chronic pancreatitis results from recurrent episodes of exacerbation, leading to fibrosis and a decrease in pancreatic function. Presence of gallstones blocking a pancreatic duct, chronic use of alcohol, post-abdominal trauma or surgery, or elevated cholesterol are associated with an increased risk of pancreatitis.

PROGNOSIS

Acute pancreatitis may be life-threatening. Pleural effusion may develop as a complication of acute pancreatitis; older patients have a greater risk of also developing pneumonia. Disseminated intravascular coagulation is another complication that may occur, affecting the body's ability to clot due to depleted clotting factors in the development of small thrombi.

HALLMARK SIGNS AND SYMPTOMS

- Epigastric pain due to inflammation and stretching of pancreatic duct
- Boring abdominal pain may radiate to back or left shoulder in acute pancreatitis
- Gnawing continuous abdominal pain with acute exacerbations in chronic pancreatitis
- Patient in knee-chest position for comfort—reduces tension on abdomen
- Nausea and vomiting
- Bluish-gray discoloration of periumbilical area and abdomen (Cullen's sign)
- Bluish-gray discoloration of flank areas (Turner's sign)
- Ascites
- Weight loss
- Blood glucose elevation
- Fatigue

INTERPRETING TEST RESULTS

- Elevated serum amylase.
- Elevated serum lipase.
- Elevated white blood cell count (WBC) due to inflammation.
- Elevated cholesterol.
- Elevated glucose due to labile effect on glucose control.
- Elevated bilirubin.
- CT scan shows inflammation.
- Chest x-ray may show pleural effusion.

TREATMENT

- NPO during acute stage to reduce release of pancreatic enzymes.
- Intravenous fluids for hydration.
- Total parenteral nutrition.
- Administer vitamin supplementation.
- Pain management with narcotics during acute stage.
- Avoid morphine that may increase pain due to spasm of the sphincter of Oddi at the opening to the small intestine from the common bile duct.
- Intravenous, patient-controlled analgesia or transdermal delivery preferable to intramuscular.
- Acute:
  - NG tube connected to suction if vomiting.
  - Surgical intervention for abscess or pseudocyst.
- Chronic:
  - Blood glucose control with insulin.
  - Administer pancreatic enzymes with meals.
  - Surgical intervention for pain control, abscess.

NURSING DIAGNOSES

- Acute pain
- Imbalanced nutrition: less than what body requires

NURSING INTERVENTION

- Assess vital signs for elevated temperature, elevated pulse, and changes in blood pressure.
- Assess pain level.
- Monitor intake and output.
- Assess abdomen for bowel sounds, tenderness, masses, ascites.
- Monitor fingerstick blood glucose.
- Assess lung sounds for bilateral equality.
- Frequent oral care for NPO patients.
- Teach patient about home care:
  - Avoid alcohol and caffeine.
  - Bland, low-fat, high-protein, high-calorie, small, frequent meals.
  - Use of blood glucose meter.
  - Medication management, schedule, side effects.
  - Plan rest periods until strength returns.

14 *Peritonitis*

WHAT WENT WRONG?

Peritonitis is an acute inflammation of the peritoneum, which is the lining of the abdominal cavity. Peritonitis may be primary or secondary to another disease process. It typically occurs due to bacterial presence within the peritoneal space. The bacteria may have passed from the gastrointestinal tract or the rupture of an organ within the abdomen or pelvis. After the introduction of the bacteria into the abdominal area, an inflammatory reaction occurs.

PROGNOSIS

It is a life-threatening disease process. Patients may develop septicemia from the bacteria within the abdomen that enter the bloodstream.

HALLMARK SIGNS AND SYMPTOMS

- Fever
- Tachycardia

- Abdominal distention
- Abdominal pain—may be localized or generalized
- Rebound pain (pain when quickly removing pressure during palpation of abdomen)
- Rigid abdomen
- Nausea, vomiting, loss of appetite
- Decreased bowel sounds
- Decreased urine output

INTERPRETING TEST RESULTS

- Elevated white blood cell count (WBC).
- Blood cultures to identify organisms.
- Abdominal x-rays to show free air from perforation.
- Ultrasound to identify causative problem (appendicitis, etc.).
- Peritoneal lavage to analyze fluid for WBC count, bacteria, bile.
- CT scan to identify causative problem (appendicitis, salpingitis, etc.).

TREATMENT

- Intravenous fluids.
- Administer broad-spectrum antibiotics.
- Surgical intervention may be necessary to correct cause of peritonitis.
- Pain management postoperatively.

NURSING DIAGNOSES

- Acute pain
- Impaired tissue integrity
- Impaired skin integrity

NURSING INTERVENTION

- Weigh daily.
- Monitor vital signs.

- Monitor intake and output.
- NPO to avoid irritation of intestinal tract, further stress on abdominal organs.
- Position for comfort, head of bed elevated.
- Assess for return of bowel sounds postoperatively.
- Teach patient about home care:
  - Pain management.
  - Wound care, drains, etc.
  - Monitor for signs of infection.

15 *Peptic Ulcer Disease (PUD)*

WHAT WENT WRONG?

An ulcer develops when there is erosion of a portion of the mucosal layer of either the stomach or duodenum. The ulcer may occur within the stomach (gastric ulcer), or the duodenum (duodenal ulcer). A break in the protective mucosal lining allows the acid within the stomach to make contact with the epithelial tissues. Gastric ulcers favor the lesser curvature of the stomach. Duodenal ulcers tend to be deeper, penetrating through the mucosa to the muscular layer. *Helicobacter pylori* infection has been associated with duodenal ulcers. Stress ulcers are associated with another acute medical condition or traumatic injury. As the body attempts to heal from the other physical condition (for example, major surgery), small areas of ischemia develop within the stomach or duodenum. The ischemic areas then ulcerate.

PROGNOSIS

The ulcerated areas may develop bleeding or may perforate. Depending on the location of the ulceration, a vessel may become exposed to the effects of the stomach acids. Damage to these vessels may result in significant bleeding. Perforation of the ulcer can occur as the ulcer continues to erode more deeply into the tissue. Perforation permits the contents of the stomach or duodenum to enter the peritoneum, leading to peritonitis, paralytic ileus, septicemia, and shock. This patient will need emergency surgery due to a life-threatening condition.

HALLMARK SIGNS AND SYMPTOMS

- Epigastric area pain:
  - Worse just after eating as acid increases with gastric ulcer
  - Worse when stomach is empty (with duodenal ulcer); may awaken during the night due to pain
  - Weight changes
    - Loss with gastric ulcer
    - Gain with duodenal ulcer
- Bleeding from ulcer causes:
  - Hematemesis (vomiting bloody fluid—red, maroon); more likely with gastric ulcer
  - Coffee-ground emesis (partially digested blood)
  - Melena (tarry stool) more likely with duodenal ulcer
- Perforation of ulcer causes:
  - Sudden, sharp pain
  - Tender, rigid, board-like abdomen
  - Knee-chest position reduces pain
  - Hypovolemic shock

INTERPRETING TEST RESULTS

- Anemia due to bleeding.
- Stool for occult blood positive due to bleeding.
- *H. pylori* testing positive.
- Upper GI or barium swallow shows areas of ulceration—not done if perforation suspected.
- Upper endoscopy shows ulcer.
- Abdominal x-rays show free air in perforation.

TREATMENT

- Administer antacids

- Administer histamine-2 blockers:
  - famotidine, ranitidine, nizatidine
- Administer proton pump inhibitors:
  - omeprazole, lansoprazole, rabeprazole, esomeprazole, pantoprazole
- Administer mucosal barrier fortifiers:
  - sucralfate
- Administer prostaglandin analogue:
  - misoprostol
- Adjust diet.
- Treat *H. pylori* infection if present with combination therapy:
  - Proton pump inhibitor plus clarithromycin plus amoxicillin *or*
  - Proton pump inhibitor plus metronidazole plus clarithromycin *or*
  - Bismuth subsalicylate plus metronidazole plus tetracycline.

NURSING DIAGNOSES

- Acute pain
- Risk for imbalanced nutrition: less than what body requires
- Risk for imbalanced nutrition: more than what body requires

NURSING INTERVENTION

- Monitor vital signs.
- Monitor intake and output.
- Assess abdomen for bowel sounds, tenderness, rigidity, rebound pain, guarding.
- Monitor stool for change in color, consistency, blood.
- Teach patient about home care:
  - Diet modification to avoid acidic foods, caffeine, peppermint, alcohol.
  - Eat more frequent, small meals.
  - Avoid nonsteroidal anti-inflammatory medication.
  - Stop smoking.

16 *Ulcerative Colitis*

WHAT WENT WRONG?

An inflammatory disease of the large intestine that affects the mucosal layer beginning in the rectum and colon and spreading into the adjacent tissue. There are ulcerations in the mucosal layer of the intestinal wall, and inflammation and abscess formation occur. Bloody diarrhea with mucous is the primary symptom. There are periods of exacerbations and remissions. Symptom severity may vary from mild to severe. The exact cause is unknown, but there is increased incidence in people with northern European, North American, or Ashkenazi Jewish origins. The peak incidences are from mid-teen to mid-twenties and again from mid-fifties to mid-sixties.

PROGNOSIS

Patients with ulcerative colitis may have an increase in symptoms with each flare-up of the disease. Malabsorption of nutrients can cause weight loss and health problems. Some patients will need surgery to resect the affected area of the large intestine, resulting in a colostomy, ileal reservoir, ileoanal anastomosis, or ileoanal reservoir. There is an increased risk of colon cancer in patients with ulcerative colitis. The patient is also at risk for developing toxic megacolon or perforating the area of ulceration.

HALLMARK SIGNS AND SYMPTOMS

- Weight loss
- Abdominal pain
- Chronic bloody diarrhea with pus due to ulceration
- Electrolyte imbalance due to diarrhea
- Tenesmus—spasms involving the anal sphincter; persistent desire to empty bowel

INTERPRETING TEST RESULTS

- Anemia—low hemoglobin and hematocrit due to blood loss and chronic disease.

- Elevated erythrocyte sedimentation rate due to inflammation.
- Electrolyte disturbance due to diarrhea and poor absorbance of nutrients.
- Double-contrast barium enema shows areas of ulceration and inflammation.
- Sigmoidoscopy or colonoscopy show ulcerations and bleeding.

TREATMENT

- Keep stool diary to identify irritating foods.
- Low-fiber, high-protein, high-calorie diet.
- Administer antidiarrheal medications:
  - loperamide
  - diphenoxylate hydrochloride and atropine
- Administer salicylate medications to reduce inflammation within the intestinal mucosa:
  - sulfasalazine
  - mesalamine
  - olsalazine
  - balsalazide
- Administer corticosteroids during exacerbations to reduce inflammation:
  - prednisone
  - hydrocortisone
- NPO for bowel rest during exacerbations.
- Administer anticholinergics to reduce abdominal cramping and discomfort:
  - dicyclomine
- Surgical resection of affected area of large intestine.

NURSING DIAGNOSES

- Acute pain
- Diarrhea
- Impaired skin integrity
- Disturbed body image

NURSING INTERVENTION

- Monitor intake and output.
- Monitor stool output, frequency.
- Weigh patient regularly.
- Sitz bath.
- Vitamin A & D ointment or barrier cream applied to skin.
- Witch hazel to soothe sensitive skin.
- Monitor for toxic megacolon (distended and tender abdomen, fever, elevated WBC, elevated pulse, distended colon).
- Teach home care for new ostomy patients or refer to enterostomal therapist for education:
  - Teach proper skin care of perianal area to avoid skin breakdown.
  - Avoid fragranced products which can be irritating.
  - Teach dietary modification, and which foods to avoid.
  - Teach medication use, schedule, and side effects.
  - Teach importance of follow-up care.
  - Teach wound care for postoperative patients.

Crucial Diagnostic Tests

Gastroscopy

This test is used to diagnose peptic, gastric, or duodenal ulcers and to obtain biopsies and specimens for *H. pylori* bacteria. An informed consent is obtained prior to any anesthesia. An endoscope is passed through the mouth to allow visualization of the pharynx, esophagus, lower esophageal sphincter, stomach, pyloric sphincter, and duodenum. Biopsies can be obtained at this time. Bleeding, ulcers, lesions, and polyps can be visually assessed. The back of the throat will be anesthetized to allow passage of the endoscope.

Before the test—The patient will be NPO.

After the test—Monitor vital signs. Assess for return of gag reflex. The patient remains NPO until the gag reflex returns.

Colonoscopy

This test is used to diagnose obstruction, bleeding, change in bowel habits, and colon cancer, among other conditions. An informed consent is obtained before the patient is given any type of anesthesia. A colonoscope is passed through the rectum to visualize the anus, sigmoid, descending colon, splenic flexure, transverse colon, hepatic flexure, ascending colon, and the ileo-cecal valve. The colon may be insufflated to aid in visualization of the structures. Biopsies are obtained as indicated. The scope is withdrawn and anesthesia is reversed. The patient may experience abdominal distention. Risks include perforation of the large intestine. The test is commonly performed as an outpatient procedure.

Before the test—A thorough colon prep is necessary to ensure complete emptying of the bowel prior to the procedure. The patient is NPO for several hours prior to the test due to the use of an anesthetic agent.

After the test—Assess the abdomen for bowel sounds and tenderness. Monitor vital signs. Assess the patient for side effects of anesthesia.

Abdominal Ultrasound

This is a noninvasive test and is usually painless. A transducer is guided over the abdomen, which produces sound waves that bounce off internal structures and produce a picture of internal organs and structures.

Before the test—The patient will need to be NPO.

After the test—No special care is needed.

Abdominal X-rays

These are plain x-rays, usually flat-plate and upright, of the abdomen, to look for obstruction, foreign bodies, gas patterns, tumors, and other abnormalities.

Before and after the test—No special care is needed.

Liver Biopsy

Here, a small sample of tissue is removed from the liver and examined under a microscope, allowing for a definite diagnosis. A thin cutting needle, through the skin of the abdomen, is used to obtain the sample. Needle biopsies are relatively simple procedures requiring only local anesthesia. Risks include bruising, bleeding, and infection.

Before the test—Informed consent will be needed.

After the test—Monitor vital signs for drop in blood pressure as well as an increase in pulse or respiration. Check the site for bruising or bleeding. Check skin for pallor or sweating.

Computerized Tomography (CT) Scan

This test uses x-rays to produce cross-sectional images of the body in two-dimensional slices. Split-second computer processing creates these images as a series of very thin x-ray beams pass through the body. A dye (contrast medium) may be injected into a vein.

Before the test—The clearer images produced with the dye make it easier to distinguish a tumor from normal tissue. A CT scan uses more radiation than do conventional x-rays, but the benefits of the test outweigh the risks.

Before the test—Ask the patient about any history of allergy to contrast dye or shellfish. The patient may need to be NPO, depending on the area that needs to be imaged.

After the test—No special care is needed.

Magnetic Resonance Imaging (MRI)

Unlike an x-ray, an MRI creates images using a magnetic field and radio waves. A contrast dye also may be used. The test can take from 15 minutes to an hour. The patient is placed in a cylindrical tube for the test. Loud banging noises are typical.

Before the test—Ask the patient about any implanted hardware such as pacemakers, or history of claustrophobia. The patient may need to be NPO, depending on the area that needs to be imaged.

After the test—No special care is needed.

Endoscopic Retrograde Cholangiopancreatiography (ERCP)

Here, a thin, flexible tube (endoscope) is passed through the pharynx, the stomach, and into the upper part of the small intestine. Air is used to inflate the intestinal tract to enable the openings of the pancreatic and bile ducts to be seen. A dye is injected into the ducts through a catheter via the endoscope. X-rays are taken of the ducts. The patient may report abdominal distention from the insufflation, and a sore throat.

Before the test—The patient is NPO.

After the test—Monitor vital signs. Assess for return of gag reflex. The patient remains NPO until gag reflex returns.

Liver Function Tests

These comprise several tests, obtained through a venipuncture, which show hepatic function. Generally includes alanine aminotransferase (ALT), alkaline phosphatase (Alk Phos), aspartate aminotransferase (AST), bilirubin, gamma-glutamyl transpeptidase (GGPT), lactate dehydrogenase (LDH), prothrombin time (PT), and partial thromboplastin time (PTT).

Alanine Transaminase (ALT)

An enzyme found mainly in liver cells, ALT helps the body metabolize protein. When the liver is damaged, ALT is released in the bloodstream.

Aspartate Transaminase (AST)

The enzyme AST plays a role in the metabolism of alanine, an amino acid. An increase in AST levels may indicate liver damage or disease.

Alkaline Phosphatase (ALP)

ALP is an enzyme found in high concentrations in the liver and bile ducts, as well as some other tissues. Higher-than-normal levels of ALP may indicate liver damage or disease.

Albumin and Total Protein

Levels of albumin—a protein made by the liver—and total protein show how well the liver is making proteins that the body needs to fight infections and perform other functions. Lower-than-normal levels may indicate liver damage or disease.

Bilirubin

Bilirubin is a red-yellow pigment that results from the breakdown of red blood cells. Normally, bilirubin passes through the liver and is excreted in stool. Elevated levels of bilirubin (jaundice) may indicate liver damage or disease.

Gamma-Glutamyl Transferase (GGT)

This test measures the amount of the enzyme GGT in the blood. Higher-than-normal levels may indicate liver or bile duct injury.

Lactate Dehydrogenase (LDH)

LDH is an enzyme found in many body tissues, including the liver. Elevated levels of LDH may indicate liver damage.

Prothrombin Time (PT)

This test measures the clotting time of plasma. Increased PT may indicate liver damage.

Hepatitis Panel

- Tests for acute viral hepatitis include:
  - Hepatitis B surface Antigen (HBsAg)
  - Hepatitis A Virus antibody (anti-HAV)
  - Hepatitis B core antibody Immunoglobulin M (IgM anti-HBc)
  - Hepatitis C Virus antibody (anti-HCV)
- Tests for chronic hepatitis include:
  - Hepatitis B surface Antigen (HBsAg)
  - Hepatitis C Virus antibody (anti-HCV)
  - Hepatitis D Virus antibody (anti-HDV)
- HAV is confirmed by detecting an IgM antibody to HAV (IgM anti-HAV).
- HBV is confirmed by detecting HBsAg and IgM anti-HBC (when Hepatitis B early Antigen (HBeAg) is detected, patient is highly infectious).
- HCV is confirmed by detecting ELISA-2 and RIBA-2.
- HDV is confirmed by detecting anti-HDV and serologic markers for HBV.
- HEV—only research-based tests are available at this time.

Helicobacter Pylori

This is a gram negative bacteria which can be detected by a serum test, discovered by gastric biopsy and ELISA for anti-*H. pylori* immunoglobulin G. A carbon isotope urea breath test can reveal the presence of *H. pylori* (which has a false-negative rate of 5 to 15 percent).

Quiz

1. An inflammatory bowel disorder in which the patient develops abdominal pain, bloody diarrhea, tenesmus and weight loss is
   (a) Crohn's disease.
   (b) diverticulitis.
   (c) ulcerative colitis.
   (d) appendicitis.

2. Chronic hepatitis C may be treated with:
   (a) sulfasalazine.
   (b) interferon and ribavirin.
   (c) metronidazole or ciprofloxacin.
   (d) acetaminophen.

3. The patient with gastroesophageal reflux disease should be taught:
   (a) to avoid coffee, tea, or other caffeine-containing beverages.
   (b) to take histamine 2 blockers, such as ranitidine, as directed.
   (c) to avoid acidic foods such as citrus or tomato.
   (d) all of the above.

4. A patient presents with abdominal pain that is initially periumbilical but over time moves to the right lower quadrant area. This pain is most likely due to:
   (a) appendicitis.
   (b) Crohn's disease.
   (c) cholecystitis.
   (d) diverticulitis.

5. On assessment of the abdomen in a patient with peritonitis, you would expect to find:

   (a) a soft abdomen with bowel sounds every 2 to 3 seconds.

   (b) rebound tenderness and guarding.

   (c) hyperactive, high-pitched bowel sounds and a firm abdomen.

   (d) ascites and increased vascular pattern on the skin.

6. Treatment of the patient with appendicitis includes:

   (a) transfusion to replace blood loss.

   (b) bowel prep for cleansing.

   (c) surgical removal of appendix.

   (d) medications to lower pH within the stomach.

7. Patients with gastrointestinal bleeding may experience an acute or chronic blood loss. Your patient is experiencing hematochezia. You recognize this as:

   (a) vomiting of bright red or maroon blood.

   (b) black, tarry stool.

   (c) coffee ground emesis.

   (d) red- or maroon-colored stool rectally.

8. Build-up of bile salts may cause the systemic symptom of:

   (a) hypotension.

   (b) pruritis (itching).

   (c) ecchymosis (bruising).

   (d) urticaria (hives).

9. Patients with gastric ulcer typically exhibit the following symptoms:

   (a) epigastric pain worse after eating and weight loss.

   (b) epigastric pain worse before meals, pain awakening patient from sleep, and melena.

   (c) decreased bowel sounds, rigid abdomen, rebound tenderness, and fever.

   (d) boring epigastric pain radiating to back and left shoulder, bluish-gray discoloration of periumbilical area, and ascites.

10. Patients with a paralytic ileus typically have:

    (a) intravenous fluid replacement and a nasogastric tube connected to suction.

    (b) surgical correction of the problem.

    (c) endoscopic injection of botulinum toxin or esophageal dilation.

    (d) endoscopy to allow biopsy followed with broad-spectrum antibiotics.

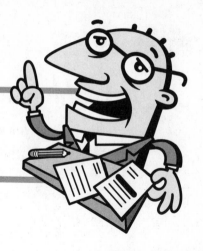

CHAPTER 8

Endocrine System

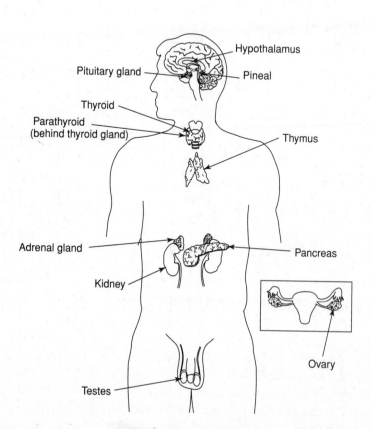

Hypothalamus

Pituitary gland

Pineal

Thyroid

Parathyroid
(behind thyroid gland)

Thymus

Adrenal gland

Pancreas

Kidney

Ovary

Testes

Learning Objectives

1	Hypothyroidism (Myxedema)		**9**	Addison's disease
2	Hyperthyroidism (Graves' disease)		**10**	Cushing's syndrome
3	Simple goiter		**11**	Primary aldosteronism (Conn's syndrome)
4	Hypopituitarism		**12**	Pheochromocytoma
5	Hyperpituitarism (Acromegaly and Gigantism)		**13**	Hypoparathyroidism
6	Hyperprolactinemia		**14**	Hyperparathyroidism
7	Diabetes insipidus		**15**	Diabetes mellitus
8	Syndrome of inappropriate antidiuretic hormone secretion (SIADH)		**16**	Metabolic syndrome (Syndrome X/Dysmetabolic syndrome)

 Key Terms

Acromegaly
Aldosterone
Antidiuretic hormone (ADH)
Catecholamines
Chvostek's sign
Conn's syndrome
Cortisol
Cortisone
Epinephrine

Gigantism
Glucocorticoids
Graves disease
Hydrocortisone
Insulin
Mineralocorticoids
Myxedema
Norepinephrine
Parathyroid hormone (PTH)

RAIU
T3
T4
Thyroid scan update test
Thyroid storm
TRH
Trousseau's sign
TSH
Vanillylmadelic acid (VMA)

How the Endocrine System Works

The endocrine system is comprised of several glands, scattered throughout the body. The glands release hormones which are chemical messengers, substances which control and regulate the activity of target cells and organs. Together, these hormones influence growth, development, digestion, and regulate metabolism and reproduction. The glands generally release the hormones into the blood due to a stimulus, another hormone, or a threshhold. The signal to turn off the hormone production is regulated by a process called direct feedback. Direct feedback is necessary to maintain homeostasis. The body receives feedback about changes in hormone levels and impacts organs or body systems to adjust the hormone production to tell the body to return to homeostasis. When the concentration of the substance reaches a threshhold, the gland and its production are turned off. The glands, the hormones they produce, and the effects are stated below.

The thyroid gland is located in the anterior neck, overlying the trachea. It makes three hormones: thyroxine (T4), triiodothyronine (T3), and calcitonin, which affects the blood calcium and phosphate release from the bones. Thyroid hormones affect metabolism, muscles, the heart, and many other body organs and systems. They help regulate carbohydrate metabolism, lipids, proteins, and growth and development. Anterior pituitary glands are controlled by hormones from the hypothyroid and by direct feedback. The adrenal glands are bilateral glands that cap each kidney. They are located in the retro peritoneum. The glands are comprised of two parts: the cortex and the aderenal medulla. The cortex secretes (1) aldosterone, which is responsible for renal reabsorption of sodium and excretion of potassium; (2) cortisol, which maintains glucose control, increases hepatic gluconeogenesis (the making of glucose), and manages the body's stress response; and (3) androgens, which are sex hormones. The adrenal medulla produces, stores, and secretes epinephrine and norepinephrine, which are called catecholamines. When they are released, heart and respiratory rate increase, blood pressure rises, airways dilate, and an increase in the metabolic rate is seen.

The parathyroid glands are composed of usually four, sometimes six or more, small glands which are found on the posterior side of the thyroid gland. Their function is to produce parathyroid hormone (PTH). PTH, also called parathormone, maintains the calcium level in the blood. It also regulates the phosphorus level in the body. If the serum calcium level falls, PTH is released, which causes bones to break down, releasing calcium into the blood. It also causes the kidneys to decrease the calcium released in the urine, and increases phosphate excretion.

Just the Facts

 ## *Hypothyroidism (Myxedema)*

WHAT WENT WRONG?

Hypothyroidism is a lack of, or too little, thyroid hormone commonly caused by Hashimoto's thyroiditis. Hashimoto's thyroiditis is a chronic disorder caused by abnormal antibodies that attack the thyroid gland. Hypothyroidism can also be caused by decreased production of the TSH hormone from the pituitary gland, a side effect of surgery, inflammation of the thyroid gland, and treatment for hyperthyroidism.

PROGNOSIS

Prognosis is excellent with replacement of thyroid hormones.

HALLMARK SIGNS AND SYMPTOMS

- Fatigue due to slow metabolism
- Hypothermia due to slow metabolism
- Brittle nails due to low levels of thyroid hormone, which helps growth and development
- Thick dry hair from lack of thyroid hormone
- Dry skin from lack of thyroid hormone
- Menstruation changes due to diminished levels of thyroid hormone
- Slow cognitive function due to slow metabolism
- Weight gain, low levels of thyroid hormone causes fatigue, sluggishness

INTERPRETING TEST RESULTS

- Increased thyroid stimulating hormore (TSH) unless the cause is due to a decreased production of TSH by the pituitary gland.
- Decreased T3, T4.
- Presence of thyroglobulin, indicating Hashimoto's thyroiditis.
- Presence of peroxidase autoantibodies in serum, indicating Hashimoto's thyroiditis.

TREATMENT

- Replacement hormone; levothyroxine is the treatment of choice.

- Serum measurements of T3 and T4 will need to be performed after 6 to 8 weeks to determine if the patient is taking the correct dose.
- The patient needs to be aware that this is a lifetime replacement.

NURSING DIAGNOSES

- Risk for imbalanced nutrition: more than what body requires
- Hypothermia related to decreased metabolic rate
- Risk for constipation related to decreased motility of the GI tract

NURSING INTERVENTION

- Monitor vital signs.
- Provide a warm environment.
- Low-calorie diet.
- Increase fluids and fiber to prevent constipation.
- Take thyroid replacement hormone each morning to avoid insomnia.
- Monitor for signs of thyrotoxcosis (an increase in T3): nausea, vomiting, diarrhea, sweating, tachycardia.
- Explain to the patient:
  - Side effects of thyroid hormone replacement.
  - Review the signs of hyperthyroidism and hypothyroidism.
  - Have patient contact health care provider if signs change.

2   *Hyperthyroidism (Graves' Disease)*

WHAT WENT WRONG?

There is an overproduction of T3 and T4 by the thyroid gland that can be caused by an autoimmune disease where the body's immune system attacks the thyroid gland. Other causes can be a benign tumor (adenomas) resulting in an enlarged thyroid gland (goiter) or an overproduction of TSH by the pituitary gland, caused by a pituitary tumor.

PROGNOSIS

The prognosis is good if the cause of hyperthyroidism is treated; however, hyper-thyroidism is a chronic disease. Signs such as bulging eyes (exophthalmos) are not reversible. Furthermore, thyroid surgery may result in complications.

HALLMARK SIGNS AND SYMPTOMS

- Enlarged thyroid gland (goiter) caused by tumor
- Protrusion of the eyeballs (exophthalmos) due to lymphocytic infiltration which pushes out the eyeball
- Sweating (diaphoresis); excess thyroid hormone raises the metabolic rate
- Increased appetite due to increased metabolism
- Nervousness due to high levels of thyroid hormone
- Weight loss due to increased metabolism
- Menstrual changes due to elevated levels of thyroid hormone

INTERPRETING TEST RESULTS

- Increased serum T3.
- Increased serum T4.
- Increased TRH and TSH if pituitary gland is the cause of hyperthyroidism.
- Presence of antibodies if cause is Graves' disease.
- Thyroid scan reveals enlarged thyroid.

TREATMENT

- For mild cases and for young patients, administer antithyroid medication such as propylthiouracil and methimazole to block synthesis of T3 and T4.
- For Graves' disease and for patients 50 years of age or older, radioactive iodine therapy is used to decrease production of thyroid hormones. Administer Lugol's solution, SSKI, or potassium iodide.
- For severe cases where the size of the thyroid gland interferes with swallowing or breathing, the thyroid gland is surgically reduced in size or removed.

- Administer beta blockers such as propranolol until hyperthyroidism diminishes to decrease sympathetic activity and control tachycardia, tremors, and anxiety.

NURSING DIAGNOSES

- Imbalanced nutrition: less than what body requires related to inadequate intake in relation to metabolic needs
- Fatigue related to sleep deprivation
- Hyperthermia related to increased metabolic rate

NURSING INTERVENTION

- Monitor vital signs.
- Provide cool environment.
- Protect the patient's eyes with dark glasses and artificial tears if the patient has exophthalmos.
- Provide a diet high in carbohydrates, protein, calories, vitamins, and minerals.
- Monitor for laryngeal edema following surgery (hoarseness or inability to clearly speak).
- Keep oxygen, suction, and a tracheotomy set near bed in case the neck swells and breathing is impaired.
- Keep calcium gluconate near the patient's bed following surgery. This is the treatment for tetany and is used to maintain the serum calcium level in normal range.
- Place the patient in a semi-Fowler's position to decrease tension on the neck following surgery.
- Support the patient's head and neck with pillows.
- Monitor for muscle spasms and tremors (tetany) caused by manipulation of the parathyroid glands during surgery.
- Check drainage and hemorrhage from incision line; red flags are frank hemorrhage and purulent, foul smelling drainage.
- Monitor for signs of hypocalcemia (tingling of hands and fingers).

- Check for Trousseau's sign (inflate blood pressure cuff on the arm and muscles contract).
- Check for Chvostek's sign (tapping of the facial nerve causes twitching of the facial muscles). Both this sign and Trousseau's sign are positive when the parathyroid glands have been manipulated during thyroid surgery, in which case they secrete too much phosphorus and not enough calcium. Since muscles, i.e. the heart, need calcium for work, a low calcium level may cause muscle spasms which are easily detected by Chvostek's sign and Trousseau's sign. The treatment is IV calcium, administered quickly.

3   *Simple Goiter*

WHAT WENT WRONG?

A lack of iodine in the patient's diet (endemic, simple goiter) causes the thyroid gland to become enlarged. This is seen less today because iodine is added to table salt. The thyroid gland can also become enlarged by ingesting large amounts of goitrogenic drugs or goitrogenic foods that decrease production of thyroxine, such as strawberries, cabbage, peanuts, peas, peaches, and spinach. This results in sporadic simple goiter. A simple goiter is not caused by inflammation or neoplasm.

PROGNOSIS

Prognosis is good if treated and patients go on to live normal lives.

HALLMARK SIGNS AND SYMPTOMS

- Difficulty in swallowing (dysphagia) due to a large thyroid pressing on the esophagus
- Enlarged thyroid gland
- Respiratory distress from the large gland, causing pressure on the trachea
- A tight feeling in the throat from a large gland
- Coughing

INTERPRETING TEST RESULTS

- Decreased or normal serum T4 level caused by an underactive thyroid.
- Increased serum TSH, by the pituitary gland, attempting to stimulate or shut off production of the thyroid in making thyroid hormone.
- RAIU uptake normal or increased—a radioactive isotope is injected into a vein. A scan of the thyroid is done to visualize the thyroid more completely.
- Ultrasound enables sound waves to bounce off the gland, giving the size and location of any nodules.

TREATMENT

- If increased TSH, administer hormone replacement with levothyroxine (T4), dessicated thyroid, or liothyronine (T3).
- If the thyroid gland is overactive, then administer small doses of Lugol's solution or potassium iodide solution.
- If the simple goiter cannot be reduced through medication, then a thyroidectomy is performed during which all or part of the thyroid is removed.

NURSING DIAGNOSES

- Imbalanced nutrition: less than what body requires; related to inadequate intake in relation to metabolic needs
- Fatigue related to sleep deprivation
- Hyperthermia related to increased metabolic rate

NURSING INTERVENTION

- Avoid goitrogenic foods or drugs in sporadic goiter since they make thyroid hormone production.
- Use iodized salt to prevent and treat endemic goiter, since the thyroid needs iodine to make thyroid hormone.
- Explain to patient:
  - The need for life-long thyroid replacement after thyroidectomy and radioactive iodine.

- The need for intermittent lab work to monitor the thyroid.
- Visits to the primary care practitioner to monitor size of thyroid gland.

4 *Hypopituitarism*
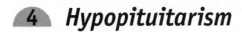

WHAT WENT WRONG?

Hypopituitarism results when the pituitary gland is unable to secrete a normal amount of pituitary hormones. Primary causes are pituitary tumors, inadequate blood supply to the pituitary gland, infection, radiation therapy, or surgical removal of a portion of the pituitary gland. Secondary causes affect the hypothalamus, which regulates the pituitary gland.

PROGNOSIS

Patients require life-long treatment and can expect a normal life span.

HALLMARK SIGNS AND SYMPTOMS

- Fatigue caused by a decreased production of ACTH
- Lethargy and diminished cognition caused by a decreased production of TSH
- Sensitivity to cold due to low TSH, which stimulates thyroid hormone
- Decreased appetite due to TSH deficiency
- Infertility due to luteinizing hormone (LH) and follicle-stimulating hormone (FSH) production
- Short stature due to diminished secretion of growth hormone
- Infertility, amenorrhea caused by decreased production of FSH and LH

INTERPRETING TEST RESULTS

- Decreased ACTH usually due to a lesion of the pituitary.
- TSH deficiency due to a mass, trauma, surgery, or idiopathic.

- Decreased prolactin due to a mass, causing diminished or lack of prolactin from the anterior pituitary.
- Presence of a pituitary tumor shown on MRI.

TREATMENT

- Administer replacement hormones (estrogen, testosterone, corticosteroids, growth hormone, and thyroid hormone).
- Surgical removal of the pituitary tumor if it exists.

NURSING DIAGNOSES

- Disturbed body image related to illness
- Sexual dysfunction related to disease

NURSING INTERVENTION

- Monitor weight daily because antidiuertic hormone (ADH) and adreno-cortiocotropic hormone (ACTH), from the pituitary, regulate fluid retention and excretion in the body.
- Monitor intake and output to ensure the balance is equal due to hormone regulation.
- Explain to the patient:
  - The need to take medication for the rest of the patient's life.
  - The need for frequent laboratory tests.

5 *Hyperpituitarism (Acromegaly and Gigantism)*

WHAT WENT WRONG?

The pituitary gland produces an excessive amount of growth hormone. If hyperpituitarism occurs before epiphyseal closure, the patient (infants and children) has gigantism, resulting in an overgrowth of all body tissues. If hyperpituitarism occurs after epiphyseal closure, which is rare, the patient has acromegaly resulting in bone thickening, growth in width (transverse growth), and enlarged organs (visceromegaly).

PROGNOSIS

Successful treatment can stop progression of the disease; however, physical changes that occur before treatment begins are permanent.

HALLMARK SIGNS AND SYMPTOMS

- Increased body size caused by overproduction of growth hormone

INTERPRETING TEST RESULTS

- Increased serum growth hormone as the pituitary gland is producing an excess of growth hormone.
- Increased prolactin; most pituitary tumors will cause on overproduction of one or more of the pituitary hormones.
- Increased glucose; diabetes is common in acromegaly.

TREATMENT

- Administer dopamine agonists such as bromocriptine and cabergoline to decrease the tumor size.
- Surgical removal of the pituitary tumor.

NURSING DIAGNOSES

- Disturbed body image related to illness or illness treatment

NURSING INTERVENTIONS

- Perform range of motion exercise to assure joint mobility.
- Provide emotional support.

- Educate the patient:
  - Don't stop taking hormone replacement suddenly.

6 *Hyperprolactinemia*

WHAT WENT WRONG

There is an overproduction of the prolactin hormone that promotes lactation. Excessive secretion is usually caused by a pituitary tumor (prolactioma) but may also be due to hypothyroidism, chronic kidney disease, and medications that affect the pituitary gland.

PROGNOSIS

Prognosis is very good once a diagnosis is made and treatment of the underlying cause is started.

HALLMARK SIGNS AND SYMPTOMS

- The primary symptom is decreased fertility.
- In females, symptoms may include decreased or absent menstruation, headache, mood changes and galactorrhea, from hormone imbalance.
- Males may experience erectile dysfunction, diminished libido, gynecomastia, headache and mood changes from too much hormone.

INTERPRETING TEST RESULTS

- Increased serum TSH as hypothyroidism can be a contributing factor to hyperprolactimenia.
- Increased creatinine/BUN as renal failure can be a contributing factor.
- Serum human chorionic gonadotropin test for pregnancy (beta hGC) as pregnancy can cause hyperprolactinemia.
- Serum AST, ALT, and bilirubin will be increased as cirrhosis has been known to cause hyperprolactinemia.

- Serum testosterone, FSH, LH, prolactin, and estradiol may be decreased in hypogonadism.
- Pituitary tumor present in MRI.

TREATMENT

- Administer dopamine agonists:
  - bromocriptine
  - cabergoline to shrink pituitary tumor and return prolactin to normal levels
- Discontinue medications that may be causing the pituitary glands to over-produce prolactin:
  - amphetamines
  - estrogens
  - methyldopa
  - narcotics
  - protease inhibitors
  - risperidone
  - selective serotonin inhibitors
  - tricyclic inhibitors
  - verapamil
- Radiation therapy to reduce the pituitary tumor.
- Surgical removal of the pituitary tumor.

NURSING DIAGNOSES

- Disturbed body image related to illness or illness treatment
- Sexual dysfunction related to disease (related to loss of libido, infertility, impotence)

NURSING INTERVENTIONS

- Monitor serum hormone levels to assure that medication is improving the patient's condition.

Diabetes Insipidus

WHAT WENT WRONG?

Either a decrease in the production of an antidiuretic hormone (ADH) by the hypothalamus or an increase in the production of ADH by the pituitary compromises the ability of the kidneys to concentrate urine. This results in the excretion of large amounts of diluted urine. The patient then drinks large amounts of fluid to replace the increased urine output.

PROGNOSIS

Treatment will eliminate the symptoms of diabetes insipidus and the patient can expect a normal life span.

HALLMARK SIGNS AND SYMPTOMS

- Increased urination as the kidneys fail to concentrate urine
- Increased thirst as the body attempts to replace lost fluid

INTERPRETING TEST RESULTS

- Normal blood glucose indicating that diabetes insipidus isn't a complication of diabetes mellitus.
- Low specific gravity in urine due to increased fluid in the urine.
- Increased BUN, indicating dehydration because the concentration of solutes to fluid is rising.
- Electrolytes indicate dehydration; Na and Cl will rise as the concentration increases.
- Vasopressin challenge test. Those patients with diabetes insipidus will note a decrease in output and thirst.
- If urine output decreases and urine specific gravity increases, then the problem is with the pituitary gland and kidneys are normal.
- If urine output remains unchanged and urine specific gravity remains low, then the pituitary gland is normal and the kidneys are the problem.
- Presence of a pituitary tumor or hypothalamus tumor appear on an MRI.

TREATMENT

- Administer replacement ADH hormone such as desmopressin to return normal urination.
- Administer a diuretic such as hyrdrochlorothiazide to decrease urination.
- Place the patient on a low-salt diet to reduce urine production in the kidneys.
- Increase fluid intake until urination returns to normal.

NURSING DIAGNOSES

- Risk for impaired urinary elimination
- Impaired oral mucous membrane related to inadequate oral secretions
- Deficient fluid volume related to excessive fluid loss or inadequate fluid intake

NURSING INTERVENTION

- Maintain fluid and electrolyte balance.
- Monitor intake and output.
- Weigh the patient each day using the same scale, at the same time of day, wearing similar clothing.
- Explain to the patient:
  - Medication must be taken every day.
  - Wear a medical alert necklace/bracelet to alert health care providers that you have diabetes insipidus.

8 *Syndrome of Inappropriate Anti-diuretic Hormone Secretion (SIADH)*

WHAT WENT WRONG?

SIADH is caused by too much ADH being secreted by the posterior pituitary gland. ADH is responsible for controlling the amount of water reabsorbed by the kidney; it prevents the loss of too much fluid. When too much water is detected, ADH production or secretion is halted. SIADH may be caused by damage to the hypothalamus or pituitary, inflammation of the brain, some medications such as selective serotonin receptor inhibitors (SSRIs), carbamazapine, cyclophosphamides, and chlorpropamide. Certain cancers, especially lung, may produce ADH.

PROGNOSIS

If sodium (Na) levels are kept within normal limits, prognosis is excellent.

HALLMARK SIGNS AND SYMPTOMS

- Headaches due to hyponatremia
- Nausea and vomiting due to hyponatremia
- Confusion due to hyponatremia
- Personality changes due to hyponatremia

INTERPRETING TEST RESULTS

- Hyponatremia (low serum sodium) due to the dilution.

TREATMENT

- Administer saline IV to replenish sodium.
- Treat underlying cause.

NURSING DIAGNOSES

- Risk for imbalanced fluid volume
- Excess fluid volume

NURSING INTERVENTION

- Monitor electrolytes to determine sodium levels.
- Restrict fluid because excess fluid dilutes sodium levels.

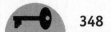

- Weigh the patient daily using the same scale, at same time of day with similar clothing.
- Monitor intake and output.

9 *Addison's Disease*

WHAT WENT WRONG?

Addison's disease is inadequate secretion of corticosteroids from the adrenal cortex, resulting from damage to the adrenal cortex. Autoimmune destruction of the adrenal gland and tuberculosis are two common causes of Addison's disease. A patient can experience Addisonian crisis when infection, surgery, or other stressful events results in a decrease in the production of cortisol and aldosterone. Addisonian crisis is a medical emergency.

PROGNOSIS

With ongoing treatment, patients can expect a normal life span.

HALLMARK SIGNS AND SYMPTOMS

- Weakness due to insufficient cortisol
- Weight loss due to insufficient cortisol
- Orthostatic hypotension due to poor fluid status from aldosterone deficiency
- Bronzing of the skin due to hyperpigmentation from the autoimmune disease

INTERPRETING TEST RESULTS

- Increased BUN due to dehydration.
- Increased serum potassium from changes in aldosterone secretion.
- Decreased serum cortisol being secreted from the adrenal cortex.
- Decreased serum glucose from decreased corticosteroids.
- Positive 24-hour urine aldosterone level due to less aldosterone being secreted.

- Positive ACTH stimulation test; ACTH acts on the adrenal cortex to stimulate adrenal hormone secretion. An infusion of ACTH is given and the test is positive if the infusion fails to raise the cortisol level.
- Abnormal adrenal glands appear on CT scan.

TREATMENT

- Administer cortisone or hydrocortisone to replace cortisol.
- Administer fludrocortisone to regulate sodium and potassium balance.
- Maintain fluid balance.

NURSING DIAGNOSES

- Fatigue related to disease state
- Risk for deficient fluid volume
- Disturbed body image related to disease state

NURSING INTERVENTION

- Monitor fluids and electrolytes.
- Weigh the patient daily.
- Suggest bone density test for osteoporosis due to decrease in mineralocorticoids.
- Explain to the patient:
  - Medication must be taken every day.
  - Wear a medical alert bracelet.
  - Keep an emergency supply of medication available.

10 *Cushing's Syndrome*

WHAT WENT WRONG?

The adrenal cortex secretes an excess of glucocorticoids or the pituitary gland an excess of ACTH as a result of either a pituitary tumor, adrenal tumor, or from ongoing glucocorticoid therapy.

PROGNOSIS

Patients can expect a normal life span once the tumor is removed; however, tumors may recur.

HALLMARK SIGNS AND SYMPTOMS

- Moon face during excess cortisol production
- Buffalo hump (fat pad located in the upper back) from excessive cortico-steroids
- Osteoporosis from an excess of corticosteroids, which weaken the bones
- Absence of menstruation (amenorrhea) from the effects of excess steroids
- Changes in mental status from excessive steroids

INTERPRETING TEST RESULTS

- Dexamethasone suppression test: A dose of glucocorticoid is given to test the hypothalamus-pituitary-adrenal axis. If there is suppression with the dose, it indicates a pituitary origin of the excess cortisol. If no suppression occurs, the etiology is an adrenal or ectopic tumor.
- Increased cortisol in 24-hour urine collection from excess production.
- Presence of a pituitary tumor or adrenal tumor on a CT; the tumor will show on a CT scan.
- Increased blood glucose due to overproduction of steroids.
- Increased sodium due to excess fluid loss.
- Decreased potassium.

TREATMENT

- Surgical removal of the pituitary tumor or adrenal tumor.

NURSING DIAGNOSES

- Disturbed body image related to illness
- Excess fluid volume related to excess water and sodium reabsorption
- Risk for infection related to immunosuppression and inadequate primary defenses

NURSING INTERVENTION

- Daily weighing to monitor fluid status.
- Monitor input and output to ensure adequate hydration.
- Monitor for glucose and acetone in urine as elevated levels of corticosteroids may produce hyperglycemia.
- Allow for adequate rest to allow the body to stabilize.
- Avoid trauma to the skin because elevated levels of corticosteroids can delay wound healing.
- Bone densitometry to assess for osteoporosis as corticosteroids can leech calcium from the bone.
- Following surgery:
  - Assist in early ambulation, deep breathing, coughing to facilitate mucous mobilization and decrease risk for emboli.
  - Monitor incision site for drainage, erythema, and signs of infection.
- Explain to patient:
  - Maintain a high-calorie, high-calcium diet to aid in wound repair and replace calcium.
  - Administer pain medication as needed.

11 *Primary Aldosteronism (Conn's Syndrome)*

WHAT WENT WRONG?

The adrenal cortex is secreting an excessive amount of aldosterone caused by an adrenal tumor, a malfunctioning adrenal cortex, or sources outside the adrenal gland producing aldosterone. Some medications, such as calcium channel blockers, can lower aldosterone levels which can confuse the diagnosis.

PROGNOSIS

The patient can expect a normal life span, if diagnosed and treated early.

HALLMARK SIGNS AND SYMPTOMS

- Increased blood pressure caused by the excess aldosterone
- Headache caused by increased blood pressure
- Muscle weakness from decreased serum potassium
- Increased thirst (polydispsia) due to high levels of aldosterone
- Increased urination (poluria) due to high levels of aldosterone

INTERPRETING TEST RESULTS

- Decreased serum potassium.
- 24-hour urine collection to monitor aldosterone, creatinine, and cortisol levels.
- Increased urinary aldosterone.
- Presence of an adrenal tumor on a CT scan.

TREATMENT

- Administer diuretics to control hypertension and raise potassium levels:
  - spironolactone
- Administer medications to block the affect of aldosterone:
  - eplerenone
- Surgically remove the adrenal tumor if present.

NURSING DIAGNOSES

- Risk for imbalanced fluid volume
- Risk for activity intolerance
- Impaired physical mobility

NURSING INTERVENTION

- Restrict sodium intake.
- Monitor intake and output.

- Weigh the patient daily.
- Explain to patient:
  - Thirst, dry mucous membranes are caused by low sodium. Allow sips of water, ice chips.

12 *Pheochromocytoma*

WHAT WENT WRONG?

A tumor on the adrenal medulla secretes excessive amounts of epinephrine and norepinephrine.

PROGNOSIS

Patients who are diagnosed and treated early can expect a normal life with close follow-up, if the tumor is benign. Patients can expect a limited prognosis if the tumor is malignant. Metastasis may develop at any time. The patient's hypertension often resolves with removal of the tumor, but may recur later in life.

HALLMARK SIGNS AND SYMPTOMS

- Uncontrollable hypertension as a result from increased epinephrine and norepinephrine
- Headaches as a result of hypertension
- Palpitations and tachycardia due to increased production of catecholamines
- Dilated pupils from increased production of epinephrine and norepinephrine

INTERPRETING TEST RESULTS

- Presences of catecholamines in serum.
- Increased catecholamines, metanephrines, and vanillylmandelic acid (VMA) in 24-hour urine collection.
- Presence of adrenal tumor shown in CT scan.

TREATMENT

- Surgical removal of the adrenal tumor.
- Administer antihypertensive medication to help lower blood pressure.
- Administer beta blockers to diminish effects of epinephrine and norepinephrine:
  - nifedipine
  - nicardipine
  - propranolol

NURSING DIAGNOSES

- Risk for delayed surgical recovery
- Ineffective tissue perfusion (cardiac)
- Anxiety

NURSING INTERVENTION

- Monitor blood pressure.
- Administer medication to control hypertension.
- Monitor urine for catecholamines.
- Decrease stress.
- Explain to patient:
  - Quit smoking to help lower blood pressure.
  - Reduce caffeine to help lower blood pressure.

13 *Hypoparathyroidism*

WHAT WENT WRONG?

Hypoparathyroidism is diminished functioning of the parathyroid glands leading to low levels of PTH, which causes hypocalcemia. The primary cause of hypoparathyroidism is destruction of the glands by an autoimmune cause. Para-thyroidectomy is no longer a major cause, since surgery now only removes the gland that is malfunctioning. Occasionally the gland(s) may be accidentally removed during thyroidectomy.

PROGNOSIS

Prognosis depends on the promptness with which a diagnosis is made and treatment started.

HALLMARK SIGNS AND SYMPTOMS

- Tetany (muscle irritability) due to abnormal levels of calcium
- Tingling of periorbital area, hands, and feet from abnormal calcium levels
- Lethargy due to low levels of parathyroid hormone
- Cataract development
- Convulsions due to acute low calcium levels

INTERPRETING TEST RESULTS

- Decreased serum calcium due to low levels of PTH.
- Increased serum phosphate due to low levels of PTH.
- Decreased serum PTH from diminished secretion from the parathyroid glands.
- Decreased urinary calcium from diminished PTH.
- Positive Chvostek's sign due to decreased calcium levels.
- Positive Trousseau's sign due to decreased calcium levels.

TREATMENT

- Initiate seizure precaution.
- Administer calcium gluconate by slow IV drip for acute hypocalcemia.

- Oral calcium—calcium gluconate, lactate, carbonate (Os-Cal).
- Large doses of vitamin D (calciferol) to help absorption of calcium.
- Aluminum hydroxide gel (Amphogel) or aluminum carbonate gel; basic (Basaljel) to decrease phosphate levels.
- Keep tracheostomy set and injectable calcium gluconate at bedside for impaired respiration from swelling as well as for emergency administration of calcium.

NURSING DIAGNOSES

- Risk for imbalanced nutrition: less than what body requires
- Ineffective health maintenance
- Impaired urinary elimination

NURSING INTERVENTION

- If the parathyroids were damaged during thyroid surgery:
  - Administer calcium to maintain the serum levels in a low normal range.
  - Testing should be done every 3 months.

14 *Hyperparathyroidism*

WHAT WENT WRONG?

Overactivity of the parathyroid glands caused by a tumor produces too much PTH, resulting in hypercalcemia and hypophosphatemia. Excess calcium is reabsorbed by the kidneys and may result in kidney stones; however, malfunction in the feedback mechanism prevents detection of excessive calcium levels in the blood, thereby failing to adjust the secretion of PTH. Parathyroid tumors are usually benign.

PROGNOSIS

Patients can expect a normal life span once the parathyroid tumor is removed.

HALLMARK SIGNS AND SYMPTOMS

- Asymptomatic
- Increased serum calcium level
- Bone pain or fracture as a result of excreting calcium from bone
- Kidney stones
- Frequent urination as a result of increased calcium in the urine (hypercalciuria)

INTERPRETING TEST RESULTS

- Increased serum calcium.
- Increased serum PTH.
- Decreased serum phosphate.
- Increased urine calcium.
- Presence of parathyroid tumor shows on ultrasound.
- Fine needle biopsy of the parathyroid tumor.

TREATMENT

- Surgical removal of the parathyroid tumor.
- Administer bisphosphonates to lower serum calcium by increasing calcium absorption in the bone.
- IV normal saline to dilute serum calcium.
- Diuretic such as furosemide to excrete excess calcium in the urine.

NURSING DIAGNOSES

- Impaired urinary elimination
- Activity intolerance
- Fatigue related to sleep deprivation

NURSING INTERVENTION

- Monitor intake and output.
- Monitor for fluid overload.
- Monitor electrolyte balance.

- Force fluids.
- Give the patient acid-ash juices such as cranberry juice.
- Strain urine for kidney stones.
- Place the patient on a low-calcium and high-phosphorus diet.
- Explain to patient:
  - Avoid over-the-counter calcium supplements.
  - Maintain daily activities.

15 *Diabetes Mellitus*

WHAT WENT WRONG?

Our body converts certain foods into glucose, which is the body's primary energy supply. Insulin from the beta cells of the pancreas is necessary to transport glucose into cells where it is used for cell metabolism. Diabetes mellitus occurs when beta cells either are unable to produce insulin (Type I diabetes mellitus) or produce an insufficient amount of insulin (Type II diabetes mellitus). As a result, glucose does not enter cells but remains in the blood. Increased glucose levels in the blood signal to the patient to increase intake of fluid in an effort to flush glucose out of the body in urine. Patients then experience increased thirst and increased urination. Cells become starved for energy because of the lack of glucose and signal to the patient to eat, causing the patient to experience an increase in hunger. There are three types of diabetes mellitus. These are Type I, known as insulin-dependent (IDDM), where beta cells are destroyed by an autoimmune process; Type II, known as non-insulin-dependent (NIDDM), where beta cells produce insufficient insulin; and gestational diabetes mellitus (DM that occurs during pregnancy).

PROGNOSIS

Patients with Type I and Type II diabetes mellitus are at risk for complications such as vision loss (diabetic retinopathy), damage to blood vessels and nerves (diabetic neuropathy), and kidney damage (nephropathy). However, complications can be minimized by maintaining a normal blood glucose level through consistent monitoring, administering insulin, and dieting. Patients with gestational diabetes mellitus will recover following pregnancy; however, they are at risk for developing Type II diabetes mellitus later in life.

HALLMARK SIGNS AND SYMPTOM

Type I:

- Fast onset because no insulin is being produced
- Increased appetite (polyphagia) because cells are starved for energy, signals a need for more food
- Increased thirst (polydipsia) from the body attempting to rid itself of glucose
- Increased urination (polyuria) from the body attempting to rid itself of glucose
- Weight loss since glucose is unable to enter cells
- Frequent infections as bacteria feeds on the excess glucose
- Delayed healing because elevated glucose levels in the blood hinders healing process

Type II:

- Slow onset because some insulin is being produced
- Increased thirst (polydipsia) from the body attempting to rid itself of glucose
- Increased urination (polyuria) from the body attempting to rid itself of glucose
- Candidal infection as bacteria feeds on the excess glucose
- Delayed healing because elevated glucose levels in the blood hinder the healing process

Gestational:

- Asymptomatic
- Some patients may experience increased thirst (polydipsia) from the body attempting to rid itself of glucose

INTERPRETING TEST RESULTS

- Increased glucose in urine (glucosuria).
- Fasting plasma blood glucose test with a serum glucose level of 126 mg/dL (7.0 mmol/l) on three different tests.
- Oral glucose tolerance test (OGTT) with plasma glucose of 200 mg/dL (11.1 mmol/l) two hours after ingesting 75 grams oral glucose.
- Random plasma glucose at or above 200 mg/dL (11.1 mmol/l).
- Glycosylated hemoglobin A1C 6.0 percent or higher.

TREATMENT

Type I:

- Regular monitoring of blood glucose.
- Administer insulin to maintain normal blood glucose levels (see Table 8-1).
- Maintain a diabetic diet.
- Administer:
  - Rapid-acting:
    - aspart
      - lispro
      - glulisine
      - human insulin—a rapid-acting insulin for before-meal control
    - inhaled insulin
  - Short-acting:
    - regular insulin
  - Intermediate:
    - human insulin—NPH
    - human insulin—zinc—lente
  - Long-acting:
    - human insulin—zinc—ultralente
    - insulin detemir
    - insulin glargine
    - combination products also available

Table 8-1   Insulin guide

Drug	Synonym	Appearance	Onset	Peak	Duration	Compatibility
Rapid-acting	Regular	Clear	<.25 hr	2 to 4 hrs	3 to 6 hrs	All insulin except lente. Aspart is not compatible.
Intermediate-acting	NPH	Cloudy	1 to 1.5 hrs	8 to 12 hrs	6 to 24 hrs	Regular insulin
Long-acting	Ultralente	Cloudy	4 to 6 hrs	16 to 20 hrs	30 to 36 hrs	Regular

Table 8-2   Oral Hypoglycemic Agents

Drug	Onset	Peak	Duration	Comments

Oral sulfonylureas
  chlorproamide
  glyburide
  glipizide
  glimepiride
  tolbutamide
  tolazamide
	1 hr
	1 hr
	15 min–1 hr
		4 to 6 hrs
		4 to 6 hrs
		2 to 8 hrs
			12 to 24 hrs
			40 to 60 hrs
			10 to 24 hrs
				chlorpropamide—use caution with renal or hepatic patients

Oral biguanides metformin	2 to 2.5 hrs		10 to 16 hrs	Decreases glucose production in liver; decrease intestinal absorption of glucose and improves insulin sensitivity

Oral alpha-glucosidose inhibitor
  acarbose
  miglitol
	Rapid	1 hr
		2 to 3 hrs
				Delays glucose absorption and digestion of carbs; lowers blood sugar; reduces plasma glucose and insulin

DPP4 inhibitors meglitinide analogs				Stimulate secretion of insulin from pancreas
D-phenylalanine derivative incretin mimetics				Stimulates insulin production Assists pancreatic insulin production; regulates liver production of glucose; decreases appetite; slows glucose transit from stomach to intestine

Type II:

- Maintain ideal body weight through diet and exercise.
- Regular monitoring of blood glucose.
- Administer oral sulfonylureas to stimulate secretion of insulin from the pancreas (see Table 8-2).
- Administer oral biguanides to reduce blood glucose production by the liver:
  - metformin
- Administer thiazolidinediones to sensitize peripheral tissues to insulin:
  - rosiglitazone

- pioglitazone
- Administer meglitinide analogs to stimulate section of insulin from the pancreas:
  - repaglinide
- Administer D-phenylalanine derivative to stimulate insulin production:
  - nateglinide
- Administer alpha-glucosidase inhibitors to delay absportion of carbohydrates in the intestine:
  - acarbose
  - miglitol
- Administer DPP4—dipeptidyl peptidase 4 inhibitors: to slow the inactivation of incretin hormones, GLP-I to assist insulin production in the pancreas:
  - sitagliptin
- Administer incretin mimetics to assist insulin production in the pancreas and help regulate liver production of glucose. It also decreases appetite and increases the time glucose remains in the stomach before entering the small intestine for absorption.
- Administer amylin analog that causes glucose to enter the bloodstream slowly; can cause weight loss:
  - pramlintide

Gestational:

- Maintain weight through diet and exercise.
- No oral diabetes medication; most are contraindicated in pregnancy.
- Administer insulin if diet and exercise fail to control blood glucose levels.

NURSING DIAGNOSES

- Risk for imbalanced nutrition: less than what body requires
- Risk for injury related to sensory alterations
- Risk for delayed surgical recovery
- Knowledge deficit for disease process
- Body image disturbance
- Nutrition self-care deficit

NURSING INTERVENTION

- Educate the patient about:
  - The disease and the importance of maintaining normal glucose levels.
  - Demonstrate blood glucose monitoring.
  - Diet and food choices, including portion sizes.
  - Encourage exercise.
  - Discuss coping skills to reduce stress.
  - Teach self-injection of insulin (Type I).
  - Urge smoking cessation.
  - Self-care.
  - Acute management.
  - Prevention of complications, such as hyperglycemia and hypoglycemia.
  - Teach importance of daily medications.
  - Explain hypoglycemia signs and symptoms and interventions.
  - Sweating, lethargy, confusion, hunger, dizziness, weakness (Type I).
  - Teach the management of hypoglycemia: glucose tablets, or 4 ounces of fruit juice, several hard candies, or a small amount of a carbohydrate.
  - Explain the signs and symptoms of hyperglycemia: fatigue, headache, blurry vision, dry itchy skin.
  - Teach the management of hyperglycemia: a change in medication or dosage, increase in regular exercise, more careful food intake and meal planning, an increase in the number of fingersticks, discussion with the MD/NP/PA.
  - Teach glucagon injection for hypoglycemic events.

16 *Metabolic Syndrome (Syndrome X/Dysmetabolic Syndrome)*

WHAT WENT WRONG?

Patients have a collection of symptoms that include high blood glucose, obesity, high blood pressure, and high triglycerides based on family history. Beta cells in the pancreas are unable to produce sufficient insulin while the liver produces a higher level of glucose. The patient is also insulin-resistant. This syndrome leads to cardiovascular disease.

PROGNOSIS

A diagnosis of metabolic syndrome puts one at high risk for the development of diabetes and heart disease. Changes in lifestyle must be made to decrease the chance of incurring these diseases.

HALLMARK SIGNS AND SYMPTOMS

- Hypertension
- Abdominal obesity

INTERPRETING TEST RESULTS

- Decreased HDL.
- Increased LDL.
- Increased triglycerides.
- Elevated fasting glucose.

TREATMENT

- Administer statin to lower LDL.
- Administer niacin to raise HDL.
- Administer fibrates to lower triglycerides.
- Administer ACE inhibitors to lower blood pressure.
- Administer angiotensin receptor blockers to lower blood pressure.
- Administer insulin sensitizers to improve the effectiveness of insulin.
- Manage weight through diet and exercise.

NURSING DIAGNOSES

- Readiness for enhanced nutritional metabolic pattern

- Risk for injury related to hyperglycemia
- Readiness for enhanced activity program

NURSING INTERVENTIONS

- Monitor blood glucose.
- Encourage weight loss.
- Explain to patient:
  - It is important to continue medication even if symptoms are not present.

Crucial Diagnostic Tests

ACTH Stimulation Test

This test measures the level of cortisol in a patient's blood after injection of synthetic ACTH. It is used to diagnose Cushing's syndrome, Cushing's disease, primary adrenal insufficiency, and ACTH insufficiency. Explain to the patient that this is a non-fasting blood test.

Aldosterone Test

This test measures the level of the hormone aldosterone in the blood. It is part of the workup for hypertension and is also used in diagnosing aldosteronism, adrenal adenoma, hyperplasia, nephrotic syndrome, Addison's Disease, Diabetes Mellitus, and acute alcohol intake. Explain to the patient that this is a non-fasting blood test.

Blood (Serum) Calcium Level Test

This test measures the level of calcium in the blood. It is used to evaluate parathyroid and renal function. Also, the level rises in certain malignancies. Explain to the patient that this is a non-fasting blood test.

Cortisol Test

This test measures the level of the hormone cortisol in the blood. It is performed to diagnose Addison's disease, nephritic syndrome, Cushing's syndrome, acute illness, trauma, septic shock, starvation, chronic renal failure, and pregnancy. Explain to the patient that this is a non-fasting blood test.

Fine Needle Biopsy/Aspiration

A small needle is passed through the skin into the area to be biopsied, retrieving a small amount of fluid or tissue to be analyzed. Depending on the organ or tissue to be studied, the procedure may be done in an outpatient or inpatient setting. The test is done to look for the presence of abnormal cells.

Before the test—An informed consent is necessary, as local anesthesia will be utilized.

After the test—A dressing will be applied to the site. Monitor the site for inflammation, drainage, bleeding, increased pain, fever, or any increase in swelling. An OTC analgesic or Rx from the practitioner may be necessary.

Follicle Stimulating Hormone (FSH) Test

This test measures the level of FSH in the blood. It is done to aid in the diagnosis of hypogonadism, precocious puberty, menstrual disorders, and the inability to conceive. Explain to the patient that this is a non-fasting blood test.

Glucose Tolerance Test

A 75–100 gram carbohydrate drink is to be swallowed by the fasting patient. Blood work and urine specimens are obtained at 30 minutes, and then hourly for 3–4 hours. The test is done to evaluate those with elevated blood sugars, those with risk factors for diabetes, and pregnant women to ascertain their risk for gestational diabetes.

Before the test—Explain to the patient the need for a 12 hour fast prior to the test and water only throughout the test.

Growth Hormone (GH), (Somatotropin) Test

A growth hormone test measures the level of GH in the blood and is part of the diagnostic workup for identifying the cause of abnormal GH production. It is performed to diagnose diminished or excessive growth, immature puberty, and pituitary abnormalities. Testing usually involves either a GH stimulation test or a GH suppression test to track GH levels over time.

Before the test—Explain to the patient that stress, exercise, and low blood sugar may increase the level of GH. Instruct the patient to fast for 10–12 hours..

Glycosylated Hemoglobin (Hgb A1C) Test

This test measures the amount of sugar that is attached to the hemoglobin in red blood cells. Because red blood cells live in the bloodstream for 100–120 days, the Hgb A1C test shows the average blood sugar level for the past several months. The test is done to evaluate the effectiveness of long–term diabetes management.

Before the test—Explain to the patient that the test is not affected by recent food intake, medication or exercise.

Luteinizing Hormone (LH) Test

This test measures the amount of LH in a sample of blood or urine. It is done to evaluate reasons for infertility, menstrual problems, precocious puberty and delayed puberty.

Before the test—Explain to the patient this is a non-fasting blood test. The patient may be asked to stop taking certain medications, including birth control pills, for up to 4 weeks before the test.

Parathyroid Hormone (PTH) Test

This test measures the level of PTH in the blood. It is used as a means of assessing the level of blood calcium, since PTH is one of the major factors affecting calcium metabolism. The test is performed to evaluate parathyroid function and to check for abnormal calcium levels.

Before the test—Explain to the patient to have nothing to eat or drink from midnight until after the test the next morning. Some prescripton drugs affect the PTH test and the patient may be asked to stop taking them prior to the test.

Prolactin Test

This test measures the level of prolactin in the blood. The test is done to determine the cause of galactorrhea (inappropriate lactation), to diagnose infertility and erectile dysfunction, and to assess for pituitary adenomas. Explain to the patient that this is a non-fasting blood test.

Triiodothyronine (T3) Test

This test measures the level of T3 in the blood in order to determine whether the thyroid is functioning properly. It is used primarily to help diagnose hyperthyroidism and is usually ordered following an abnormal TSH or T4 test. Explain to the patient that this is a non-fasting blood test.

Thyroxine Total (T4) Test

This test measures the amount of T4 in the blood and is ordered to evaluate the thyroid function and to help diagnose hyperthyroidism and hypothyroidism. Explain to the patient that this is a non-fasting blood test.

Thyroid Stimulating Hormone (TSH) Test

This blood test measures the level of TSH in the blood and is used to check for thyroid gland problems. It may be done at the same time as tests to measure T3 and T4. Explain to the patient that this is a non-fasting blood test.

Thyroid Scintiscan (Thyroid Scan)

A radioactive substance is orally given to the patient, who returns at a designated time for a thyroid scan. The test is done to assess nodules as either hot (functioning) which often indicates a goiter or a benign mass or cold (non-functioning) which may indicate a cancer, thyroiditis or other disease process.

Before the test—Find out whether the patient has any allergies to iodine or shellfish. Speak to the practitioner about withholding thyroid medications before the test. It is a non-invasive test.

Urinary Catecholamines

This test, a 24-hour urine test, measures the amount of the hormones epinephrine, norepinephrine, and dopamine in the body. The test is done to assess for pheochromocytoma (tumor of the adrenal gland) as the cause of elevated blood pressure.

Before the test—Instruct the patient to collect urine in a special container for a 24-hour period. Explain to the patient that the test is started in the morning. Discard the first voided specimen, then save subsequent specimens, ending with the first voided specimen the following day. A preservative has been added to the container and it must be refrigerated.

Vasopressin Challenge Test

This test is performed assess the ability of the kidneys to concentrate urine and to help determine which type of diabetes insipidus is present. Vasopressin is injected subcutaneously. Serum and urine samples are collected at 1 to 2-hour intervals after the injection, and the osmolality of these samples is measured in the laboratory.

Before the test—Explain to the patient that fluids are restricted the evening before the test and the patient must be NPO after midnight. Any extra fluid or food intake invalidates the test.

Quiz

1. Annabelle has been referred to an endocrinologist for evaluation of the following symptoms: infertility, hypogonadism, and delayed puberty. Which hormone from the pituitary is lacking in Annabelle?

   (a) FSH and LH.

   (b) ACTH.

   (c) TSH.

   (d) Growth hormone.

2. Twenty-eight-year-old Alicia has recently been diagnosed with hyperthyroidism. Signs and symptoms regarding hyperthyroidism include:

   (a) tachycardia, sweating, and tremors.

   (b) fatigue, lethargy, and weight gain.

   (c) muscle twitching, tetany, and galactorrhea.

   (d) scotoma, alopecia, and hirsutism.

3. You are providing patient teaching for 46-year-old Anthony about his new medication levothyroxine. Treatment for hypothyroidism depends on:

   (a) length of time to make the diagnosis.

   (b) gender.

   (c) symptoms.

   (d) etiology of the disease.

4. You explain to Anthony that his symptoms should resolve as the medication reaches an appropriate level. Presenting signs and symptoms of hypothyroidism include:

   (a) fatigue and cold intolerance.

   (b) weight loss and hyperglycemia.

   (c) polydipsia and polyphagia.

   (d) tachycardia and diarrhea.

5. Antoinette has gone to her primary care provider for a routine physical. Some of her lab results indicated an endocrine disorder. In hyperparathyroidism which test results are typical?

   (a) Decreased WBC and increased alkaline phosphatase.

   (b) Increased calcium and decreased phosphate.

   (c) Decreased parathyroid hormone and increased magnesium.

   (d) Increased parathyroid hormone and decreased calcium.

6. Addison's disease frequently causes skin pigment changes. When teaching the patient about medications used for Addison's disease, it is important that he or she understands:

(a) medication for hypertension.

(b) cholesterol medication.

(c) that they continue for life.

(d) that they can be stopped when symptoms abate.

7. Addie has recently been diagnosed with Cushing's syndrome. The symptoms for which the primary care provider most likely tested the patient include:

(a) buffalo hump, moon facies, and central obesity.

(b) diarrhea, confusion, and exophthalmos.

(c) weight loss, low blood pressure, and tachycardia.

(d) nausea, low hemoglobin, and shortness of breath.

8. Alison is being treated for hyperthyroidism. In reviewing her lab results, you would expect to see:

(a) diminished thyroid hormone.

(b) elevated thyroid hormone.

(c) diminished parathyroid hormone.

(d) elevated parathyroid hormone.

9. Adam has just been diagnosed with diabetes insipidus. The most common presenting sign is:

(a) body wasting.

(b) hyperglycemia.

(c) hypoglycemia.

(d) increase in urination.

10. Alexa, a 32-year-old female, has been diagnosed with metabolic syndrome. Your nursing interventions would include teaching her about the typical accompanying signs and symptoms, such as:

(a) weight loss, malar rash, and pharyngitis.

(b) hypothyroidism, podagra, and elevated fasting glucose.

(c) violaceous rash, pittting peripheral edema, and palpitation.

(d) hypertension, low HDL, and elevated triglycerides.

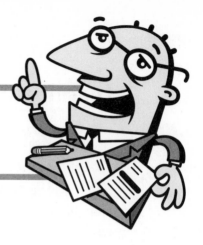

CHAPTER 9

Genitourinary System

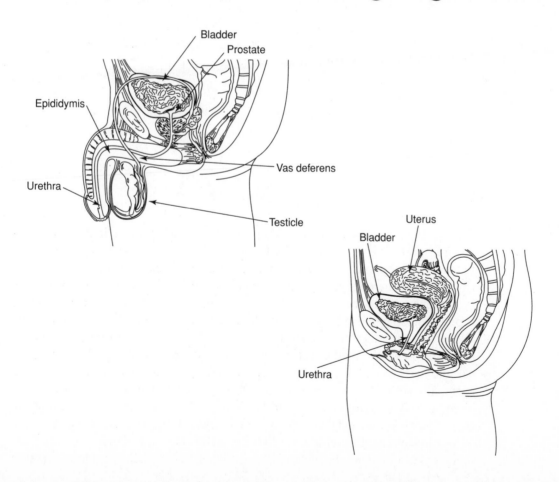

Learning Objectives

1 Benign prostatic hypertrophy (BPH)
2 Bladder cancer
3 Acute glomerulonephritis
4 Kidney cancer
5 Kidney stones

6 Prostate cancer
7 Pyelonephritis
8 Renal failure
9 Testicular cancer
10 Urinary tract infection

Key Terms

Azotemia
Bacilli Calmette-Guérin
Bladder biopsy
Cystoscopy
Glomerular filtration rate
Hematuria

Nephrectomy
Nephritic syndrome
Nephrolithiasis
Nocturia
Oliguria
Peripheral edema

Renal calculi
Transrectal ultrasound
Urinary frequency
Urinary hesitancy
Urinary urgency
· Urography

How the Genitourinary System Works

The genitourinary system refers to the parts of the body involved in the production and transport of urine, as well as the surrounding structures. The kidneys are found in the posterior part of the upper abdominal area, relatively protected by the lower ribs. They are lateral to the spinal column. The left kidney is found higher than the right kidney due to the location of the liver within the abdomen. The renal artery supplies blood to the kidneys. The nephron is the functional unit of the kidney, the area where urine is formed. Within the nephron, there is a long tubule. This initially surrounds the glomerulus in an area called Bowman's capsule. Bowman's capsule narrows into a proximal convoluted tubule which has many curves and eventually straightens into a downward loop of Henle, which makes a sharp turn to come back up into the cortex of the kidney. The initial upward portion of the loop of Henle is thin and then becomes thick, which is the distal convoluted tubule.

The kidneys are responsible for filtering wastes from the bloodstream; they aid in the control of fluid and electrolyte balance, acid-base balance, blood pressure control through production of renin, and red blood cell production through the production of erythropoetin. As urine is produced within the kidneys, it travels through the ducts (ureters) to the bladder. Once the body senses the urge to empty the bladder, the detruser muscles contract and the sphincter at the bladder neck relaxes to aid in emptying the urine. The urine passes through the urethra to the outside. Male patients have a prostate gland located under the bladder, surrounding the urethra. Prostatic fluid is secreted from the gland into the urethra.

Just the Facts

1   *Benign Prostatic Hypertrophy (BPH)*

WHAT WENT WRONG?

The prostate gland is found just below the bladder in men, surrounding the urethra. As men age, the prostate enlarges, putting pressure on the surrounding structures and causing symptoms such as frequent urination and urinary retention. The enlargement of the prostate causes narrowing of the urethra and upward pressure on the lower border of the bladder. Urinary retention may develop, as the body has a harder time emptying the bladder. Hydronephrosis and dilation of the renal pelvis and ureter are complications of the urinary retention due to overgrowth of the prostate.

PROGNOSIS

The symptoms of BPH are the same as those for prostate cancer. It is important for the patients to have regular check-ups to evaluate for risk of prostate cancer and conduct periodic screenings for prostate cancer. Renal function may be temporarily effected by hydronephrosis secondary to urinary retention.

HALLMARK SIGNS AND SYMPTOMS

- Urinary hesitancy—difficulty initiating stream of urine due to pressure on urethra and bladder neck
- Urinary frequency—need to urinate frequently due to pressure on bladder
- Urinary urgency—need to get to bathroom quickly to urinate due to pressure on bladder

- Nocturia—need to get up at night to urinate due to pressure on bladder
- Decrease in force of urinary stream
- Intermittent stream of urination
- Hematuria

INTERPRETING TEST RESULTS

- Urography shows high volume of post-void residual urine.
- PSA (prostate-specific antigen) may be mildly elevated.
- Prostate ultrasound shows hypertrophy.
- Digital rectal exam reveals fullness of prostate and loss of median sulcus (midline groove between the two lateral lobes of the prostate).
- Urinalysis may show microscopic hematuria.
- BUN and creatinine levels may elevate, if renal function is impaired.

TREATMENT

- Administer alpha$_1$-blockers for symptom relief:
  - doxazosin
  - tamsulosin
  - terazosin
- Monitor blood pressure; hypotension may be side effect of some alpha$_1$-blockers.
- Administer finasteride to relieve symptoms by shrinking prostate gland.
- Monitor PSA levels periodically.
- Monitor renal function.
- Surgical removal of prostate tissue to relieve pressure.
- Continuous bladder irrigation postoperatively.
- Administer antispasmodics for patients experiencing bladder spasms.

NURSING DIAGNOSIS

- Risk for impaired urinary elimination
- Urinary retention
- Risk for urge urinary incontinence

NURSING INTERVENTIONS

- Maintain the 3-port catheter postop. One port is for irrigation, another is for drainage, and the third to inflate a balloon that holds the catheter in position.
- Monitor intake and output.
- Monitor vital signs for changes.
- Monitor postoperative patient's bladder irrigation:
  - Monitor the amount of fluid instilled and the amount of fluid returned and subtract the amount of fluid instilled from the amount returned to determine the actual urine output.
- Document color of urinary output postoperatively; the greatest risk of hemorrhage is the first day after the operation.
- Monitor for bladder spasms which may indicate blocked catheter drainage postoperatively.
- Teach patient:
  - Avoid caffeine, alcohol, decongestants, anticholinergics which may increase symptoms of BPH.
  - Proper home care of urinary catheter.
  - Monitor for signs of urinary tract infection.

2 *Bladder Cancer*

WHAT WENT WRONG?

Bladder cancer is typically a nonaggressive cancer that occurs in the transitional cell layer of the bladder. It is recurrent in nature. Less frequently, bladder cancer is found invading deeper layers of the bladder tissue. In these cases the cancer tends to be more aggressive. Exposure to industrial chemicals (paints, textiles), history of cyclophosphamide use, and smoking increase the risks for bladder cancer.

PROGNOSIS

The more aggressive the cancer cell type, the greater the risk of metastasis of the disease. Patients may have advanced disease at the time of diagnosis. The more advanced the disease at the time of diagnosis and the more aggressive the tumor, the greater the risk of death for the patient.

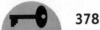

HALLMARK SIGNS AND SYMPTOMS

- Fatigue—due to chronic process
- Hematuria—blood in urine, may be microscopic
- Change in urinary pattern—color, frequency, or amount of urine

INTERPRETING TEST RESULTS

- Urinalysis shows red blood cells in urine.
- Cystoscopy to identify tumor site and obtain biopsy.
- Bladder biopsy shows cancer cell type.
- CT scan shows metastasis or invasion of tumor.

TREATMENT

- Surgical removal of tumor:
  - May be removal of superficial tumor from bladder wall with transurethral approach; removal of part or all of the bladder.
  - If all of the bladder is removed, a stoma is created on the surface of the abdomen or an ileal reservoir is created internally to collect the urine.
- Instillation of BCG (bacilli Calmette-Guérin) into bladder to decrease chance of recurrence.
- Radiation therapy.
- Chemotherapy.

NURSING DIAGNOSIS

- Risk of impaired urinary elimination
- Disturbed body image
- Fear
- Powerlessness

NURSING INTERVENTIONS

- Monitor vital signs.
- Monitor intake and output:
  - Document amount and color of drainage from all drains.

- Monitor color of urine.
- Monitor stoma for color, checking adequate blood flow to tissue.
- Monitor abdomen for bowel sounds, pain, distention.
- Monitor skin for signs of breakdown, redness.
- Monitor for side effects of medications.
- Teach patient:
  - Proper skin care postoperatively.
  - Catheterization of ileal reservoir if needed.

3 *Acute Glomerulonephritis*

WHAT WENT WRONG?

Glomerulonephritis, also known as acute nephritic syndrome, is typically preceded by an ascending infection or occurs secondary to another systemic disorder. Infectious causes include group A beta-hemolytic Streptococcus, measles, mumps, cytomegalovirus, varicella, coxsackievirus, pneumonia due to mycoplasma, chlamydia psittaci, or pneumococcal infection. Systemic disorders include systemic lupus erythematosus, viral hepatitis B or C, thrombotic thrombocytopenia purpura, or multiple myeloma.

PROGNOSIS

Depending on the cause, the acute episode may completely resolve. Patients should be monitored during the occurrence; signs of renal function need to be checked.

HALLMARK SIGNS AND SYMPTOMS

- Hematuria
- Peripheral edema
- Elevated blood pressure, compared with patient's norm
- Oliguria—decrease in urine output
- Nausea, vomiting, loss of appetite as renal function declines

INTERPRETING TEST RESULTS

- Urinalysis shows red blood cells and red blood cell casts.
- Glomerular filtration rate will be decreased.
- 24-hour urine collection for protein will be elevated.
- BUN level will be increased.
- Serum albumin will be decreased.
- Renal biopsy to determine cause.

TREATMENT

- Monitor renal function.
- Monitor electrolyte levels.
- Monitor vital signs.
- Administer diuretics to remove excess fluids.
- Monitor urinary output.
- Restrict fluid intake—measure output, intake should match 24-hour output plus 500 cc.
- Plasmapheresis if due to autoimmune cause.

NURSING DIAGNOSIS

- Impaired urinary elimination
- Excess fluid volume

NURSING INTERVENTIONS

- Monitor vital signs.
- Monitor intake and output.
- Weigh daily.
- Assess respiratory system for lung sounds, difficulty breathing, crackles in lungs suggesting fluid overload.
- Assess cardiovascular status, heart rate, heart sounds, presence of S_3 suggesting fluid overload.

- Assess extremities for edema.
- Teach patient about medications, disease process.

4 *Kidney Cancer*

WHAT WENT WRONG?

Kidney cancer occurs when cancer cells create a tumor within the kidney. Exposure to chemicals, lead, and smoking all increase the risk of developing kidney cancer.

PROGNOSIS

Identification of renal cancer is integral to a favorable outcome. Patients often have vague symptoms and may not seek healthcare until later in the disease when the cancer is well developed. Metastatic disease has the worst prognosis.

HALLMARK SIGNS AND SYMPTOMS

- Weight loss
- Anemia due to altered erythropoetin production
- Hematuria
- Elevated blood pressure due to increase in renin production
- Flank pain, dull or aching, occurs in small amount of patients

INTERPRETING TEST RESULTS

- CBC may show either anemia or erythrocytosis.
- Urinalysis shows red blood cells.
- Erythrocyte sedimentation rate elevated.
- Ultrasound shows renal mass.
- CT scan with contrast shows renal mass.
- MRI shows renal mass.

TREATMENT

- Surgical removal by nephrectomy.
- Tumor destruction by radiofrequency ablation.
- Chemotherapy.

NURSING DIAGNOSIS

- Fear
- Impaired skin integrity
- Risk of impaired urinary elimination

NURSING INTERVENTIONS

- Monitor vital signs for changes.
- Monitor intake and output.
- Monitor operative site for redness, swelling, and bleeding.
- Monitor pain level postoperatively.
- Hourly urine output monitoring for first 24 to 48 hours postoperatively.
- Monitor hemoglobin and hematocrit as scheduled.
- Monitor for signs of infection postoperatively.

5 *Kidney Stones*

WHAT WENT WRONG?

Kidney stones, also known as renal calculi or nephrolithiasis, occur within the kidneys. Stones can also form elsewhere within the urinary tract. The patient may not have any symptoms from kidney stones until the stone attempts to move down the ureter towards the bladder. Patients develop crystals within the urine. A slow flow of urine gives the crystals time to form a stone. Crystals may be formed from calcium, uric acid, cystine, or struvite. Medications such as diuretics can increase the risk of kidney stone formation in some patients.

PROGNOSIS

A stone may lodge in the ureter blocking the flow of urine. Hydronephrosis and swelling of the ureter may follow. Kidney stones typically recur, especially in those with a family history of nephrolithiasis.

HALLMARK SIGNS AND SYMPTOMS

- Hematuria
- Unilateral spasms of pain in the flank area (renal colic)
- Pain may radiate to lower abdomen, groin, scrotum or labia
- Nausea, vomiting, and sweating associated with occurrence of pain
- Elevated blood pressure with pain
- Extreme flank pain that comes slowly or quickly

INTERPRETING TEST RESULTS

- Urinalysis shows red blood cells.
- Ultrasound shows stones.
- X-ray of kidneys, ureters, and bladder (KUB) shows stones.
- CT scan shows stones.
- MRI shows stones.

TREATMENT

- Provide pain relief:
  - narcotics such as morphine
  - non-narcotics such as ketorolac, a nonsteroidal anti-inflammatory
- Administer antispasmodics as adjuncts for pain control.
- Increase fluid intake to flush through the urinary tract.
- Lithotripsy—shock waves are used to break the stone into very small pieces that can pass more easily.
- Stent placement to allow free flow of urine and passage of small stones or stone pieces.
- Surgical removal of stone.

NURSING DIAGNOSIS

- Risk of impaired urinary elimination
- Acute pain

NURSING INTERVENTIONS

- Monitor intake and output.
- Monitor pain level and response to pain medications.
- Strain urine to obtain stone for analysis in lab.
- Teach patient about:
  - Adequate fluid intake.
  - Medications used to reduce chance of recurrence.
  - Dietary modifications needed based on content of stone.

6 *Prostate Cancer*

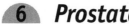

WHAT WENT WRONG?

Cancer of the prostate typically is found in the peripheral area of the prostate gland. Nodules may be palpable on digital rectal exam. There is a greater incidence as men age. African-American males and those with a family history of the disease have a higher risk for prostate cancer. The symptoms of prostate cancer are the same as those of benign prostatic hypertrophy.

PROGNOSIS

Prostate cancer is the most common cancer found in American males, and the second leading cancer-related cause of death. The number of cases of prostate cancer found on autopsy are even higher than those found clinically. Screening for prostate cancer has increased the number of cases identified.

HALLMARK SIGNS AND SYMPTOMS

- Urinary hesitancy—difficulty initiating stream of urine due to pressure on urethra and bladder neck

- Urinary frequency—need to urinate frequently due to pressure on bladder
- Urinary urgency—need to get to bathroom quickly to urinate due to pressure on bladder
- Nocturia—need to get up at night to urinate due to pressure on bladder
- Decrease in force of urinary stream
- Intermittent stream of urination
- Hematuria
- Palpable nodule on digital rectal examination
- Urinary retention due to enlargement of the tumor, blocking flow of urine
- Back pain due to metastasis

INTERPRETING TEST RESULTS

- PSA elevates as tumor size increases.
- Digital rectal exam may reveal nodule.
- Transrectal ultrasound used to identify prostate cancer and determine the stage.
- MRI to identify prostate lesions and involvement of surrounding tissue or lymph nodes.
- Biopsy to identify cell type.
- Alkaline phosphatase elevates with metastasis to bone.

TREATMENT

- Radiation therapy:
- External beam.
- Brachytherapy—insertion of radioactive substance into prostate.
- Surgery—radical prostatectomy.
- Chemotherapy.
- Cryosurgery—freezing of tissue with ultrasound guidance.
- Watchful waiting—monitoring PSA and ultrasound depending on patient's age and cell type of cancer and any comorbidities.
- Hormonal treatment to suppress natural androgen production:
- leuprolide
- goserelin
- estrogen
- Orchiectomy to reduce natural androgen production.

NURSING DIAGNOSIS

- Fear
- Impaired urinary elimination
- Pain

NURSING INTERVENTIONS

- Monitor vital signs.
- Monitor intake and output.
- Assess abdomen for signs of bladder distention due to urinary retention.
- Assess for pain in back.
- Assess skin for signs of redness or breakdown if undergoing radiation treatments.
- Monitor for side effects of medications.

7   *Pyelonephritis*

WHAT WENT WRONG?

Pyelonephritis is an infection involving the kidneys. Inflammation of the tissue accompanies the infectious process. The most common bacteria are *E. coli*, *Klebsiella*, *Enterobacter*, *Proteus*, *Pseudomonas*, and *Staphylococcus saprophyticus*. Typically the infection begins in the lower urinary tract and ascends upward. Identification of infections and initiation of treatment is important to prevent the infection from getting worse.

PROGNOSIS

Older patients and patients with comorbidities have a greater chance of complications from pyelonephritis. Impaired renal function may complicate recovery in some patients. Septic shock may occur.

HALLMARK SIGNS AND SYMPTOMS

- Flank pain
- Fever due to infection

- Chills
- Frequency, urgency, dysuria due to urinary tract infection
- Nausea, vomiting, and diarrhea due to infection
- Increased heart rate due to fever
- Costovertebral angle (CVA) tenderness

INTERPRETING TEST RESULTS

- Urinalysis shows leukocytes, bacteria, nitrites, and red blood cells; may see white blood cell casts.
- Urine culture identifies organism.
- Sensitivity shows which antibiotics the organism is most responsive to.
- CBC shows leukocytosis.

TREATMENT

- Administer antibiotics to treat infection—intravenous or oral depending on severity of infection and comorbidities of patient:
  - nitrofurantoin
  - ciprofloxacin
  - levofloxacin
  - ofloxacin
  - trimethoprim-sulfamethoxazole
  - ampicillin
  - amoxicillin
- Administer antipyretics for fever.
- Administer fluids for dehydration due to vomiting and diarrhea.
- Administer phenazopyridine for relief of dysuria symptoms.
- Repeat urine culture after completion of antibiotic course.

NURSING DIAGNOSIS

- Impaired urinary elimination
- Nausea
- Hyperthermia

NURSING INTERVENTIONS

- Monitor vital signs.
- Monitor intake and output.
- Assess for side effects of medication.
- Teach patient that phenazopyridine will cause orange-colored urine.

8 Renal Failure

WHAT WENT WRONG?

A decrease in renal function can occur in an acute (sudden) or a chronic (progressive) manner. Acute renal failure can be broken down into pre-renal, renal, and post-renal. Prerenal causes result from diminished renal perfusion. Hypovolemia due to blood or fluid losses, diuretic use, third-spacing of fluids, reduced renal perfusion due to NSAID use or CHF can cause pre-renal failure. Renal failure in acute care patients most commonly results from acute tubular necrosis. Drug-related reactions, particularly to antibiotics, may cause an allergic interstitial nephritis. Pylenonephritis or glomerulonephritis may also cause renal failure. Post-renal failure is due to some type of urinary tract obstruction, bladder outlet obstruction, stone, prostate hypertrophy, or compression of ureter due to abdominal mass.

Chronic renal failure is an irreversible disease due to damaging effects on the kidneys caused by diabetes mellitus, hypertension, glomerulonephritis, HIV infection, polycystic kidney disease, or ischemic nephropathy.

PROGNOSIS

In acute renal failure, kidneys start working following intensive treatment and rectifying the underlying condition that caused the problem. In chronic renal failure, the patient can die as a result of complications of the disease.

HALLMARK SIGNS AND SYMPTOMS

- Azotemia—elevated BUN and creatinine
- If hypovolemic (pre-renal), tachycardia, orthostatic hypotension, dry skin, and mucous membranes

- Weight loss due to chronic disease
- Abdominal bruit with ischemic nephropathy
- Peripheral edema with third spacing of fluids
- Decreased urinary output
- Uremic pruritis—see excoriations from scratching
- Anemia in chronic disease—kidneys produce erythropoetin

INTERPRETING TEST RESULTS

- BUN elevated.
- Creatinine elevated.
- BUN/creatinine ratio elevated.
- Urinalysis may show casts (hyaline or granular in acute prerenal; RBC, WBC in renal), proteinuria.
- Glomerular filtration rate decreases in chronic disease.
- Creatinine clearance decreases.
- Renal ultrasound shows decrease in renal size in chronic renal failure; dilation and fluid build up in post-renal failure.

TREATMENT

Treatment needs to address the underlying disease process. What will correct one cause may make another cause worse.

- Administer intravenous fluids to correct hypovolemia.
- Administer inotropic agents for patients with CHF to enhance cardiac output.
- Administer antibiotics for pyelonephritis.
- Stent placement or catheter (urethral, suprapubic, nephrostomy) to allow for drainage of urine if blockage present.
- Dialysis.
- Administer erythropoetin to treat anemia.
- Restrict potassium, phosphate, sodium, and protein in diet.
- Administer phosphate binders to reduce phosphate levels.
- Administer sodium polystyrene sulfonate to reduce potassium levels.
- Monitor electrolyte levels.

- Control blood pressure.
- Control blood glucose levels.

NURSING DIAGNOSIS

- Impaired urinary elimination
- Ineffective tissue perfusion (renal)
- Fear

NURSING INTERVENTIONS

- Monitor vital signs for changes in heart rate or blood pressure.
- Monitor intake and output.
- Assess intravenous site for redness, swelling, or pain.
- Check dialysis access site for signs of infection.
- Check AV shunt for thrill (palpable turbulence of bloodflow; gently feel for flow of blood through shunt) and bruit (audible turbulence of bloodflow; listen with stethoscope for sound of bloodflow through shunt).
- No contrast dye tests.
- No nephrotoxic medication.
- Monitor patient very closely.

9 *Testicular Cancer*

WHAT WENT WRONG?

Cancer involving the testicle typically occurs in males in their teens or twenties. The cancer is hormonally dependent and tends to metastasize fairly quickly to lungs or to bone. A painless nodule may be found by the patient. There is an increased incidence in patients with a history of cryptorchism.

PROGNOSIS

Prognosis is better for patients with solitary nodules that have not had a chance to metastasize. Tumors that have already metastasized to other locations have a poorer prognosis. The diagnosis will also have varied degrees of psychological impact on the patient.

HALLMARK SIGNS AND SYMPTOMS

- Painless enlargement of the testis
- Palpable mass on surface of testis
- Unilateral feeling of heaviness in the scrotum
- Testicular pain due to bleeding within the testis in a small percentage of patients
- Back pain due to metastasis
- Cough or shortness of breath due to pulmonary metastasis

INTERPRETING TEST RESULTS

- Scrotal ultrasound shows mass on testis.
- CT scan of pelvis, abdomen, and chest may be needed to check for metastasis.
- Human chorionic gonadotropin (hCG) elevated.
- Fetoprotein (AFP) elevated.
- Lactate dehydrogenase (LDH) elevated.
- CBC shows anemia later in disease.

TREATMENT

- Orchiectomy.
- Chemotherapy, combination medications.
- Radiation therapy to reduce chance of recurrence.
- Monitor tumor markers periodically.
- Monitor follow-up CT scans periodically.
- Depending on treatments planned, some patients may want to bank sperm, if fertility will be a concern after treatment.

NURSING DIAGNOSIS

- Fear
- Anxiety
- Disturbed body image

NURSING INTERVENTIONS

- Monitor vital signs.
- Monitor intake and output.
- Assess patient's coping abilities.
- Teach patient testicular self-exam.

10 *Urinary Tract Infection*

WHAT WENT WRONG?

Urinary tract infection occurs when an infecting organism, typically a gram negative bacteria such as *E. coli*, enters the urinary tract. Inflammation of the local area occurs, followed by infection as the organism reproduces. Often the bacteria is present on the skin in the genital area and enters the urinary tract through the urethral opening. The organism can also be introduced during sexual contact. The infection occurs as an uncomplicated, community-acquired infection in this setting. Patients with a urinary catheter in place may also develop an infection due to the presence of the catheter which allows a pathway for the bacteria to enter the bladder. Instrumentation of the urinary tract, e.g. cystoscopy, also allows a pathway for bacteria to enter the bladder. Some of the instruments are not completely sterilized between patients; they are treated with a high-level disinfectant due to fiberoptics and lenses within because they would not withstand the high temperatures needed to sterilize. These infections would be considered nosocomial.

PROGNOSIS

Urinary tract infections that are identified are typically treated and resolve. Some bacteria have become resistant to certain antibiotics, so testing the urine to be sure the infection has cleared after treatment is a good idea. Infections that are left untreated can progress and travel upward through the urinary tract to involve the kidneys or become a systemic infection or sepsis, especially in elderly or infirm patients.

HALLMARK SIGNS AND SYMPTOMS

- Frequency due to irritation of bladder muscles
- Urgency due to irritation of bladder muscles

- Dysuria due to irritation of mucosal lining
- Feeling of fullness in suprapubic area
- Low back pain

INTERPRETING TEST RESULTS

- Urinalysis shows leukocytes, nitrites, and red blood cells.
- Urine culture and sensitivity indicates the infecting organism and the appropriate antibiotic to treat the infection.

TREATMENT

- Administer antibiotics:
  - nitrofurantoin
  - ciprofloxacin
  - levofloxacin
  - ofloxacin
  - trimethoprim-sulfamethoxazole
  - ampicillin
  - amoxicillin
- Encourage fluids, to make urine less concentrated.
- Administer phenazopyridine for symptoms of dysuria.
- Repeat urine testing after antibiotics are completed.

NURSING DIAGNOSIS

- Risk of impaired urinary elimination
- Risk of urge urinary incontinence

NURSING INTERVENTIONS

- Monitor intake and output.
- Monitor vital signs for changes, signs of fever.
- Encourage fluid intake.
- Encourage cranberry juice to acidify urine.
- Teach patient that phenazopyridine will cause orange-colored urine.

Crucial Diagnostic Tests

Culture and Sensitivity Tests

The culture test checks for the presence of bacteria in the urine. The sensitivity test determines what antibiotics can be used to eliminate the bacteria. The laboratory divides the urine specimen in half; one part is cultured to determine which bacteria grow. A preliminary report should be available in 24 hours. The second half is is used to determine to which antibiotics the organism(s) are sensitive.

Before the test—Explain to the patient that the specimen must be obtained before an antibiotic can be started or the results will be altered.

Cystoscopy

This test examines the bladder walls to check for tumors and growths. It is also used as a therapeutic tool to remove small tumors, stones, and foreign bodies and to dilate the urethra and ureters. A cystoscope is inserted into the urethra to the bladder, which allows structures to be actually visualized; i.e. urethra, bladder, ureters, and prostate.

Before the test—Explain to the patient that this test may be performed under general, light or local anesthesia. It will be uncomfortable if the patient is awake. Obtain informed consent.

After the test—Advise the patient to increase fluids to flush out bacteria that may have been introduced with the cystoscope. Bladder muscle spasms may result. The patient should expect some pink urine following the test. Frank, red blood warrants a call to the physician. Observe for signs of a UTI—chills, fever, frequent, uncomfortable voiding, pelvic discomfort.

Kidney, Ureter, Bladder (KUB) X-ray Study

The KUB study is an abdominal x-ray used to detect kidney stones, abdominal abscesses, paralytic ileus or obstruction. Explain to the patient that this is not an invasive procedure.

Prostate Specific Antigen (PSA) Test

This test measures the level of PSA in the blood. The level will be elevated in patients with BPH (benign prostatic hypertrophy) or prostate cancer. Elevated PSA levels alone do not give doctors enough information to distinguish between benign prostate conditions and cancer; however, the doctor will take the test results into account when deciding whether to order additional screening for prostate cancer. The test is also used to monitor treatment and to test for recurrences of prostate cancer.

Before the test—Explain to the patient that rectal and prostate exams, ejaculation, UTI, and prostatitis will all elevate a PSA level.

24-Hour Urine Collection

This is a diagnostic test that involves collecting a patient's urine for 24 hours. It is typically used to measure volume and various other factors of kidney function as well as to determine the daily elimination of such substances as proteins, electrolytes, etc.

Before the test—Explain to the patient that the test is started in the morning. Discard the first voided specimen, then save subsequent specimens, ending with the first voided specimen the following day. The urine collection jug should be kept on ice or under refrigeration.

Urinalysis

Urinalysis is the physical, chemical, and microscopic examination of urine. It involves a number of tests to evaluate the urine specimen for appearance, color, clarity, pH, specific gravity, and the presence of bacteria, blood, casts, glucose, ketones, leukocytes, proteins, RBCs, and WBCs. The tests are used to confirm symptoms of a UTI, to check diabetics for excess glucose levels, and to monitor the kidney function of renal patients.

Before the test—Explain to the patient that many drugs affect a urine specimen. Some samples, as when ascertaining the presence of an infection, may need to be "clean catch" or "midstream clean" collection. The perineum or urethral opening should be cleansed, and the voiding stream started. Without stopping the stream, position the sterile container into the flow of urine. When the container is more than half full, withdraw from the flow of urine. Allow the patient to finish emptying the bladder. Tightly cap and send to the laboratory immediately.

Urine Flow Studies

Urine flow studies, also known as uroflowmetry, measure the strength and volume per second of urine flow from the bladder when a patient urinates into a test machine. They help identify an obstruction or abnormality of the urinary tract and assist in evaluating how well or poorly a patient is urinating.

Before the test—Explain to the patient not to urinate for a few hours before the test and to drink enough fluids to develop an urge to urinate . It is not an invasive test. They will need to void into a flowmeter.

Voiding Cystogram

This test involves taking an x-ray image of the bladder and urethra during urination. A radiopaque contrast material is instilled into the bladder via a Foley catheter. After x-rays are taken, the catheter is removed. The patient voids while more x-rays are obtained. This test is performed to look for defects of the urinary system, for tumors of the bladder, ureters, and urethra, or for reflux of urine from the bladder to the ureters.

Before the test—Explain to the patient that the presence of the catheter will feel like the urge to urinate. Obtain informed consent. Check for allergies to contrast material. Advise the patient to increase po fluids before and after test to aid the kidneys in removal of contrast material.

Quiz

1. Patients with nephrolithiasis or kidney stones need to increase fluid intake. This is to:
   (a) concentrate the urine.
   (b) help flush the stones through the urinary tract.
   (c) crystallize the struvite from the renal tubules.
   (d) break down the stones into smaller pieces that will more easily pass through the urinary tract.

2. You are caring for a patient with a urinary tract infection. You would expect the plan of care to include:

(a) antibiotics and phenazopyridine.

(b) erythropoetin and stent placement.

(c) hormonal therapy and intravenous fluids.

(d) hourly urine output measurements and antibiotics.

3. Patients with bladder cancer typically exhibit symptoms of:

(a) weight loss and low back pain.

(b) fatigue and anemia.

(c) hematuria and change in urinary pattern.

(d) difficulty initiating urinary stream and nocturia.

4. Teach a patient at risk for testicular cancer to:

(a) restrict potassium, phosphate, sodium, and protein in diet.

(b) self-catheterize ileal reservoir.

(c) perform testicular self-exam.

(d) monitor change in color of urine.

5. Care of the postoperative nephrectomy patient includes:

(a) assessing the wound site for redness, swelling, or drainage.

(b) giving diuretics to enhance urinary output.

(c) monitoring urinary output every 2 hours.

(d) encouraging intake of cranberry juice to acidify the urine.

6. You are caring for a patient who has had a transurethral resection of the prostate for benign prostatic hypertrophy. There is a continuous bladder irrigation set up. You would notify the physician if you noted:

(a) any signs of hematuria.

(b) a decrease in the amount of blood in the urine.

(c) a change from clear red output to thicker, bright red output.

(d) the development of uremic pruritis.

7. One of your patients is awaiting lab results for kidney function. The patient has recently recovered from a streptococcal throat infection. The patient has most likely developed symptoms of:

(a) pyelonephritis.

(b) nephrolithiasis.

(c) chronic renal failure.

(d) glomerulonephritis.

8. Symptoms of prostate cancer include:

   (a) nocturia and intermittent stream of urination.

   (b) diminished force of urinary stream and urgency.

   (c) difficulty initiating stream of urine and frequency.

   (d) all of the above.

9. Acute renal failure due to a decrease in circulating blood volume causing diminished renal perfusion is treated with:

   (a) intravenous fluids.

   (b) inotropic agents.

   (c) erythropoetin.

   (d) diuretics.

10. Dialysis is used to manage patients with:

   (a) acute glomerulonephritis.

   (b) renal failure.

   (c) nephrolithiasis.

   (d) pyelonephritis.

CHAPTER 10

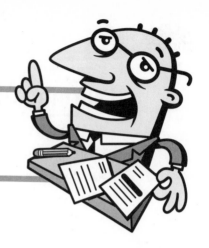

Integumentary System

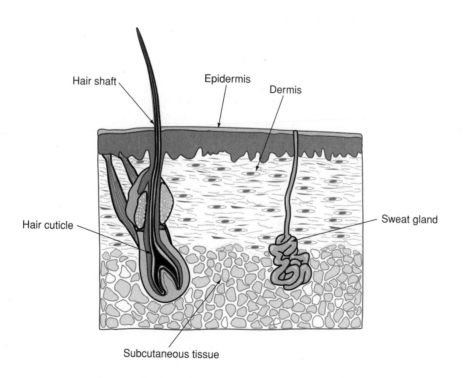

Hair shaft

Epidermis

Dermis

Hair cuticle

Sweat gland

Subcutaneous tissue

Learning Objectives

1 Burns

2 Dermatitis

3 Skin cancers

4 Cellulitis

5 Pressure ulcers

6 Wounds and healing

Key Terms

Atopy	Fibroblastic phase	Proliferative phase
Basal cell carcinoma	First-degree burn	Pruritis
Braden scale	Hydrocolloids	RAST testing
Cryosurgery	Hyperpigmentation	Second-degree burn
Debrided	Immunosuppressant	Squamous cell
Eczema	Lymphedema	Third-degree burn
Erythema	Melanoma	Vesicles
Eschar	Mohs' surgery	

How the Integumentary System Works

The outside covering of the body, or the skin, serves three major purposes. It prevents dehydration, regulates body temperature, and is the major deterrent of infection in the body. When this barrier is broken, whether by surgical incision, wound, cut, or scrape, the primary defense is no longer intact. Superficial breaks in the skin may be treated on an outpatient basis. However, deeper wounds, and those involving the face and neck, may need more intense care with IV antibiotics. Skin is comprised of several layers and is waterproof. Many skin manifestations are described using common terms. Macules are small, flat-topped lesions, less than 1 cm in diameter, similar to a freckle. Papules are elevated lesions, also smaller than 1 cm in diameter. A wheal is a raised area filled with fluid and usually temporary, such as in hives. A vesicle is a fluid-filled blister, often seen in shingles. Bullae are larger than 1 cm in diameter and are fluid-filled blisters. A plaque (sticky deposits that attaches to the inner lining of an artery) is greater than 1 cm in diameter, raised, and shallow. A nodule is a solid lesion, up to 1 cm in diameter with depth. A tumor is larger than 1 cm in diameter, and is solid with depth. A pustule is an elevation containing purulent material. Petechiae are smaller than 1 cm in diameter and are usually round areas of deposits of blood. A purpura is a large petechia.

Just the Facts

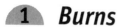 *Burns*

WHAT WENT WRONG?

Burns are damage to the skin and body tissues caused by flames, heat, cold, friction, radiation (sunburn), chemicals, or electricity. Burns are generally divided into three categories, depending on the damage. First-degree burns are those with injury to the outer layer of skin called the epidermis. They will be red, and painful, with some swelling. A second-degree burn is when the epidermis is burned, as well as the next layer, the dermis. Severe pain, white and reddened areas, swelling, blisters, and perhaps drainage will be seen. A third-degree burn goes through all the layers of the skin and could involve underlying tissues. It is often painless due to destruction of the nerves in the area. The area will look black (termed eschar) and/or reddened. Many drugs may make the skin more sensitive to the sun, producing the effect of a sunburn with little exposure. Common medications with this effect include: amiodorone, carbamazepine, furosemide, naproxen, oral contraceptives, piroxicam, quinidine, quinolones, sulfonamides, sulfonulureas, tetracyclines, and thiazides, among others.

PROGNOSIS

Prognosis depends on the severity of the burn plus the amount of surface area involved. When large portions of the face, chest, hands, feet, genitalia, or joints have sustained a large second- or third-degree burn, prompt medical attention is necessary. Serious burns can lead to death. If smoke inhalation has occurred, or if the nasal hairs are singed, or if quantities of soot are present around the face, assess for adequacy of breathing and damage to the respiratory tract. CPR may need to be started. Infants and elderly patients with burns require prompt medical attention.

HALLMARK SIGNS AND SYMPTOMS

- Redness, no break in skin—indicates a first-degree burn from damage to the epidermis
- Deeper red, with clear fluid blisters—indicates a second-degree burn as the epidermis and dermis are burned

- Charred black or dry white—indicates death of the tissue from the burn (third-degree burn)

INTERPRETING TEST RESULTS

- Pulse oximetry—a sensor is placed on the finger, toe, or earlobe to assess the amount of oxygen in the blood to ensure adequate oxygenation.
- Pulmonary function tests show how well the lungs are working. The patient breathes into a machine, a spirometer, which records changes in the lung size with inhalation and exhalation and the time it takes to perform this test.
- Rule of nines—a way of measurement to estimate the total body surface area burned: head, 9 percent; anterior torso, 18 percent; posterior torso, 18 percent; each leg, 18 percent; each arm, 9 percent; perineum, 1 percent.

TREATMENT

The objective of burn treatment is to prevent infection, decrease inflammation and pain, and promote healing of the areas. Treatment choices depend on the degree of burn and the amount of body surface area that was burned. Any second-degree burn greater than 5 to 10 percent of surface area and all third-degree burns belong in a hospital, preferably within a specialized burn unit. All electrical burns and burns of the ears, eyes, face, hands, feet, and perineum require hospital care, as do chemical burns and burns in infants or the elderly.

- Check the area for any exposed electrical wires, if you are present on the scene.
- Use cold water to decrease the temperature of the area for a first-degree burn or a small second-degree burn and to stop the burning.
- For chemical burns, ensure that all the chemical has been flushed away.
- For electrical burns, look for entrance and exit wounds.
- Cover the area with dry gauze.
- If the skin is broken (second-degree burn), use a topical antibiotic ointment such as silvadene to prevent a secondary bacterial infection before applying the gauze.
- Administer pain medications (ibuprofen, acetaminophen) as needed.
- For third-degree burns, the eschar needs to be debrided (cut away) to allow new tissue to grow.
- These wounds are often covered in moist sterile saline gauze, as new tissue grows best in this environment. When the gauze dries; it adheres to the dead tissue. The area is mechanically debrided when the gauze is removed.

- Oral antibiotics may be necessary.
- Administer pain medications (oxycodone, morphine) as needed, especially before dressing changes that may be painful.
- Prevent heat loss due to large areas of tissue exposed from lack of skin coverage.
- Maintain fluid levels since fluid loss is common from evaporation and wound drainage.

NURSING DIAGNOSES

- Risk of fluid volume deficit
- Pain, discomfort
- Risk of altered body temperature

NURSING INTERVENTION

- Anticipate pain medication needs to make the patient more comfortable.
- Assist in range of motion to avoid contracture development due to pain with movement.
- Encourage family visitation.
- Assist with activities of daily living.
- Isolation may be needed to protect the patient from bacteria, especially if a large amount of skin is not intact.
- Teach the patient to look for signs and symptoms of infection: fever, increased redness, increase in drainage, or change in color of drainage.

2 *Dermatitis*

WHAT WENT WRONG?

Inflammation of the skin as a result of contact with an irritating substance such as a chemical, foreign substance, medication, or contact with a plant, such as poison ivy. The skin may become reddened, irritated, and itchy. The usual causes are allergic reactions. Often the patient has a history or a family history of asthma, allergy, or eczema. Some later symptoms may be the result of scratching of the skin. Often the cause may be a drug reaction, the body's immune system reacting to a medication.

PROGNOSIS

Resolution of the rash occurs within one to two weeks once the offending substance is identified and removed. However, if the patient is atopic, frequent exacerbations and remissions may occur with unknown etiology.

HALLMARK SIGNS AND SYMPTOMS

- Rash on the affected skin area from contact with the offending substance
- Pruritis from histamine release from mast cells
- Erythema and edema
- Vesicles where the substance came in contact with the skin
- Hyperpigmentation from irritation from scratching

INTERPRETING TEST RESULTS

- RAST testing may be done to determine allergens.
- Patch testing.

TREATMENT

Treatment involves determining, if able, the triggers that began the flare, and avoidance of the same. Treatment aimed at each symptom will help to decrease discomfort. If the dermatitis is widespread, IV medications, steroids, or antihistamines may be necessary to resolve the flare. Topical corticosteroid cream, gel, or lotions will decrease the symptoms.

NURSING DIAGNOSES

- Body image disturbance
- Risk of altered skin integrity
- Pain, discomfort

NURSING INTERVENTION

- Avoid irritants that caused the dermatitis to prevent recurrence.
- Allow for healing and prevent bacterial infections.
- Cool compresses.
- Use protective gloves and clothing.
- Wash hands often.
- Explain to patient:
  - Keep the skin moist.
  - Keep nails short to diminish scratching.
  - Warm, not hot, showers.
  - Use mild soap.
  - Apply moisturizers.

3 *Skin Cancers*

Cancers of the skin are the most common type of cancer. The incidence of skin cancer is one of the fastest growing. Early detection is of the utmost importance because a cure is obtainable in the early stages. Heredity may also be a factor. Skin cancer is usually divided into three major subtypes: basal cell, the most common; squamous cell, which is the second most common; and melanoma, the most fearsome. Basal cell carcinomas are directly related to sun damage, with most lesions occurring in sun-exposed areas. This type recurs frequently. Squamous cell carcinomas are often due to sun-exposure, may be difficult to distinguish from some changes in the skin, and spread more readily. Melanoma is the most deadly form of skin cancer; it usually occurs on the face or upper back. A mnemonic to aid in melanoma characteristics may be helpful: A—asymmetrical shape; B—borders that are irregular; C—change in color; D—diameter larger than a pencil eraser; E—ever changing.

WHAT WENT WRONG?

New skin cells are made in the epidermis, which then push the older cells toward the surface where they are shed. Solar exposure can interrupt this process, causing cells to divide at an unusual rate, which may lead to a cancer. Those individuals with a large amount of exposure to ultraviolet radiation, which appears to be cumulative, are more at risk to develop cancerous tumors. Exposure to greater amounts of x-rays also increase the risk for skin cancers, as does arsenic which is a metal found in the environment and in our food. People who take immunosuppresant medications are at a greater risk for skin cancers as are fair-skinned people and those with a family history of skin cancer.

PROGNOSIS

If the lesion is identified and treated early, prognosis is excellent. Follow-up care with frequent skin assessments is mandatory. Basal cell cancers are unlikely to have a poor prognosis. Squamous cell tumors may spread if left unchecked. Melanoma is staged by determining thickness of the lesion, and the extent to which it has spread. Stage 0 is a confined tumor. The other stages mean the cancer has spread to other tissues, and organs.

HALLMARK SIGNS AND SYMPTOMS

- Basal cell—pearly white, waxy-appearing papule or a flat, brown patch
- Squamous cell—firm red nodule; a flat scaly lesion; a change in a scar
- Melanoma—any mole that is new, that has changed, and/or that meets any of the ABCDE criteria

INTERPRETING TEST RESULTS

- Biopsy with an interpretation by a pathologist.

TREATMENT

Treatment is dependent upon the type of cancer, location, and size of the tumor.
- Surgical excision involves removing the tumor and surrounding healthy tissue to ensure all the cancerous tissue has been extracted.
- Cryosurgery in which the cells are killed by freezing with liquid nitrogen.
- Mohs' surgery where the tumor is removed layer by layer. Each surface area is evaluated microscopically, to ascertain that no cancer cells are present in the remaining tissue.
- Laser treatments to vaporize the cancer cells.
- Topical creams and ointments.

- Radiation used to kill cancer cells in melanoma.
- Chemotherapy, using drugs to kill the melanoma cells.

NURSING DIAGNOSES

- Impaired skin integrity
- Body image disturbance

NURSING INTERVENTION

- Stay out of the sun when its rays are the strongest.
- Avoid tanning salons.
- Wear sunscreen.
- Wear sun-protective clothing.
- Check the skin regularly for new moles, as well as changes in existing moles, freckles, and birthmarks.
- Medications may make the skin more sensitive to sunlight.

4 *Cellulitis*

WHAT WENT WRONG?

Cellulitis is an infection of the skin, caused by bacteria that enter the skin through an opening. The legs are the most common site of cellulitis, although it may occur anywhere bacteria enters. The most common bacteria are streptococcus and staphylococcus. Bacteria may enter through fissures in the feet from fungal infections, through cracks in dry skin, from insect bites, or cuts from shaving. The elderly, immunocompromised patients, and patients with lymphedema, diabetes, or poor circulation are at greatest risk.

PROGNOSIS

If treatment is started early, the prognosis is good. If the symptoms don't begin to resolve or the infection is on the face or widespread, hospitalization and IV antibiotics are needed. A severe cellulitis of deep tissue, necrotizing fasciitis, is caused by a streptococcal bacteria and is considered a medical emergency.

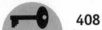

HALLMARK SIGNS AND SYMPTOMS

- Hot, red skin over the area of infection
- Swollen and painful skin and tissue due to the infection

INTERPRETING TEST RESULTS

- CBC to check on the white blood cell count.
- Culture of the wound to identify the organism causing the cellulitis.
- Ultrasound of the leg to rule out a DVT—deep vein thrombosis.

TREATMENT

Treatment for a beginning infection is oral antibiotics. If fever and body aches accompany the infection or if the face is involved or the area is extensive, hospitalization may be necessary. Empiric treatment is started immediately and is effective against the most common bacteria.

- Cephalexin.
- Dicloxacillin.
- Levofloxacin.
- Tetanus booster if needed.
- Drainage of abscess by a surgeon if necessary.
- Pain medications.

NURSING DIAGNOSES

- Pain, discomfort
- Risk of infection
- Impaired skin integrity

NURSING INTERVENTION

- Explain to the patient the importance of good hygiene.
- Wash the affected area daily.
- Use a topical antibiotic ointment and a dry dressing twice daily.
- Elevate the area if possible.

- Monitor for temperature, enlarging area of redness, increase in drainage.
- Explain to the patient how to prevent openings in the skin by using proper skin care interventions.
- Monitor feet and legs daily for cracks, fissures.
- Use care in trimming nails, or visit podiatrist.
- Use moisturizing lotions regularly.

 ## *Pressure Ulcers*

WHAT WENT WRONG?

A pressure ulcer starts on the skin and often progresses to deeper tissue; it is caused by impaired circulation to the tissue from pressure over a period of time. Without adequate blood flow and the nutrition it brings, the tissue will die. Those often affected are confined to a wheelchair or bed, and unable to move themselves, not reducing the pressure frequently enough. It can take as little as a few hours in one position for a stage one pressure ulcer to develop. The usual sites of pressure ulcers, or bedsores, are on bony prominences, such as the buttocks, sacrum, heels, knees, and hips. Friction from linens can impair the integrity of the skin as can the shear force, when the skin moves in one direction and the deeper structures don't move. Assessment tools are available to predict the risk of pressure ulcers developing. A commonly used scale is the Braden scale which includes such criteria as friction, the nutritional status of the patient, mobility and activity levels, moisture exposure of the skin and any limitations of sensory perception.

PROGNOSIS

Unfortunately, prognosis is poor. The very factors that caused the pressure ulcer are the same factors that interfere with healing. Resolution often is very involved and slow. Setbacks are common, such as wound infection, cellulitis, and sepsis, which can lead to death.

HALLMARK SIGNS AND SYMPTOMS

- Stage I:
  - Firm warm areas of skin from poor circulation
  - Spongy, reddened tissue from increased pressure

- Stage II:
  - Opening in the skin with surrounding erythema from pressure
- Stage III:
  - The ulcer is deep, down to the dermis, with red base and some drainage
- Stage IV:
  - A deep ulcer involving muscle and bone, with visible signs of tissue death

INTERPRETING TEST RESULTS

- Culture to check for bacteria content.
- CBC to evaluate the hemoglobin and hematocrit for oxygen-carrying capabilities.
- Albumin and pre-albumin levels to check on nutrition.
- Chemistry to evaluate fluid status.

TREATMENT

Treatment is based on relieving pressure and providing adequate nutrition. Wound treatment is aimed at preventing infection and encouraging healing. Stage I and stage II wounds may heal with conservative treatments. However, stage III and stage IV wounds often require surgical debridement and skin grafting. Treatment choice depends on the stage of the wound.

- Clean wound with soap and water or saline.
- Debridement to clean away dead, devitalized, and infected tissue. Debridement methods include surgery, topical enzymatics, and mechanical debridement.
- Dressings to protect the wound and keep it moist, which promotes healing.
- Hydrocolloids which keep moisture in.
- Nonadherant dressings, such as aquaphor.
- Bulk dressings to absorb copious drainage.
- Semipermeable dressings which allow for transfer of gases but are impermeable to liquids.
- Antibiotic ointment for infected wounds.
- Oral antibiotics.
- Specialized matresses.
- Whirlpool treatments.

NURSING DIAGNOSES

- Impaired skin integrity
- Impaired physical mobility
- Nutrition altered: less than what body requires

NURSING INTERVENTION

- Prevention is the key to pressure ulcers.
- Mobility or repositioning of patients unable to move themselves; every 1 to 2 hours.
- Proper nutrition to encourage healing.
- Adequate fluid intake.
- Remove pressure from stage I areas.
- Use pillows to reduce pressure.
- Use specialized wheelchair cushions to reduce pressure.
- Daily skin inspection.
- Stop smoking in order to increase oxygen to tissues.
- Daily measurement of wounds to assess status including length, width, and depth.

6   *Wounds and Healing*

A wound is any break in the skin. It may be intentional, as with surgery, or unintentional, as a result of trauma. Types of wounds include surgical, penetrating (such as a knife), crushing, burn, lacerations, bites, (human, animal), ulcers, and pressure ulcers. Immediately after a wound occurs, inflammation begins with platelet aggregation. Next, leukocytes travel to the area for infection surveillance. A proliferative phase starts when the epidermal cells move toward the wound, and cover the approximated wound edges, usually by the third day. The fibroblastic phase occurs with collagen and fibroblasts forming a scar.

Wound healing occurs in various ways. Primary intention happens when edges are closely approximated and new tissue, or granulation, knits the close edges together. Wound healing by secondary intention occurs in a larger wound where the edges are further apart. This is often intentional when the wound is infected, dirty, or from a bite. The granulation tissue builds across the surface of the wound forming a large clot and sequentially, a larger scar.

PROGNOSIS

Prognosis depends on the size, location, and cause of the wound. Items which need to be assessed in patients with wounds include chronic disease, such as diabetes, impaired circulation; nutrition; hydration status; and immunosuppression, such as corticosteroid or chemotherapeutic agents. Epithelialization of wound occurs within 48 hours, wound strength is 60 percent of previous strength within 4 months.

HALLMARK SIGNS AND SYMPTOMS

- Pain from injury to nerves
- Drainage from injury to tissues and cells migrating to the site of injury
- Bleeding from injury to blood vessels
- Foreign body—look for penetrating objects
- Deeper tissue trauma—assess for nonintact tendons, ligaments, and pieces of bone
- Debris—look for dirt, fragments
- Signs and symptoms of infection include increased erythema; purulent, foul-smelling drainage; and fever
- Wounds may be accompanied by pain, drainage, bleeding, infection, a foreign body, or deeper tissue trauma. Assessment of the wound, including deeper structures if necessary, is imperative.

INTERPRETING TEST RESULTS

- CBC to assess for leukocytoses for infection.
- Chemistry to assess hydration status.

TREATMENT

- Assess circulation if the wound is in a limb. Check distal pulses.
- Tetanus prophylaxis as needed. A booster is indicated if the last one was not within the past ten years.
- Irrigation of the wound with large amounts of saline to flush away all dirt, debris, and foreign bodies.

- Wound closure, either by sutures, steri strips, or dressings.
- Dirty wounds are usually left open to heal by secondary intention.
- Antibiotics if necessary, usually 7 to 10 days.

NURSING DIAGNOSIS

- Impaired tissue integrity
- Risk of infection
- Impaired skin integrity

NURSING TREATMENT

- Explain to the patient:
  - Disease process.
  - Signs of infection, i.e., swelling, redness, increase in pain, fever, chills, drainage, bleeding, foul odor, or reopening of wound.
  - Medication, including indication for, frequency of use, and side effects.
  - Demonstrate proper dressing change techniques, including frequency, proper hand washing, cleansing of wound, and application of topicals if ordered.
  - Adequate nutrition and hydration.
  - Elevation of affected limb, if indicated.
  - Rest, decrease in activities.
  - Proper immunization schedules

Crucial Diagnostic Tests

Allergy Skin Testing

An allergy skin test is used to confirm whether such symptoms as sneezing, wheezing, and skin rashes are caused by allergies. The test is performed by exposing an area of the skin to the extract of an allergen and then evaluating the skin's reaction. A wheal and/or erythema indicate confirmation of the allergy. An intradermal test, where the allergen is injected just under the skin, or a patch test, where an allergen patch is placed on the skin, may also be used.

Before the test—Instruct the patient to withhold antihistamines, steroids, and leukotriene modulator medications which would interfere with the results of the test. Explain to the patient what to expect.

Skin Biopsy

A skin biopsy is usually done to diagnose an abnormal area of the skin, such as a growth or mole for cancer It is also used to diagnose a bacterial or fungal skin infection or other abnormal skin condition. A sample of tissue is taken for analysis by a pathologist to determine if cellular changes have occurred. There are several types of biopsy as follows:

- Punch biopsy where a small cylindrical fragment of tissue is removed from the affected area, by a sharp cookie-cutter-like tool (punch).
- Shave biopsy where a superficial piece of skin is removed from the affected area with a sharp, sterile blade
- Excisional biopsy where a larger area of skin is removed, allowing for analysis of deeper skin structures or removal of the entire lesion. A local anesthetic is typically used.

After the test—Monitor the area for healing.

Gram Stain

Gram stain or Gram's method is a way of differentiating bacterial species into two large groups, Gram-positive and Gram-negative based on properties of their cell walls. A stain is added to a culture on a slide which will show blue for Gram-positive cells or red for Gram-negative cells. This is the first step in determining the identity of a particular bacterial sample and can be used to allow empiric antibiotics to be started, before the final culture is ready.

Herpes Simplex Virus (HSV) Culture

The test is performed by taking a fluid sample from the lesions within 3 days of appearance. The virus, if present, can be detected in this fluid sample in a few days.

Blood testing can also be performed to identify antibodies for the particular type of Herpes virus.

Potassium Hydroxide Preparation (KOH)

This test is done to provide a rapid, differential diagnosis of fungal infections of the hair, skin, or nail. A solution of KOH mixed with a blue-black dye is added to a slide containing cells from the infected tissues, and the slide is viewed under a microscope.

Radioallergosorbent Test (RAST)

This is a blood test used to screen for an allergy to a specific substance or substances. It measures the amount of IgE antibody that reacts specifically with the suspected allergen.

Additional Blood Test

Rapid plasma regain (**RPR**), Venereal Disease Research Laboratory (**VDRL**), fluorescent treponema antibody test (**FTA-ABS**), treponema pallidum partiate agglutinate (**TP-PA**) are blood tests used to diagnose syphilis.

Quiz

1. When assessing a suspicious skin lesion, you are looking for A—asymmetry, B—irregular borders, C—variegated colors, D—diameter, and E—
    (a) edema.
    (b) erythema.
    (c) elevation.
    (d) ever-changing.

2. Patient teaching for risk reduction of skin cancer should include:

(a) having suspicious moles checked by a dermatologist.

(b) daily sun exposure every one-half hour.

(c) daily sun exposure of 1 hour to build tolerance.

(d) applying moisturizer.

3. A patient with a second-degree burn has a greater risk for:

(a) constipation.

(b) infection.

(c) hypotension.

(d) hyperglycemia.

4. When staging a pressure ulcer, you correctly recognize a stage II ulcer as:

(a) redness, with no break in the skin.

(b) shallow ulcer with red base.

(c) dermis involvement with eschar.

(d) bone visible with no drainage.

5. Appropriate treatment for a patient with cellulitis includes:

(a) petrolatum and vitamin A and D ointment.

(b) antibiotics, such as cephalexin, and over-the-counter analgesics.

(c) weight-bearing exercises and diuretics, such as furosemide.

(d) wet to dry dressings and steroids.

6. You are caring for a patient with an infected wound. You would expect:

(a) to prepare for sutures, to close the wound.

(b) the use of steri-strips, to hold the edges together.

(c) to leave the wound open.

(d) to cover with a loose, fluffy dressing.

7. Steps to prevent a pressure ulcer may include:

(a) not disturbing the patient.

(b) changing the position of a bed-bound patient every 4 hours.

(c) vigorously rubbing the skin with alcohol.

(d) avoiding pressure on the heels of a bed-bound patient.

8. For your patient with a mild dermatitis rash, you would encourage:
   (a) washing the area with an antiseptic soap frequently to keep the area clean.
   (b) the use of an antifungal ointment.
   (c) talcum powder to soothe the inflamed skin.
   (d) the use of a mild steroidal cream.

9. Your postoperative patient develops cellulitis in the leg. Your nursing treatments would include:
   (a) keeping both the legs elevated as much as possible.
   (b) encouraging ambulation as much as possible to help the blood flow.
   (c) application of ice four times a day for one hour each to reduce inflammation.
   (d) application of moisturizing lotion three times daily to keep the skin moist.

10. To clean a wound, it is best to use:
   (a) hydrogen peroxide to bubble away the debris.
   (b) tap water.
   (c) saline.
   (d) it is best not to disturb a healing wound.

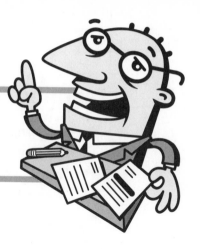

CHAPTER 11

Fluids and Electrolytes

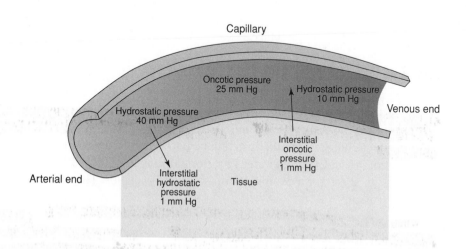

Capillary

Oncotic pressure
25 mm Hg

Hydrostatic pressure
10 mm Hg

Venous end

Hydrostatic pressure
40 mm Hg

Interstitial
oncotic
pressure
1 mm Hg

Arterial end

Interstitial
hydrostatic
pressure
1 mm Hg

Tissue

Learning Objectives

1 Hyponatremia
2 Hypernatremia
3 Hypocalcemia
4 Hypercalcemia
5 Hypokalemia
6 Hyperkalemia
7 Hypomagnesemia

8 Hypermagnesemia
9 Metabolic acidosis
10 Metabolic alkalosis
11 Hypophosphatemia
12 Hyperphosphatemia
13 Dehydration

Key Terms

Acid base balance
Aldosterone
Angiotensin
Antidiuretic hormone
 (ADH)
Diffusion

Edema
Extracellular
Hypertonic
Hypotonic
Interstitial space
Intracellular

Isotonic
Natriuretic peptides
Osmolarity
pH
Renin
Third space

How Fluids and Electrolytes Work

Fluids in the body are found in three basic places: within the cells (intracellular), outside the cells (extracellular), and within the tissue spaces (interstitial space or third space). A balance should be maintained to keep concentrations of both fluids and electrolytes in the proper areas for normal function. The cell walls are semi-permeable to allow for movement (diffusion) of molecules. This helps to maintain osmotic pressure.

Edema occurs when too much fluid enters the interstitial space. Peripheral edema usually collects in subcutaneous areas. The higher hydrostatic pressure in the vessel causes fluids to move into the interstitial areas which have lower pressure, allowing the fluid to build up.

Normal osmolarity of plasma is 270 to 300 mOsm/L. Isotonic or normotonic fluids have similar concentrations. This prevents fluids from shifting into spaces they do not belong. Hypertonic solutions have a concentration greater than 300 mOsm/L and exert a greater pressure, which pulls water from the isotonic area to the hypertonic solution in an attempt to equalize the osmolarity. Hypotonic solutions have a concentration of less than 270 mOsm/L and exert less pressure, which allows water to be pulled from the hypotonic area into the isotonic area.

HORMONAL REGULATION OF FLUIDS AND ELECTROLYTES

Aldosterone is secreted by the adrenal cortex in response to sodium changes. Where sodium goes, water follows. Aldosterone signals the tubules within the nephrons in the kidneys to reabsorb sodium and therefore water. This increases blood osmolarity. Aldosterone also aids in control of potassium levels.

Renin is secreted by the kidneys in responses to changes in sodium or fluid volume. In the circulation, renin acts on a plasma protein called renin substrate (also called angiotensinogen), converting it to angiotensin I. In the pulmonary circulation, angiotensin-converting enzyme converts angiotensin I to angiotensin II. This causes vascular constriction and aldosterone secretion.

Antidiuretic hormone (ADH) is produced in the brain and stored in the posterior pituitary. It is released when there is a change in the osmolarity of the blood. ADH acts on the renal tubules, causing them to reabsob more water, which decreases blood osmolarity. When the osmolarity gets too low, the release of ADH is not needed and the water is excreted in the urine.

Natriuretic peptides are secreted in response to increases in blood volume and blood pressure. When atrial natriuretic peptide (ANP) and brain natriuretic peptide (BNP) are secreted, kidney reabsorption of sodium is inhibited and the glomerular filtration rate is increased. Blood osmolarity is decreased and urine output is increased.

IV fluids		
Solution	Osmolarity (mOsm/L)	Hypo-, Iso-, or Hypertonic
0.9% saline (normal saline, NS)	308	Isotonic
0.45% saline (1/2 normal saline)	154	Hypotonic
5% dextrose in water (D_5W)	272	Isotonic
10% dextrose in water ($D_{10}W$)	500	Hypertonic
5% dextrose in Ringer's lactate	525	Hypertonic
5% dextrose in 0.45% saline	406	Hypertonic
5% dextrose in 0.9% saline	560	Hypertonic
Ringer's lactate	273	Isotonic

ACID BASE BALANCE

Maintaining acid-base balance will keep the pH level within the normal range of 7.35 to 7.45. The lungs and the kidneys are integral in maintaining the normal acid-base balance. The body constantly monitors the pH level and makes adjustments in an attempt to correct any abnormalities. $pHCO_3$ is regulated by the kidneys. pCO_2 is regulated by the lungs. If the patient develops acidosis there will be a low pH and either a drop in $pHCO_3$ (metabolic) or a rise in pCO_2 (respiratory). If the patient develops alkalosis there will be an increase in pH and either an increase in $pHCO_3$ (metabolic) or a drop in pCO_2 (respiratory). In an attempt to maintain as normal an internal environment as possible, the body will attempt to compensate for the changes that are occurring. The lungs are able to correct much more rapidly than the kidneys.

Just the Facts

1 *Hyponatremia*

WHAT WENT WRONG?

Hyponatremia is an abnormally low amount of sodium in the blood. Low levels of sodium may be due to loss of sodium from the body, movement of sodium from the blood to other spaces, or dilution of sodium concentration within the plasma. Some causes include increased excretion or abnormal excretion of sodium, water imbalance, hormonal imbalance (such as excess ADH), ecstasy (methylenedioxymethylamphetamine) use, hypothyroidism, renal failure, diuretics, diarrhea, vomiting, and wound drainage.

PROGNOSIS

Identification and correction of the underlying cause is important in treatment of hyponatremia. Water restriction of all patients with hyponatremia will help to prevent further dilution of the plasma concentration of sodium. Seizure and death may occur if the electrolyte imbalance is not identified and corrected.

HALLMARK SIGNS AND SYMPTOMS

- Hypotension, especially orthostatic (with position changes—from lying to sitting) due to decrease in cardiac output in setting of hypovolemia

- Nausea
- Diarrhea due to increased gastrointestinal motility
- Increased bowel sounds due to increased gastrointestinal motility
- Malaise or excessive activity
- Muscle weakness
- Decreased deep tendon reflexes
- Personality changes due to cerebral edema and increased intracranial pressure
- Altered level of consciousness
- Seizure

INTERPRETING TEST RESULTS

- A blood serum sodium level < 135 mEq/L (normal sodium level is 135 to 145 mEq/L).
- Spot urine for sodium level.

TREATMENT

- Water restriction.
- Administer saline solution IV if patient has fluid deficit (hypovolemic).
- Furosemide if fluid-overloaded.
- Treat underlying cause to correct problem.

NURSING DIAGNOSES

- Deficient fluid volume
- Excess fluid volume
- Risk for disturbed thought processes
- Decreased cardiac output

NURSING INTERVENTION

- Record fluid intake and output to monitor fluid status.
- Monitor vital signs.
- Weigh patient daily.

- Monitor for signs of dehydration: decreased skin turgor (elasticity), dry mucous membranes, decreased sweating, neurologic changes.
- Appropriate oral hygiene for dry mucous membranes.
- Proper skin care is especially important if the patient is experiencing diarrhea or dehydration.
- Explain to the patient fluid restriction and dietary modifications.
- Increase sodium in diet appropriately, considering comorbidities.

2 *Hypernatremia*

WHAT WENT WRONG?

Hypernatremia is an abnormally high amount of sodium in blood. Fluid volume may be altered as a result of changes in the levels of sodium. A mild rise in sodium levels causes tissue that is normally excitable to become more irritable—for example, cardiac muscle. The osmolarity of extracellular fluid also increases as the sodium level increases. This is in attempt to correct the sodium increase by bringing more fluid from the cells into the extracellular area. These dehydrated, more irritable cells have a decreased ability to respond to stimuli.

Causes may include insufficient water intake (patients who are NPO), insufficient sodium excretion due to hormone imbalance, renal failure, corticosteroids, increased sodium intake or increased water loss due to fever, hyperventilation, increased metabolism, and dehydration due to sweating, vomiting, or diarrhea.

PROGNOSIS

Identification and correction of the cause is necessary to return the patient to a normal fluid and electrolyte balance. IV fluids are carefully monitored during this treatment period to avoid overcorrection of the sodium level, causing hyponatremia. If the sodium level is severely elevated, the patient may need hemodialysis. Hypervolemia associated with hypernatremia in some patients may cause heart failure and pulmonary edema.

HALLMARK SIGNS AND SYMPTOMS

- Weight gain due to fluid retention
- Restlessness, irritability, and agitation due to increase in neural activity with normal or low fluid volume

- Decreased level of consciousness due to decrease in neural activity with hypervolemia
- Muscle twitching due to irregular muscle contractions
- Muscle weakness bilaterally
- Blood pressure increased—compare with normal for patient
- Decreased myocardial contractility, resulting in less effective pumping action of heart muscle
- Distended neck veins in hypervolemic patients
- Less cardiac output, especially with hypovolemic patients
- Increased thirst in an attempt to increase fluid intake

INTERPRETING TEST RESULTS

- A blood serum sodium level > 145 mEq/L. Normal sodium is 135 to 145 mEq/L.
- Spot urine for sodium level.

TREATMENT

Hypotonic IV fluids are typically given to correct hypernatremic patients who are volume-depleted. Diuretics are also used to help correct the sodium balance.

- Administer 0.225 percent sodium chloride, 0.33 percent sodium chloride, or 0.45 percent sodium chloride to correct fluid and sodium status.
- Administer diuretics to remove excess fluids and promote sodium loss:
  - furosemide, bumetanide

NURSING DIAGNOSES

- Disturbed thought process
- Excess fluid volume
- Deficient fluid volume

NURSING INTERVENTION

- Monitor vital signs, check pulse rate and rhythm, check blood pressure, and compare with prior.

- Weigh daily and compare.
- Record fluid intake and output to check balance of fluid.
- Monitor IV site for patency, signs of infiltration such as redness or induration.
- Consult with dietician.
- Explain to the patient:
  - Restrict salt in the diet.
  - Fluid intake restriction.
  - Proper oral hygiene to avoid irritation due to fluid restriction.

3 *Hypocalcemia*

WHAT WENT WRONG?

Hypocalcemia is an abnormally low level of calcium in the blood. Decreased levels of calcium may be due to inadequate intake or absorption (vitamin D deficiency, malabsorption), excess loss (associated with burns, renal disease, diuretics, or alcoholism), endocrine disorders (such as hypoparathyroidism), decreased serum albumin, hyperphosphatemia, or sepsis.

PROGNOSIS

Identification and correction of the cause is necessary to return the patient to a normal fluid and electrolyte balance. As the calcium level becomes more abnormal, the risk to the patient is greater. Seizures and cardiac arrhythmias may develop, which may become life-threatening.

HALLMARK SIGNS AND SYMPTOMS

- Irritability
- Paresthesia of lips (circumoral) and extremities
- Muscle spasm and cramping
- Tetany—intermittent painful tonic spasms, usually involving the arms and legs
- Abdominal pain due to muscle cell cramping within the gastrointestinal tract
- Laryngospasm and stridor (abnormal high-pitched breathing sound) as airway becomes narrowed

- Seizures due to irritation of nervous system tissue
- Cardiac arrhythmias due to increased excitation of cardiac muscle cells
- Prolonged QT interval will predispose to ventricular arrhythmias
- Contraction of facial muscle after tapping facial nerve anterior to ear (Chvostek's sign) due to increased excitation of nerve and muscle cells
- Carpal spasm after inflation of blood pressure cuff to upper arm—occludes brachial artery and applies pressure to nerves (Trousseau's sign)

INTERPRETING TEST RESULTS

- Blood serum calcium level of less than 9 mg/dL.

TREATMENT

- Maintain intravenous access.
- High calcium diet to replenish lost calcium.
- Administer vitamin D if patient has deficiency; helps with absorption of calcium:
  - ergocalciferol (vitamin D_2)
- Administer calcium gluconate 10 percent IV (emergency treatment for seizure, tetany, cardiac arrhythmia).
- Administer calcium chloride (emergency treatment).

NURSING DIAGNOSES

- Imbalanced nutrition: less than what body requires
- At risk for injury

NURSING INTERVENTION

- Monitor vital signs for changes.
- Monitor intake and output.
- Monitor neurologic status for change, irritability, and disorientation.
- Monitor cardiovascular status for changes, irregularity of heartbeat, pulse deficit (difference between heartbeat and peripheral pulse checked at the same time), and cardiac rhythm.

- Monitor for signs of hypercalcemia when administering medication (can over-medicate with calcium):
  - nausea
  - vomiting
  - anorexia
- Explain to the patient:
  - Avoid dependence on laxatives—these medications can alter bowel patterns, causing altered absorption and excess elimination of calcium and other electrolytes.
  - Avoid dependence or overuse of antacids—these medications cause excess intake of calcium (or other electrolytes, depending on composition).

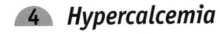 **4**   *Hypercalcemia*

WHAT WENT WRONG?

Hypercalcemia is an abnormally high amount of calcium in the blood. Excess intake of calcium (such as supplements or antacids) or altered excretion of calcium (such as in patients with renal failure or those taking thiazide diuretics) may cause hypercalcemia. Patients may also develop elevated calcium levels with prolonged immobility, glucocorticoid use, hyperthyroidism, hyperparathyroidism, lithium use, dehydration, or malignancies with metastasis to the bone.

PROGNOSIS

Correction of the calcium level is necessary to control the signs and symptoms. Correction or management of the underlying disorder is necessary to correct the abnormal calcium level. High calcium levels cause altered excitability of heart, skeletal, and smooth muscle tissues of the gastrointestinal tract, and nervous tissues.

HALLMARK SIGNS AND SYMPTOMS

- Increased heart rate initially
- Bounding peripheral pulses

- Bradycardia later as electrical conduction is slowed
- Sinus arrest then cardiac arrest due to altered response of cardiac tissue to normal stimuli
- Shallow respirations due to skeletal muscle weakness
- Muscle weakness due to changes in neuromuscular response to normal stimuli
- Cardiac arrhythmias
- Nausea and vomiting due to decrease in peristaltic activity
- Constipation due to decrease in peristaltic activity
- Dehydration
- Kidney stones form as excess calcium deposits in kidneys; may be excreted in urine

INTERPRETING TEST RESULTS

- Blood calcium level of greater than 10.5 mEq/L.
- Increased calcium level in urine.
- EKG shows shortened ST segment, widened T-waves.

TREATMENT

Medications are typically used to reduce calcium levels. When levels are highly elevated or patients are having life-threatening problems, dialysis may also be utilized to reduce calcium levels.

- Stop all calcium-containing medications (supplements, antacids).
- Monitor cardiac rhythm.
- Maintain intravenous access.
- Administer 0.9 percent normal saline solution to ensure adequate hydration status; sodium aids in urinary excretion of calcium.
- Administer Loop diuretics to enhance the excretion of calcium:
  - furosemide
- Administer plicamycin, a calcium binder, to lower calcium levels.
- Administer calcitonin, phosphorus, bisphosphonates (etidronate, pamidronate —to inhibit calcium resorption from the bone).

NURSING DIAGNOSES

- Ineffective breathing pattern
- Decreased cardiac output
- Impaired urinary elimination

NURSING INTERVENTION

- Monitor vital signs for changes.
- Monitor cardiovascular status for irregularity of heart rhythm, pulse deficit.
- Monitor intake and output.
- Assess muscle strength—hand grips, foot pushes bilaterally for strength and equality.
- Assess abdomen for bowel sounds, distention, and pain.
- Encourage mobilization, assist with ambulation if necessary to decrease bone resorption due to immobility.
- Assist with range-of-motion exercises.
- Low-calcium diet to reduce intake.
- Strain urine for stones.
- Explain to patient:
  - High calcium foods.
  - Avoid calcium supplements.
  - Avoid calcium-based antacids.
  - Weight-bearing exercise is important to avoid bone resorption.

5 *Hypokalemia*

WHAT WENT WRONG

Hypokalemia is a lower-than-normal level of potassium in the blood. A balance between the amount of potassium within the cell (intracellular) and outside the cell (extracellular) is necessary. This allows the resting potential of the cell membrane to be maintained. When there are low potassium levels, a greater-than-normal stimulus is needed to depolarize the cell membrane. Many cells become more sluggish, especially nerve cells. However, cardiac cells become more excitable. Fluid losses due to diuretics or diarrhea, endocrine disorders (such as hyperthyroidism, hyperaldosteronism), insufficient intake of potassium, and low magnesium levels can all contribute to low potassium levels. Dietary intake is the main source of potassium, so patients with poor nutritional intake or prolonged NPO status are also at risk for hypokalemia.

PROGNOSIS

Low potassium levels may range from minor to life-threatening. The more abnormal the level, the greater the chance the patient will develop a cardiac arrhythmia. Correction or management of the underlying cause is necessary to help restore the electrolyte balance.

HALLMARK SIGNS AND SYMPTOMS

- Muscle weakness due to need for greater stimulation of cell due to low potassium level
- Muscle cramps
- Malaise and lethargy
- Decrease in deep tendon reflex response due to lack of response of nerve tissue to normal stimuli
- Anorexia and constipation due to decrease in peristaltic activity
- Palpitations due to cardiac arrhythmias caused by excitability of cardiac muscle
- Rhabdomyolysis (destruction or degeneration of muscle tissue) in severe hypokalemia
- Cardiac arrest in severe hypokalemia

INTERPRETING TEST RESULTS

- Serum potassium level less than 3.5 mEq/L.
- EKG shows development of U-waves, ST depression, premature ventricular contractions, AV block.

TREATMENT

- Correct fluid imbalance.
- Stop or change medications that contribute to potassium loss, if possible (for example, Loop diuretics).

- Encourage potassium-rich foods.
- Administer potassium supplements.
- Administer potassium in intravenous fluids:
  - Avoid glucose in fluid which will shift potassium into cells.
  - Potassium concentration of no more than 40 mEq/L in peripheral lines.
- Monitor cardiac rhythm.

NURSING DIAGNOSIS

- Activity intolerance
- Decreased cardiac output
- Fatigue

NURSING INTERVENTIONS

- Monitor vital signs for change.
- Monitor cardiac system for rate, rhythm, and pulse deficit.
- Monitor intake and output.
- Monitor intravenous site for redness, swelling, warmth, and pain.
- Teach patient about medication and diet changes:
  - Foods rich in potassium (bananas, tomatoes, orange juice)

6 *Hyperkalemia*

WHAT WENT WRONG

Hyperkalemia is an elevated level of potassium in the blood. Dietary intake is the main source of potassium. Patients are at risk for hyperkalemia when there is excessive ingestion of potassium-rich foods or salt substitutes, they are on medications that cause potassium retention (ACE inhibitors, angiotensin receptor blockers, potassium-sparing diuretics such as amiloride or spironolactone, NSAIDs, trimethoprim, pentamidine), or there is excess release of potassium from the cells (hemolysis, acidosis, low insulin levels, beta blocker use, digoxin overdose, succinylcholine, or rhabdomyolysis).

PROGNOSIS

As potassium levels rise, the risk of cardiac arrhythmias also increases. An extreme elevation creates a medical emergency. Correction or management of the underlying cause is necessary to help restore the electrolyte balance.

HALLMARK SIGNS AND SYMPTOMS

- Weakness and dizziness due to neuromuscular changes
- Abdominal distention
- Nausea, vomiting, diarrhea due to change in membrane potential on GI system
- Palpitations due to arrhythmias
- Arrhythmias due to changes in normal cardiac conduction
- Cardiac arrest

INTERPRETING TEST RESULTS

- Potassium level > 5 mEq/L.
- EKG shows peaked T-waves, widened QRS-waves, ventricular asystole, cardiac arrest.

TREATMENT

The treatment choices will depend on the severity of the potassium elevation. Decreasing further intake, enhancing renal excretion, and cellular uptake are all goals of treatment.

- Monitor cardiac rhythm.
- Administer intravenous insulin and glucose to move potassium from extracellular fluid to intracellular fluid.
- Administer calcium gluconate intravenously.
- Administer $NaHCO_3$ to move potassium from extracellular fluid to intracellular fluid.
- Administer diuretics to remove potassium from body.
- Administer kayexalate to remove potassium from body via GI tract.
- Monitor electrolyte levels.

- Restrict potassium intake.
- Dialysis for severe elevations.

NURSING DIAGNOSIS

- Decreased cardiac output
- Risk for imbalanced fluid volume
- Activity intolerance
- Altered bowel elimination

NURSING INTERVENTIONS

- Monitor vital signs.
- Monitor cardiac rhythm.
- Monitor cardiovascular status for regularity of rhythm, rate, heart sounds, and peripheral pulses.
- Monitor abdomen for bowel sounds, distention, and pain.
- Monitor intravenous site for redness, swelling, and pain.
- Teach patient about medications and diet:
  - Avoid foods that are high in potassium.
  - Avoid salt substitutes (most are potassium-based).

7 *Hypomagnesemia*

WHAT WENT WRONG?

Hypomagnesemia is a lower-than-normal magnesium level in the blood. Low serum levels of magnesium can be due to lack of sufficient intake or absorption (malnutrition, vomiting, diarrhea, celiac disease, Crohn's disease), excess excretion of magnesium (renal loss, chronic alcohol intake, diuretic use, aminoglycoside antibiotics, antineoplastics), or intracellular movement of magnesium (ascites, hyperglycemia, insulin administration). The cell membranes become more excitable in the setting of low magnesium levels. Patients may also have associated imbalances of potassium and calcium.

PROGNOSIS

Correction of the magnesium level is necessary to return normal electrolyte balance to the patient. Correction or management of the underlying condition may be necessary to correct the magnesium level. Nerve impulse transmission is increased in patients with hypomagnesemia. As the magnesium level drops, the patient may develop seizures or cardiac arrhythmias.

HALLMARK SIGNS AND SYMPTOMS

- Painful paresthesia (numbness and tingling)
- Hyperactive deep tendon reflexes—using a reflex hammer, strike tendon at specific site to elicit response (patellar tendon, Achilles tendon, brachioradialis, bicep, or tricep)
- Muscle twitching
- Seizures due to irritability of nervous tissue in brain
- Confusion due to Central Nervous System (CNS) irritability
- Headaches
- Mood changes or irritability
- Decreased appetite, nausea, and constipation due to decreased gastrointestinal motility
- Decreased bowel sounds and abdominal distention
- Arrhythmia, ectopic beats, ventricular arrhythmias
- Contraction of facial muscle after tapping facial nerve anterior to ear (Chvostek's sign) due to increased excitation of nerve and muscle cells if concurrent hypocalcemia
- Carpal spasm after inflation of blood pressure cuff to upper arm—occludes brachial artery and applies pressure to nerves (Trousseau's sign) if concurrent hypocalcemia

INTERPRETING TEST RESULTS

- Blood serum magnesium level < 1.5 mEq/L.
- EKG shows depressed ST segments, tall T-waves.

TREATMENT

- Administer magnesium sulfate intravenously to increase levels.
- Monitor deep tendon reflexes.
- Monitor cardiac rhythm.
- Increase magnesium in the patient's diet.
- May need to correct calcium and potassium concurrently.

NURSING DIAGNOSES

- Impaired gas exchange
- Risk for injury
- Decreased cardiac output

NURSING INTERVENTION

- Monitor intake and output.
- Monitor vital signs for changes.
- Monitor cardiovascular status for changes in heart rhythm, pulse deficit.
- Explain to the patient:
  - Eat whole grains, legumes, fish, and dark green leafy vegetables that are high in magnesium.
  - No laxatives.

8   *Hypermagnesemia*

WHAT WENT WRONG?

Hypermagnesemia is a greater-than-normal amount of magnesium in the blood. Patients with poor renal function or long-term abuse of magnesium-containing compounds have difficulty excreting magnesium. The excess of magnesium in the blood causes the cell membranes to become less excitable than normal, requiring a greater stimuli than would normally be needed to cause a required effect. As the magnesium level continues to rise, the cell membrane becomes more resistant to its natural stimuli.

PROGNOSIS

Correction of the magnesium level is necessary to prevent life-threatening complications. Patients are at significant risk for cardiac arrest as the magnesium levels continue to rise.

HALLMARK SIGNS AND SYMPTOMS

- Bradycardia due to slowed cellular response to normal stimuli
- Hypotension due to vasodilation
- Drowsiness or lethargy
- Weakness
- Less-than-normal deep tendon reflexes
- Confusion
- Urinary retention
- Cardiac arrest when level severely elevated

INTERPRETING TEST RESULTS

- Blood serum magnesium levels > 2.5 mEq/L.
- EKG shows widened QRS complex, prolonged PR intervals.
- BUN elevation if there is renal insufficiency.

TREATMENT

- Administer magnesium antagonist intravenously:
  - calcium chloride
- Administer Loop diuretic to reduce magnesium level:
  - furosemide
- Dialysis—hemodialysis or peritoneal, to remove excess magnesium (especially in patients with renal failure).
- Reduce magnesium in diet (avoid meat, legumes, dark green leafy vegetables, fish, whole grains, nuts).
- Increase fluid intake to maintain hydration.

NURSING DIAGNOSES

- Impaired gas exchange
- Risk for injury
- Reduced cardiac output

NURSING INTERVENTION

- Monitor intake and output.
- Monitor vital signs for changes.
- Monitor cardiovascular status for changes in heart rate, rhythm.
- Monitor labs for electrolyte balance.
- Explain to the patient:
  - Avoid foods high in magnesium.
  - Avoid magnesium-based medications.

9 *Metabolic Acidosis*

WHAT WENT WRONG?

The acid-base balance of the blood is thrown off, causing it to become more acidic. There is an arterial pH of less than 7.35. There may be an overproduction of hydrogen ions (lactic acidosis in fever or seizures, diabetic ketoacidosis, starvation, alcohol or aspirin intake), deficient elimination of hydrogen ions (renal failure), deficient production of bicarbonate ions (renal failure, pancreatic insufficiency), or excess elimination of bicarbonate ions (diarrhea).

PROGNOSIS

Correction or management of the underlying cause is necessary to help restore the acid-base balance.

HALLMARK SIGNS AND SYMPTOMS

- Lethargy due to increased hydrogen ion concentration in blood
- Muscle weakness bilaterally due to neuromuscular manifestations

- Tachycardia early in acidosis; later, cardiac electrical conduction slows, causing bradycardia and increasing risk for heart block or arrhythmia
- Hypotension due to vasodilation
- Rapid, deep breathing (hyperventilation) as body attempts to compensate

INTERPRETING TEST RESULTS

- Arterial blood gas showing pH < 7.35 and bicarbonate < 22 mEq/L, normal $PaCO_2$.
- Ketones in urine possible.
- Potassium level elevated.
- Chloride level normal or elevated.

TREATMENT

- Administer intravenous fluids for hydration as necessary.
- Monitor arterial blood gas levels.
- Administer supplemental oxygen as necessary.
- Administer bicarbonate if bicarbonate levels are low.
- Correct the underlying condition that is causing the imbalance.
- Administer insulin and fluids in diabetic ketoacidosis.
- Mechanical ventilation if necessary.
- Hemodialysis if necessary to restore normal balance in system or remove offending substance.

NURSING DIAGNOSES

- Disturbed thought processes
- Ineffective breathing pattern

NURSING INTERVENTION

- Monitor intake and output.
- Monitor vital signs for changes.

- Monitor lab test results.
- Monitor ABG results.

10 *Metabolic Alkalosis*

WHAT WENT WRONG?

The acid-base balance of the blood is basic because of either a decrease in acidity or an increase in bicarbonate. Alkalosis is often associated with decreased levels of potassium or calcium. Metabolic alkalosis may be due to excess intake of antacids, blood transfusions, long-term parenteral nutrition, prolonged vomiting or nasogastric suctioning, Cushing's disease, use of thiazide diuretics, or excess aldosterone.

PROGNOSIS

Correction or management of the underlying cause is necessary to help restore the acid-base balance.

HALLMARK SIGNS AND SYMPTOMS

- Muscle weakness due to neuromuscular changes and hypokalemia
- Muscle cramping and twitching due to electrolyte changes
- Anxiety and irritability
- Tetany and seizures, as alkalosis worsens
- Positive Chvostek's sign due to hypocalcemia
- Positive Trousseau's sign due to hypocalcemia
- Increased reflexes due to neuromuscular irritability
- Increased heart rate and myocardial irritability

INTERPRETING TEST RESULTS

- Arterial blood gas showing pH > 7.45, bicarbonate > 28 mEq/L, pCO_2 elevated.
- Serum potassium low, chloride low.

TREATMENT

- Monitor arterial blood gases and electrolyte levels.
- Administer fluids and electrolytes as necessary.
- Administer supplemental oxygen if necessary.
- Administer electrolyte replacement as indicated.

NURSING DIAGNOSES

- Risk for injury
- Disturbed thought process

NURSING INTERVENTION

- Monitor vital signs for changes.
- Monitor cardiovascular status for changes in heart rate, rhythm.
- Monitor intake and output.
- Assess intravenous site for signs of infiltration.
- Check neurological status for changes.

11 *Hypophosphatemia*

WHAT WENT WRONG?

Hypophosphatemia is a lower-than-normal amount of phosphorus in the blood. Chronic alcohol use, chronic obstructive pulmonary disease, asthma medications (loop diuretics, corticosteroids, adrenergic agonists, xanthine derivatives) are associated with low phosphate levels. Vitamin D is important in the intestinal absorption of phosphate. Parathyroid hormone stimulates the release of phosphate from the bone tissue. An overproduction can lead to hypophosphatemia.

PROGNOSIS

Correction or management of the underlying cause is necessary to help restore the electrolyte balance. Proper treatment cannot be given without identification of the underlying cause.

HALLMARK SIGNS AND SYMPTOMS

- Muscle weakness due to impairment in oxygen delivery to the tissues
- Rhabdomyolysis with breakdown of muscle tissue
- Paresthesia (tingling sensations)
- Hemolytic anemia due to fragility of red blood cells
- Encephalopathy (irritability, confusion, disorientation, seizures, coma)
- Respiratory failure or trouble weaning from ventilator due to changes in oxygen delivery to cells
- Weakening of bone structure seen in chronic, severe hypophosphatemia due to phosphate leaving bones
- Petechiae due to poorly functioning platelets

INTERPRETING TEST RESULTS

- Phosphorus < 1.7 mEq/L in blood serum.
- Spot urine sampling for diminished phosphate.
- Parathyroid (PTH) levels elevated.
- In anemia, low hemoglobin and hematocrit.
- Elevated creatine kinase in rhabdomyolysis.

TREATMENT

- Administer potassium phosphate to replace phosphate:
  - Oral for mild to moderate loss, or intravenous for severe loss.
- Monitor for hypotension if intravenous replacement of phosphate.
- Monitor serum phosphate, calcium, potassium, and magnesium levels every 6 to 8 hours during initial replacement.
- Diet high in phosphorus for chronic hypophosphatemia.

NURSING DIAGNOSES

- Risk for injury
- Imbalanced nutrition

NURSING INTERVENTION

- Monitor intake and output.
- Monitor vital signs; may see hypotension with intravenous phosphate infusion.
- Explain to the patient:
    - Diet of turkey, skim milk and milk products, and dried fruits.

12 *Hyperphosphatemia*

WHAT WENT WRONG?

Hyperphosphatemia is a higher-than-normal amount of phosphorus in the blood. Patients may develop increased phosphate levels as a result of renal insufficiency, increase in phosphorus intake (supplements, laxatives, enemas, excess vitamin D), hypoparathyroidism, rhabdomyolysis, or as a result of cell destruction from chemotherapy. As phosphate levels increase, calcium levels decrease.

PROGNOSIS

Correction or management of the underlying cause is necessary to help restore the electrolyte balance.

HALLMARK SIGNS AND SYMPTOMS

- Asymptomatic
- Symptoms of underlying disorder, such as renal disease
- May see symptoms of coexisting electrolyte disorders, such as hypocalcemia

INTERPRETING TEST RESULTS

- Phosphorus > 4.6 mEq/L in blood serum.

TREATMENT

- Administer medications orally in divided doses during the day to bind phosphate:
  - calcium acetate
  - aluminum hydroxide
  - lanthanum
- Dialysis to remove excess phosphate.
- Diet low in phosphorus to avoid excess intake.
- Monitor labs for correction of electrolytes.

NURSING DIAGNOSES

- Risk for injury
- Imbalanced nutrition

NURSING INTERVENTION

- Monitor intake and output.
- Monitor vital signs.
- Explain to the patient:
  - No over-the-counter medications (i.e. laxatives) that contain phosphorus to avoid recurrence.
  - Medication use and schedule.

13 *Dehydration*

WHAT WENT WRONG?

A state of having less-than-normal body fluids, due to an excess loss of fluids or an inadequate intake of fluids. Dehydration may be actual or relative. A relative dehydration exists when the amount of fluid and electrolytes in the body is correct, but the placement is not correct. If fluid shifting has occurred and the fluid is now in the interstitial areas rather than in the circulating blood volume, the patient may actually be experiencing a relative dehydration. Even though there is adequate fluid within the body, it cannot be utilized at this time. More commonly, dehydration is actual and due to loss of fluid from the body or lack of adequate hydration.

PROGNOSIS

Adequate replacement of fluids with the appropriate fluid type is essential to ensure adequate circulating blood volume.

HALLMARK SIGNS AND SYMPTOMS

- Thirst as the body wants more fluids
- Poor skin turgor due to fluid loss
- Tachycardia—heart rate increases to circulate remaining volume faster
- Tachypnea—respiratory rate increases in an attempt to obtain more oxygen
- Decreased urinary output—less volume available to leave the body
- Increased BUN as volume depletes
- Hypotension due to decrease in circulating blood volume

INTERPRETING TEST RESULTS

- BUN elevated.
- Elevated hemoglobin and hematocrit as blood hemoconcentrates.

TREATMENT

- Intravenous and oral fluid replacement.
- Monitor serum electrolytes, BUN, creatinine, urine electrolytes.
- Monitor cardiac rhythm if there is an electrolyte disturbance.

NURSING DIAGNOSIS

- Deficient fluid volume
- Risk for impaired urinary elimination
- Impaired oral mucous membrane

NURSING INTERVENTION

- Monitor vital signs; check for orthostatic hypotension.
- Monitor intake and output.
- Assess intravenous access site for signs of redness, swelling, or pain.
- Assess skin and mucous membranes for dryness.
- Assess cardiovascular status—heart rate, heart sounds, peripheral pulses.
- Assess respiratory status—lung sounds, respiratory rate.
- Encourage oral fluid intake.
- Increase frequency of mouth care.

Crucial Diagnostic Tests

Blood Tests

Blood is removed from the patient and sent to the lab. The lab determines if the levels of any critical elements of the blood are abnormal. These are:

- Red blood cell count (RBC): decreased in anemia, bleeding, SLE, chronic infection, Addison's disease, Hodgkin's disease, leukemia, multiple myeloma; increased in polycythemia; relative increase in dehydration, severe burn, shock. Normal range $3.71–5.25 \times 10^6/mm^3$
- White blood cell count (WBC): decreased in viral infection, bone marrow depression or disorder, heavy metal intoxication, irradiation, hypersplenism; increased in bacterial infection. Normal range $3.8–10.8 \times 10^3/mm^3$
- Prothrombin time (PT): High means blood less likely to clot; increases with anticoagulants (coumadin), deficiency in vitamin K, factors II, V, VII, X, liver disease, DIC. Normal range 9.9–13.1 seconds
- International normalized ratio (INR): High means clotting ability is diminished; spontaneous bleeding is possible with INR level greater than 6.0. Normal range 0.69–1.37
- Partial thromboplastin time (PTT): Low in early DIC and in extensive cancer; high means blood is thin due to clotting disorder or medication such as heparin. Normal range 25.8–34.6 seconds
- Platelet count: Low means diminished clotting ability, very low counts mean spontaneous bleeding may occur; high means increased clotting ability, potential for platelet clumping. Normal range $132–413 \times 10^3/mm^3$

- Hematocrit (Hct): decreased in anemia, chronic disease, hemolytic reaction, adrenal insufficiency, leukemia, lymphoma. Normal range 34.3–44.4%

- Hemoglobin (Hgb): decreased in anemia, cancer, hemolytic reaction, liver disease, kidney disease, hyperthyroidism, SLE; increased in chronic obstructive pulmonary disease, hemoconcentration, polycythemia, burns. Normal range 11.5–15.2 g/dL

- Erythrocyte sedimentation rate (ESR): Low means anti-inflammatories (steroids, aspirin), blood sample not processed in timely manner (allowed to sit); high means inflammation, hormonal effect (pregnancy, menses, oral contraceptives). Normal range 0–30

- Sodium (Na): Low means diarrhea, vomiting, edema, excess water intake, diuretic use, nasogastric suction, Addison's disease, hypothyroidism; high means dehydration, bronchitis, Cushing's disease, diabetes insipidus, insufficient water intake. Normal range 136–146 mmol/L

- Calcium (Ca): Low means decreased albumin levels, hyperphosphatemia, hypoparathyroidism, vitamin D deficiency, acute pancreatitis; high means cancer, hyperparathyroidism, hyperthyroidism, prolonged immobilization, Paget's disease. Normal range 8.5–10.5 mg/dL

- Phosphorus: Low means hyperparathyroidism, elevated insulin level, diabetic coma, vomiting, renal tubular acidosis; high means renal insufficiency, hypothyroidism, hypocalcemia, excess intake of alkali, Addison's disease, healing fractures.

- Magnesium: Low means hemodialysis, blood transfusion, hypoparathyroidism, malabsorption, chronic disease, chronic pancreatitis; high means renal failure, diabetic acidosis, Addison's disease, hypothyroidism, antacid use.

- Chloride (Cl): Low means vomiting, nasogastric suctioning, chronic respiratory acidosis, metabolic alkalosis, Addison's disease, SIADH, excess water intake; high means dehydration, diarrhea, metabolic acidosis, hyperparathyroidism, Cushing's syndrome, renal tubular acidosis. Normal range 99–108 mmol/L

- Potassium (K): Low means GI loss, renal loss, diuretic use, eating disorders, wound drainage, respiratory alkalosis, licorice intake; high means dehydration, renal failure, metabolic acidosis, diabetic ketoacidosis, sickle cell anemia, interstitial nephritis. Normal range 3.4–5.2 mmol/L

- Blood urea nitrogen (BUN): Low means fluid overload, low muscle mass, with low protein, low carbohydrate diet; high means renal disease, dehydration, acute MI, ketoacidosis, excess protein intake. Normal range 8–25 mg/dL

Quiz

1. Bernadette's morning lab results have just come in. Her serum potassium level is currently 5.4 mEq/L. You recognize this as:

    (a) hypokalemia.

    (b) hyperkalemia.

    (c) hypocalcemia.

    (d) hypercalcemia.

2. Rob has a history of using ectasy. He is exhibiting symptoms of hypotension, nausea, diarrhea, personality change, diminished level of consciousness, and decreased deep tendon reflexes. Lab results confirm your suspicion of hyponatremia. Treatment would include:

    (a) water restriction.

    (b) 0.33 percent sodium chloride intravenously.

    (c) use of salt substitute.

    (d) calcium carbonate orally.

3. Derek has recently converted his outdoor garage to a gym. He has been exercising frequently in his new gym due to the convenience, even in the extreme heat. He has started taking salt tablets. You think his current symptoms may be due to hypernatremia. You recognize these as:

    (a) cardiac arrhythmias, palpitations, and sinus arrest.

    (b) weakness, dizziness, abdominal distention, nausea, vomiting, and diarrhea.

    (c) weight gain, irritability, muscle twitching, and decreased myocardial contractility.

    (d) muscle cramps, malaise, constipation, rhabdomyolysis, and pupilary constriction.

4. Rocco was admitted to the hospital with a diagnosis of hypomagnesemia. He is complaining of painful paresthesia. Which of the following do you recognize as part of his treatment plan?

    (a) Dialysis and removal of legumes and whole grains from the diet.

    (b) Monitoring cardiac rhythm and checking deep tendon reflexes.

    (c) Monitoring urinary output and auscultating bowel sounds.

    (d) Palpating peripheral pulses and checking pupil reactions.

5. When performing a neurological assessment on Ken, you notice that there is contraction of his facial muscle after tapping the facial nerve anterior to his ear. You recognize this as Chvostek's sign. This is seen in:

    (a) hyponatremia.

    (b) hypokalemia.

    (c) hypocalcemia.

    (d) hypomagnesemia.

6. Grace was diagnosed with hyperparathyroidism after a work-up to determine the cause of her elevated calcium levels. The greatest concern in a patient with hypercalcemia would be:

    (a) cardiac arrhythmia and sinus arrest.

    (b) nausea and vomiting.

    (c) constipation and dehydration.

    (d) kidney stones and muscle weakness.

7. Brendan has chronic obstructive pulmonary disease, causing a constant state of respiratory acidosis. He has a history of chronic trimethoprim and NSAID use, leading to hyperkalemia. Which of the following are associated with hyperkalemia?

    (a) Irritability, circumoral paresthesia, muscle spasms, tetany, abdominal pain, laryngospasm, and prolonged QT intervals.

    (b) Muscle cramps, malaise, diminished deep tendon reflexes, anorexia, constipation, palpitations, and rhabdomyolysis.

    (c) Cardiac arrhythmia, nausea, vomiting, constipation, dehydration, kidney stones, muscle weakness, and sinus arrest.

    (d) Weakness, dizziness, abdominal distention, nausea, vomiting, diarrhea, palpitations, and cardiac arrhythmias.

8. You are monitoring intravenous fluids for Tom who is currently being treated for metabolic acidosis. You monitor his signs and symptoms typical of metabolic acidosis which include:

    (a) elevated blood pressure, bradycardia, elevated respiratory rate, and muscle twitching.

    (b) hypotension, altered heart rate, elevated respiratory rate, and muscle weakness.

    (c) hypertension, tachycardia, slowed respiratory rate, and muscle spasms.

    (d) hypotension, hypoxia, irritability, and paresthesia.

9. Vince has been taking excessive amounts of over-the-counter antacid tablets. He has been exhibiting signs of irritability, anxiety, muscle cramping, and weakness, and has recently developed tetany. You have initiated seizure precautions. You recognize that the patient is being monitored and treated for:

   (a) hyperkalemia.

   (b) hyperphosphatemia.

   (c) metabolic acidosis.

   (d) metabolic alkalosis.

10. Liz is an elderly woman brought in by concerned family members. After physical examination, she was diagnosed with dehydration. What assessment findings would you expect to see?

   (a) Bradycardia, slowed respirations, low body temperature, and weight gain.

   (b) Rales, peripheral edema, palpitations, and diaphoresis.

   (c) Tachypnea, tachycardia, hypotension, poor skin turgor, and decreased urinary output.

   (d) Malaise, lymphadenopathy, fever, shortness of breath, and nausea.

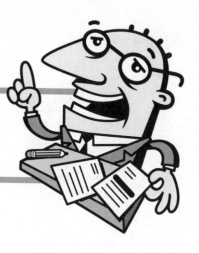

CHAPTER 12

Mental Health

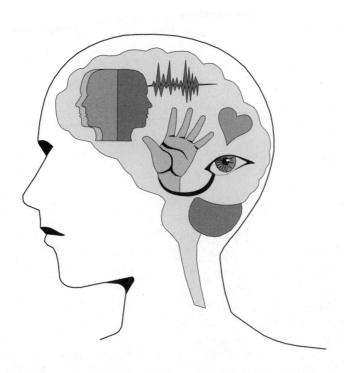

Learning Objectives

1. Anxiety
2. Panic disorder
3. Depression
4. Bipolar disorder

5. Schizophrenia
6. Anorexia nervosa
7. Bulimia nervosa
8. Delirium

Key Terms

Affect
Cognition
Content of thought
Delusions
Impairment in judgment

Insight
Judgment
Mood
Paranoid ideation

Selective serotonin
   reuptake inhibitors
Suicidal ideation
Thought process

A Look at Mental Health

Alterations in mental health can be more difficult to diagnose because there is no definitive laboratory test or radiological study with which to isolate the disorder. Patients may initially seek treatment from primary care practitioners for a variety of complaints: anxiety, insomnia, generalized aches, or other somatic complaints.

A thorough patient history should include past medical conditions, any prior mental health conditions and their treatment course, current medications, social history (including habits, work, exercise, and substance use), cultural background, environmental factors, family history, and changes in libido, appetite, or sleep. Physical examination focuses on the chief complaint from the patient's point of view and traces the progression of symptoms in a chronological order from the time of onset. Mental status examination is completed focusing on the patient's appearance, activity and behavior, affect, mood, speech, content of thought, thought process, cognition, judgment, and insight.

The majority of patients are cared for on an outpatient basis. Hospitalization should be considered for those who:

- Are too sick to care for themselves.
- Present a serious threat to themselves or to others.
- Neglect to care for themselves.
- Are violent or have bizarre behavior.
- Have suicidal ideation.
- Have paranoid ideation.
- Have delusions.
- Have a marked impairment in judgment.

Patients with a coexisting mental health disorder are also admitted to a medical surgical floor only if the medical condition warrants medical management. Caring for the patient admitted with a medical or surgical condition does not preclude the need to care for the patient's depression or schizophrenia as well. Patients may also develop medical conditions as a result of their mental health issues. Patients with inadequate nutritional intake due to an eating disorder may have significant electrolyte imbalances or cardiac dysfunction.

Just the Facts

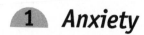 1 *Anxiety*

WHAT WENT WRONG?

Patients exhibit symptoms when an imbalance develops between the number of open receptor sites and the number of available neurotransmitters. Neurotransmitters are released from one side of a synapse and land on a specific receptor site across the synapse. A second mechanism exists (a reuptake mechanism) to remove excess neurotransmitters left within the space between where they are released and where they fill the receptor sites. When there are insufficient neurotransmitters available to fill the open neurotransmitter receptor sites, the patient develops symptoms. Patients experience an uncontrollable feeling of anxiousness which is present more days than not.

Symptom onset is typically in late teens through early thirties. Anxiety is more common in women and in patients with a family history of anxiety.

PROGNOSIS

Without proper treatment the anxiety will continue, and symptoms may even progress. The patient's quality of life is adversely affected. Social functioning becomes impaired and in some cases the patient becomes more socially isolated. Physical symptoms continue, at times necessitating visits to a primary care provider or even the emergency room. With proper treatment, the symptoms are controlled, neurotransmitter balance is restored, and remission is achieved. The symptoms will typically recur at a later point, even when properly treated. It may be months or years after a successful course of treatment before the symptoms recur. The treatment that was effective in the past will typically be effective again in the future. A longer treatment course is recommended for subsequent treatment cycles when using SSRIs (selective serotonin reuptake inhibitors).

HALLMARK SIGNS AND SYMPTOMS

- Fear, tension, apprehension due to alteration in neurotransmission
- Persistent worry
- Trouble concentrating
- Irritability and restlessness
- Tachycardia, palpitations, elevated blood pressure due to autonomic nervous system stimulation
- Hyperventilation due to fear, elevated heart rate, and palpitations
- Sweating, tremors due to autonomic nervous system stimulation
- Sleep disturbance and fatigue due to alteration in neurotransmission
- Headache due to nervous system irritability and lack of sleep

INTERPRETING TEST RESULTS

- Normal lab results

TREATMENT

- Administer anxiolytics for acute management:
  - alprazolam, clonazepam, clorazepate, diazepam, lorazepam, oxazepam

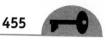

- Monitor for respiratory depression or decrease in blood pressure.
- Have benzodiazepine antagonist (flumazenil) on hand to reverse effect if needed.
- Administer antidepressants:
  - selective serotonin reuptake inhibitors—paroxetine
  - selective serotonin and norepinephrine reuptake inhibitors—venlafaxine
  - tricyclics
- Administer buspirone.
- Administer beta-blockers for symptom control.
- Psychotherapy.
- Cognitive-behavioral therapy.
- Relaxation techniques such as biofeedback.
- Desensitization—repeated exposures to graded doses of the object or situation that produces the anxiety.
- Group therapy.
- Family therapy.
- Emotive therapy.

NURSING DIAGNOSIS

- Sleep pattern disturbance
- Anxiety
- Fear
- Impaired social interaction
- Ineffective role performance

NURSING INTERVENTION

- Monitor medication intake.
- Discuss patient response to therapy.
- Monitor vital signs, watch for elevation in blood pressure with some medications.

- Monitor weight; some medications are associated with changes in weight.
- Monitor sleep; ask patient about restful sleep during the night or difficulty falling asleep.
- Teach patient to avoid alcohol intake with benzodiazepine use.

2 *Panic Disorder*

WHAT WENT WRONG?

Patients experience intermittent episodes that have a sudden onset and no predictable pattern, causing intense anxiety associated with pronounced physical symptoms. These episodes are short in duration and recurrent in nature. The disorder tends to present before the age of 25, is twice as common in women as it is in men, and tends to be familial. Some patients will choose to self-medicate with alcohol in an attempt to escape the disease, diminish symptoms, or decrease the occurrence of the episodes. Others become dependent on tranquilizing medications. Panic attacks can impede a person's life and restrict activity, especially in anticipation of a panic attack.

PROGNOSIS

With proper treatment, the frequency and intensity of the episodes will decrease. Some patients may not experience complete resolution of symptoms, even with appropriate medications.

HALLMARK SIGNS AND SYMPTOMS

- Depersonalization, as if the symptoms are happening to someone else
- Sense of doom, fear of dying due to the intensity of the physical symptoms
- Fear of losing control due to the unpredictable nature of the episodes
- Worry about future attacks due to the unpredictable nature of the episodes
- Change in behavior due to anxiety about being in a place where an attack might occur

- Palpitations, tachycardia, and chest pain
- Dyspnea
- Choking sensation
- Nausea
- Dizziness
- Diaphoresis
- Numbness

INTERPRETING TEST RESULTS

- EKG normal.
- Cardiac monitor normal.
- Lab results normal.
- Pulse oximetry normal.

TREATMENT

- Cognitive-behavioral therapy.
- Relaxation therapy.
- Administer antidepressants:
  - selective serotonin reuptake inhibitors
  - tricyclics
  - monoamine oxidase inhibitors
- Administer benzodiazepines as adjunctive treatment:
  - clonazepam, alprazolam, lorazepam
- Provide reassurance to patient.

NURSING DIAGNOSIS

- Powerlessness
- Fear
- Social isolation

NURSING INTERVENTION

- Provide reassurance to patient.
- Reduce anxiety.
- Monitor vital signs.

3 *Depression*

Patients with depression have a persistent sense of sadness, more days than not, often associated with somatic complaints. The medical work-ups for varied physical complaints will be negative. Patients typically have a loss of interest in normal activities and alterations in sleep and eating habits. Up to one-third of patients will seek care from primary care providers. Patients can also present as unkempt, dirty, withdrawn, and unwilling to engage in conversation. They see life as a state of hopelessness. The patient's depression must be treated seriously, since it can lead to suicide. A patient's request for help might be his or her last recourse.

WHAT WENT WRONG?

Several different theories exist involving the cause of depression. Genetic factors may lead to changes in the normal functioning of neurotransmitters. Neurotransmitters are released from one side of a synapse and land on a specific receptor site on the other side of the synapse. When a balance is maintained between the amount released and the amount needed to fill the receptor sites, normal function continues. When there is an imbalance, the neurotransmission is altered. Developmental factors can often be traced back to childhood. Personality disorders may begin during school age or adolescence. Psychosocial stressors are another factor linked to the development of depression. Major life changes such as the death of a family member, unemployment, or moving away from family and friends may lead to the onset of depression. A sense of sadness or grief is considered a normal response to this type of loss and should resolve as the person progresses through the normal stages of grieving. Depression, however, is not a normal response to loss. A grieving person will have a sustained sense of self-esteem, whereas a person with depression will have a sense of worthlessness.

PROGNOSIS

Proper treatment can help control the symptoms of depression. Adequate treatment can cause remission of symptoms. It is not unusual for there to be a recurrence of symptoms at some point in the future, even with appropriate treatment.

HALLMARK SIGNS AND SYMPTOMS

- Intense feeling of sadness
- Depressed mood
- Anhedonia (loss of interest in usual activities)
- Hopelessness or worthlessness
- Difficulty concentrating
- Indecision
- Changes in sleep (more or less than usual), eating (more or less than usual), and activity (more or less than usual)
- Social withdrawal and isolation
- Decreased libido
- Thoughts of death
- Physical complaints include headache, malaise, decreased libido, and changes in sleep, activity, and eating

INTERPRETING TEST RESULTS

- Diagnostic testing results normal, unless co-existing disease present.

TREATMENT

- Ask patient about suicidal thoughts.
- Ask patient about suicidal plan.
- Psychotherapy.
- Cognitive-behavioral therapy.
- Support groups.

- Antidepressant medications:
  - SSRIs
  - venlafaxine
  - nefazodone
  - bupropion
  - mirtazapine
  - tricyclics
  - monoamine oxidase inhibitors
- Electroconvulsant therapy (ECT) in refractory cases.

NURSING DIAGNOSIS

- Hopelessness
- Risk for suicide
- Dysfunctional grieving
- Impaired social interaction
- Social isolation
- Disturbed self-esteem

NURSING INTERVENTION

- Monitor patient frequently when first admitted.
- One-to-one observation if patient is a suicidal risk.
- Develop a level of sensitivity and trust with the patient.
- Ask patient about suicidal ideation; do they have a plan, have they attempted to carry out a plan.
- Monitor medication intake.
- Discuss patient response to therapy.
- Monitor vital signs; watch for elevation in blood pressure with some medications.
- Monitor weight; some medications are associated with changes in weight.
- Monitor sleep; ask patient about restful sleep during the night, and difficulty falling asleep.

Bipolar Disorder

Patients suffering from mood disorders often have difficulty with interpersonal interactions. Substance abuse occurs as patients attempt to self-medicate.

WHAT WENT WRONG?

Some patients experience episodes of depression alternating with episodes of mania or hypomania. These episodes may occur in a mixed or cyclic manner. There tends to be a high comorbidity with substance abuse in these patients. Depressive episodes tend to last longer than the manic episodes. During mania the patients are overenthusiastic, elated, hyperactive, and often engage in activities that they later regret. Others may be drawn to the patient during manic episodes due to their outgoing, engaging behavior. Later the patient's behavior tends to alienate due to mood swings, irritability, aggression, and grandiosity. There is a positive correlation between creative behavior and mood disorders. During the manic phase, the patient has grandiose ideas.

PROGNOSIS

Proper medication management is necessary to control the symptoms of bipolar disorder. Initial diagnosis and treatment of depression without recognition of the coexisting mania can lead to the onset of mania due to the antidepressant treatment. It is important to treat both components of the disorder to effectively manage the patient. Ongoing treatment is often necessary to prevent the patient from cycling into another manic or depressive episode. Some patients may have psychotic symptoms as part of the disease process.

HALLMARK SIGNS AND SYMPTOMS

- Elation
- Hyperactivity
- Increased irritability
- Flight of ideas
- Grandiosity

- Diminished need for sleep
- Rapid speech
- Easily distracted
- Excessive spending
- Hypersexuality
- Episodes of depression
- The patient may stray from medication regimen because he or she feel weighed down

INTERPRETING TEST RESULTS

- Lab results normal.

TREATMENT

- Mood stabilizers:
  - lithium
  - valproic acid
  - carbamazapine
  - lamotrigine
- Antipsychotic medications:
  - olanzapine
  - risperidone
  - aripiprazole
- Psychotherapy.
- Assess suicide risk.
- Antidepressants.

NURSING DIAGNOSIS

- Powerlessness
- Social isolation

- Risk for loneliness
- Altered sexuality patterns

NURSING INTERVENTION

- Monitor patient frequently when first admitted.
- Ask about suicidal ideation.
- Monitor medication intake.
- Discuss patient response to therapy.

5 *Schizophrenia*

WHAT WENT WRONG?

The exact cause of schizophrenia is not known. There is a familial tendency to the disease, and genes have been identified that are associated with the disease. Dysfunction of the neurotransmitter dopamine seems to be partially responsible for the development of the symptoms of psychosis associated with schizophrenia. NMDA receptors may also be involved in the disease.

PROGNOSIS

Patients with schizophrenia typically need long-term medication to control symptoms. Medication compliance can be difficult for some patients, whether due to accessibility of medications, side effects, symptoms of disease, or desire not to take daily medication. Symptom recurrence is likely.

HALLMARK SIGNS AND SYMPTOMS

- Impairment in reality testing
- Flat affect
- Disorganized speech
- Disorganized thought process
- Unusual behavior

- Delusions
- Auditory hallucinations

INTERPRETING TEST RESULTS

- Diagnostic test normal.

TREATMENT

- Antipsychotic medications:
  - clozapine
  - aripiprazole
  - ziprasidone
  - loxapine
  - risperidone
  - olanzapine
  - quetiapine
  - thiothixene
- Psychotherapy.
- Behavioral therapy.
- Structured environment.

NURSING DIAGNOSIS

- Impaired environmental interpretation syndrome
- Disturbed thought process
- Disturbed auditory sensory perception

NURSING INTERVENTION

- Monitor medication intake.
- Discuss patient response to therapy.
- Discuss importance of medication compliance.

Anorexia Nervosa

Anorexia nervosa is a disease process that exists within the developed world, where access to adequate amounts of nutritious food is not an issue. An unrealistic expectation of body size may be part of the process, due to society's expectations as depicted in the media. There is an alteration of normal eating behaviors, resulting in a refusal to maintain body weight at or above that which is minimally expected.

WHAT WENT WRONG?

Patients have a fear of gaining weight, even though they appear underweight to those around them. Patients may restrict the intake of calories or binge and purge to rid the body of the calories consumed. Anorexia affects females much more frequently than males, with onset typically in the teen or preteen years. The patient has an altered perception of body image.

PROGNOSIS

There is an increased mortality rate for patients with untreated anorexia nervosa. The majority of these patients succumb to cardiovascular or renal problems. Patients may need to be treated periodically for electrolyte disturbances, cardiac rhythm disturbances, or renal dysfunction. The medical management of the patient needs to be incorporated with the cognitive behavioral therapy to best meet the needs of the patient. The symptoms of disease may recur.

HALLMARK SIGNS AND SYMPTOMS

- Disturbance in self-perception of body shape
- Refusal to maintain minimal normal body weight
- Abnormalities in eating behaviors
- Electrolyte imbalances due to nutritional deficiency
- Amenorrhea (absence of menstrual flow) or oligomenorrhea (very light menstrual flow) due to lack of body fat
- Dental caries or periodontitis due to nutritional deficiency

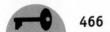

- Temporal wasting, visible ribs, and other bony prominences due to lack of body fat
- Cardiovascular abnormalities due to electrolyte disturbance
- Gastrointestinal abnormalities due to nutritional deficiency
- Dizziness due to lack of calorie intake
- Bradycardia (heart rate below 60 beats per minute)
- Hypotension (low blood pressure)

INTERPRETING TEST RESULTS

- CBC—may see anemia of chronic disease if iron, B_{12} and folate levels are not sufficient to keep up with RBC production.
- Electrolytes—abnormalities of Na (sodium), K (potassium), Cl (chloride), and CO_2 (carbon dioxide).
- Calcium—abnormality as stores are depleted and intake is insufficient.
- Magnesium—abnormality as stores are depleted and intake is insufficient.
- Phosphorus—abnormality as stores are depleted and intake is insufficient.
- BUN (blood urea nitrogen) elevated if fluid depleted.
- TSH (thyroid stimulating hormone) to rule out thyroid dysfunction as cause of weight loss.
- FHS and LH to monitor hormone function to stimulate ovulation.
- Elevated amylase and normal lipase if vomiting.
- EKG shows abnormal heart rhythm.

TREATMENT

- Psychotherapy:
  - Interpersonal therapy.
- Cognitive-behavioral therapy.
- Family therapy.
- Antidepressant medications—selective serotonin reuptake inhibitors.
- Medical management of electrolyte imbalance—replacement as needed.

- Monitor cardiac rhythm for rate and presence of arrhythmia.
- Calorie replacement; monitor for problems with initial refeeding.
- Monitor vital signs.
- Monitor weight.
- Monitor fluid and calorie intake.

NURSING DIAGNOSIS

- Disturbed body image
- Imbalanced nutrition: less than what body requires
- Altered dentition

NURSING INTERVENTION

- Monitor vital signs.
- Monitor calorie intake.
- Monitor cardiac rate and rhythm.
- Monitor lab results; report abnormalities.

7   *Bulimia Nervosa*

The ideal body type depicted in the media has affected the perception of body image of many adolescents and young adults. Some of them may have an associated biologic vulnerability that makes this societal pressure more pronounced. Peer issues or family problems may compound this, setting the stage for development of symptoms.

WHAT WENT WRONG?

Patients have recurrent episodes in which they eat a much larger quantity of food than would be expected within a given time frame; this is accompanied by a lack of control over eating, followed by some compensatory mechanism to prevent weight gain. This compensatory mechanism may include self-induced vomiting, excessive exercise, laxative use, diuretic use, enema use, or fasting. While eating disorders overall are much more common in women, males are more likely to have bulimia than anorexia.

PROGNOSIS

Patients may need to be treated periodically for electrolyte disturbances, cardiac rhythm disturbances, or renal dysfunction. The medical management of the patient needs to be incorporated with the cognitive behavioral therapy to best meet the needs of the patient. The symptoms of disease may recur.

HALLMARK SIGNS AND SYMPTOMS

- Repeated binge eating followed by compensatory behavior (vomiting, excessive exercise, laxative use, fasting)
- Electrolyte imbalances
- Amenorrhea or oligomenorrhea due to loss of body fat
- Cardiovascular disturbance
- Erosion of enamel on back of teeth due to repetitive vomiting
- Callus formation on knuckles from self-induced vomiting
- Gastrointestinal disturbances due to repetitive purging

INTERPRETING TEST RESULTS

- Electrolytes—abnormalities of Na (sodium), K (potassium), Cl (chloride), and CO_2 (carbon dioxide).
- Calcium—abnormality as stores are depleted and intake is insufficient.
- Magnesium—abnormality as stores are depleted and intake is insufficient.
- Phosphorus—abnormality as stores are depleted and intake is insufficient.
- BUN (blood urea nitrogen) elevated if fluid depleted.
- Elevated amylase and normal lipase if vomiting.

TREATMENT

- Psychotherapy:
  - Interpersonal therapy.
- Cognitive-behavioral therapy.
- Family therapy.
- Medical management of electrolyte imbalance—replacement as needed.
- Monitor cardiac rhythm for rate and presence of arrhythmia.
- Monitor vital signs.
- Monitor weight.
- Monitor fluid and calorie intake.

NURSING DIAGNOSIS

- Disturbed body image
- Imbalanced nutrition: less than what body requires
- Altered dentition

NURSING INTERVENTION

- Monitor vital signs.
- Monitor calorie intake.
- Monitor cardiac rate and rhythm.
- Monitor lab results; report abnormalities.

8 *Delirium*

WHAT WENT WRONG?

Patients exhibit a global disturbance in cognitive functions that may develop rapidly, sometimes within hours. Symptom severity may vary during the course of the day, depending on cause of symptoms. The patient with a sudden onset of disorientation and behavioral changes, especially the elderly patient, is often sent for a psychiatric evaluation.

PROGNOSIS

Delirium is often due to an underlying infection, ischemic change, or metabolic disturbance. Rapid identification and intervention for the underlying cause is essential for the patient. Without proper treatment the cause may prove to be fatal.

HALLMARK SIGNS AND SYMPTOMS

- Confusion
- Disorientation
- Behavioral changes
- Inappropriate words or dress
- Agitation

INTERPRETING TEST RESULTS

- EEG shows generalized slowing.
- WBC elevated in bacterial infection.
- Glucose abnormalities in hyper- or hypoglycemia.
- EKG abnormalities in myocardial ischemia or infarction.
- CT scan of brain shows ischemic changes.
- Electrolyte abnormalities if causative.

TREATMENT

- Monitor vital signs.
- Monitor neurologic status, orientation, level of consciousness, eye opening, and pupil response.
- Treatment of underlying cause.
- Supplemental oxygen delivery if hypoxic.

NURSING DIAGNOSIS

- Risk for falls

NURSING INTERVENTION

- Protect patient from injury.
- Monitor intravenous site for signs of infiltration.
- Perform neurological checks.

Quiz

1. Alex is a 78-year-old married man with sudden onset of confusion and disorientation. He is exhibiting combative behavior, which is upsetting to his wife because it is so unlike his normal, easy-going nature. A psychiatric consult has been called. He has no previous psychiatric history. You suspect Alex has:

   (a) delirium.

   (b) psychosis.

   (c) depression.

   (d) panic disorder.

2. Appropriate treatment for Alex would include:

   (a) selective serotonin reuptake inhibitors.

   (b) monoamine oxidase inhibitors.

   (c) atypical antipsychotic medication.

   (d) identification and treatment of the underlying disorder.

3. Karen has been dieting and exercising daily. Her weight is well below the recommended minimum for her height. Assessment for Karen would include looking for:

   (a) ecchymosis and extraocular movements.

   (b) temporal wasting and irregular heart rhythm.

   (c) peripheral edema and rales.

   (d) periorbital edema and chorea.

4. Ongoing management of Karen would include monitoring of:
   (a) electrolyte levels.
   (b) thyroid studies, FSH, LH.
   (c) caloric intake.
   (d) All of the above.

5. Felicia's family brings her in for an evaluation. They are concerned because she states that she is hearing voices. You recognize this as symptomatic of:
   (a) bipolar disorder.
   (b) panic disorder.
   (c) schizophrenia.
   (d) bulimia nervosa.

6. Teresa was recently started on fluoxetine, a selective serotonin reuptake inhibitor for treatment of her depression. After just a few days she is hardly sleeping, hyperactive, easily distracted, and appears elated. You would expect her treatment to include:
   (a) continuation of the selective serotonin reuptake inhibitor.
   (b) switching to a tricyclic antidepressant.
   (c) starting a mood stabilizer.
   (d) adding a monoamine oxidase inhibitor.

7. Mandy is a 17-year-old female. On physical examination you note partial erosion of her tooth enamel and callus formation on the posterior aspect of the knuckles of her hand. This is indicative of:
   (a) a connective tissue disorder and she should be referred to dermatology.
   (b) self-induced vomiting and she likely has bulimia nervosa.
   (c) self-mutilation and correlates with anxiety.
   (d) a genetic disorder and her siblings should also be tested.

8. Joan presents with signs and symptoms of Bipolar Disorder. What medication would you anticipate the physician prescribing to stabilize Joan's mood?
   (a) Aripiprazole
   (b) Lithium
   (c) Bupropion
   (d) Tricyclics

9. Sam presents with impairment in reality testing, flat affect, deluisions and auditory hallucinations. What medical diagnoses would you expect to find in Sam's chart?

(a) Biopolar Disorder

(b) Schizophrenia

(c) Delirium

(d) Anxiety

10. Mick arrived in the ER showing signs of fear, tension, apprehension and persistent worry. He reports trouble concentrating. Mick is showing signs of:

(a) Biopolar Disorder

(b) Schizophrenia

(c) Delirium

(d) Anxiety

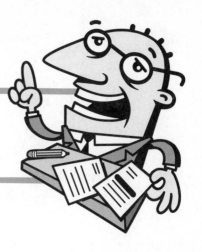

CHAPTER 13

Perioperative Care

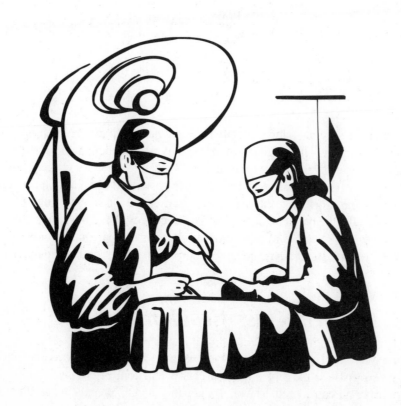

Learning Objectives

1. Surgical classifications
2. The preoperative period
3. The intraoperative period
4. The postoperative period
5. Cardiovascular complications
6. Respiratory complications
7. Infection
8. Gastrointestinal complications

Key Terms

Anatomical location
Anesthesia
Degree of urgency
Extent of the surgery
Informed consent
Intraoperative

Postoperative
Postoperative complications
Postanesthesia care unit
Preoperative
Preoperative clearance
Preoperative teaching

Risk for injury
Reason for surgery
Surgical procedures
Surgical team
Transfer of the patient

Perioperative Care

The care of the surgical patient ideally begins when the patient is first informed of the need for surgery. The surgical procedure may be a sudden, unexpected event for the patient, resulting in stress and anxiety, such as necessary surgery following trauma, or may be something that the patient has planned, such as a liposuction, far in advance. The more time the patient has to prepare for surgery, both physically and emotionally, the better able the patient is to cope with the physiological stresses of the surgery. Nurses are in a position to care for the patient, provide necessary education, act as patient advocate, and encourage health promotion behaviors.

1 *Surgical Classifications*

The American Society of Anesthesiology categorizes surgical procedures based on the degree of risk to the patient. The urgency, location, extent, and reason for the procedure are all considered, as well as the patient's age; preexisting cardiovascular, respiratory, and neurologic status; endocrine disorders; malignancies; nutritional, fluid, and electrolyte status; abnormal laboratory findings; abnormal vital signs; and presence of infection. The risks of doing the surgery are weighed against the risks of not doing the surgery. There are some cases in which the risk of surgery is very high, but the patient may certainly die if the surgery is not performed (patients with uncontrolled internal bleeding following a gunshot or stabbing, for example).

The anatomical *location* of the surgery will affect the degree of risk to the patient. Surgical procedures performed within the thoracic cavity or skull are a greater risk to the patient than procedures performed on the extremities. Surgical procedures involving vital organs such as the heart, lungs, or brain carry a higher risk. The procedures that involve a greater potential for blood loss, such as vascular surgery, also involve greater risk.

The degree of *urgency* of the procedure is described as emergent, urgent, or elective. Emergent procedures need to be performed immediately after identifying the need for surgery. Examples include surgery to stop bleeding from trauma, shooting, or stabbing, or a dissecting aortic aneurysm. Urgent procedures are scheduled after the determination of surgical need is made. Examples include tumor removal and removal of kidney stones. Elective procedures are scheduled in advance at a time that is convenient for both patient and surgeon. Postponement of the surgery for several weeks or even months will not cause harm to the patient. Examples include joint replacement procedures and cosmetic procedures.

The *extent* of the surgery will affect the risk to the patient. The more extensive the surgical procedure, the greater the potential risk to the patient. More extensive surgical procedures cause more physical insult to the body and typically require a longer duration of anesthesia. The anesthesia can also cause stress to the patient's system, interact with medications in the patient's system, and must be metabolized out of the body.

The *reason* for surgery is another way that surgical procedures are classified. The purpose may be diagnostic, curative, restorative, palliative, or cosmetic. Diagnostic procedures are performed to obtain a biopsy for definitive diagnosis of a mass. Curative procedures are performed to remove a diseased area, such as a lumpectomy for breast cancer or an appendectomy. Restorative procedures are performed to restore function, such as joint replacements. Palliative procedures are procedures are performed primarily for comfort measures, such as tumor debulking. Cosmetic procedures are typically performed at the patient's request; at times some cosmetic procedures may fall into restorative (repairing damage or a congenital defect), curative, or diagnostic (in the setting of skin cancer).

The perioperative period can be broken down into the *preoperative* (time before the surgery), *intraoperative* (time during the surgery), and the *postoperative* (time following the surgery until recovery) periods.

The Preoperative Period

The preoperative period, the time prior to surgery, is used to prepare the patient for surgery both physically and psychologically. Ideally there is time to correct as many abnormalities as possible prior to the surgical procedure. For patients having a scheduled procedure with a significant anticipated blood loss, this is the time to donate blood to be banked for use in their surgery and begin to take iron, folic acid, vitamin B_{12}, and vitamin C to aid in red blood cell production. Preoperative clearance is given, informed consent is obtained, and preoperative teaching occurs during this time.

PREOPERATIVE CLEARANCE

The patient's primary care provider typically gives preoperative clearance for surgery. This physician, nurse practitioner, or physician's assistant is familiar with the patient's medical history and current medications and is able to adequately assess the impending risk of the surgery to the patient. Things to consider when providing clearance for the patient include the type of surgical intervention planned, the potential for blood loss during surgery, the patient's age, general health and comorbidities, past medical and surgical history, current medications, use of herbal remedies or supplements, alcohol use, smoking history, substance use, allergies, family history including problems with surgery, and diagnostic testing results. Diagnostic studies often include a CBC (to identify anemia or signs of infection), a chemistry panel (to identify electrolyte imbalance, abnormal glucose, liver or renal function), a urinalysis (to identify infection, protein, glucose), PT/INR/PTT (to identify blood clotting disorders), an EKG (to identify abnormal cardiac rhythms or damage to myocardium), chest x-ray (to identify pulmonary pathology or enlargement of cardiac silhouette), or pulmonary function testing (for patients with respiratory disorders such as asthma or emphysema). CT scans, MRIs, PET scans, or stress testing may be ordered for individual patients depending on their medical history, type of surgical procedure planned, and results of other diagnostic studies.

INFORMED CONSENT

An informed consent is obtained prior to any invasive or dangerous procedure. The reason for the surgery, type and extent of surgery to be performed, the risks of the procedure, the person to perform the procedure, alternative options and their associated risks, and the risks associated with anesthesia are all explained to the patient. It is the surgeon's responsibility to make sure this information is explained to the patient. The patient must be a competent adult in order for his or her signature to be valid. If the patient has been given medications that alter his or her ability to reason or to make judgments, the consent will not be valid. The nurse witnesses the patient's signature on the consent form.

PREOPERATIVE TEACHING

Explaining normal preoperative routines to the patient can be very helpful, so the patient knows what to expect. The nurse needs to be familiar with the types of surgical procedures and what the expected postoperative course will entail. The extent of the procedure, type of incision, presence of any tubes or drains, and anticipated pain level after the surgery will help guide the type of teaching necessary for the patient.

Preoperatively the patient can expect to be NPO, or not allowed to eat or drink anything for several hours prior to the procedure. The time frame will depend on the extent and location of procedure, the type of anesthesia, and the scheduled time of surgery. An exception to this nothing-by-mouth rule would be for patients who need to take oral medications the morning of surgery. Cardiovascular, diabetic, and certain other medications may need to be taken even though the patient is not to eat or drink anything else.

An intravenous access site will be obtained prior to the surgery. Fluids can be administered to the patient in this way. The access also allows for giving the patient medications intravenously for rapid action. Fluids are routinely given in the operating room and in the immediate recovery period. The patient may have continued intravenous fluids for more extensive procedures.

Skin preparation may only involve washing of the surgical site in the operating room with an antimicrobial solution. Other patients may need to have removal of hair from the surgical site. This may be with a razor or a depilatory agent. It is important not to cut the skin if you are shaving a surgical site; small cuts or abrasions on the skin allow for potential sites of infection. Depilatory agents can be caustic on the skin of some patients, causing irritation or a rash. A small spot test away from the surgical area is a good idea in a patient with known skin sensitivity or history of allergies.

For patients having planned surgery involving the intestinal tract, a bowel preparation will be completed prior to the surgery. This is done to decrease the bacterial count within the intestinal tract. Cleansing of the bowel is also completed to empty the intestine of stool before the surgeon plans on cutting into either the small or large intestine. Both of these preparations help to reduce the possibility of infection in the postoperative period. For patients who will have tubes or drains in place in the postoperative period, a simple explanation of what to expect can help to alleviate some anxiety.

Availability of pain medication in the postoperative period should be explained to the patient. In many instances the patient is able to manage his or her own pain medication. For outpatient procedures, patients may be given a prescription for an oral pain medication prior to the procedure. This way the medication is available when the patient gets home from the surgery. For postoperative patients in the hospital, many patients have an intravenous patient-controlled analgesia, known as PCA, for pain management, where pain medication is delivered via a pump. Typically a small basal dose of narcotic is delivered all the time. These patients also have the ability to press a button whenever they are experiencing pain. The pump will monitor the amount and timing of each dose of pain medication. If the patient is due for medication, a dose will be administered; if the patient is not due for medication, no dose will be administered.

TRANSFER OF THE PATIENT

Most facilities have a preoperative checklist to assist the nurse to make sure that all the needed components have been checked prior to sending the patient to the operating room (OR). All pertinent documentation—the signed consent form, the patient's chart, and current lab results—accompanies the patient to the OR.

3 *The Intraoperative Period*

The intraoperative period is the time involved with the surgical procedure. The focus during this time is on asepsis and protection of the patient. Within the operative suite, the staff wears scrub suits. They change into the scrub shirt and pants when they get to the locker room within the surgical area. A surgical cap covers hair. Shoe covers are worn to prevent tracking bacteria or dirt from other areas into the operating rooms.

THE SURGICAL TEAM

Members of the surgical team include the surgeon, a surgical assistant, an anesthesiologist or anesthetist, a circulating nurse, a scrub nurse or surgical tech, and a holding area nurse. The *surgeon* is the doctor who will perform the surgery. The *surgical assistant* may be another surgeon, a surgical resident, an RN first assist, or a physician's assistant. The person providing anesthesia and monitoring the vital signs of the patient is either an *anesthesiologist* (a physician) or a certified registered nurse *anesthetist* (CRNA). The *circulating nurse* is a registered nurse who acts as the patient advocate, obtains the necessary supplies for the procedure, makes sure diagnostic studies and blood products are available if necessary, prepares the operative table, positions the patient (padding bony prominences if necessary), and cleanses the skin in the operative area before positioning surgical drapes. The *scrub nurse* or *surgical tech* sets up the sterile field, assists with draping the patient, and hands sterile supplies into the operative field and takes used instruments from the surgeon. The circulating nurse and scrub nurse (or surgical tech) together count all instruments, sponges, and sharps used in the surgical field. The count is performed before, during, and after the procedure. The *holding area nurse* cares for the patients who have been brought into the operating room suite but who are not yet ready to go into the operating room. The holding area nurse may be managing several patients at one time and can also help to transport and transfer the patient.

Before entering the operating room, the members of the surgical team scrub at the sink just outside the room in which the surgery will be performed. Prior to starting the scrub, the team member applies a mask with face shield or goggles. The surgical scrub is usually timed and covers the area from the fingertips to 2 inches above the elbows. The surgical scrub renders the skin clean, not sterile. After the scrub, the skin is dried with a sterile towel. A sterile gown, then sterile gloves are applied. The front of the gown is considered sterile in the front from two inches below the neck to the waist and from the elbow to the wrist. The circulating nurse applies the gown and gloves unassisted, and then assists the other members of the team into their gown and gloves as they enter the room.

RISK FOR INJURY

During the surgery, the patient is anesthetized and cannot tell you if there is pressure anywhere. The patient is positioned to allow for maximal access to the operative site. This sometimes causes unnatural positioning of the patient or the patient's extremities. The operative table is padded to decrease pressure on the patient. There may be additional padding added to areas of flexion or bony prominences to reduce the risk of pressure ulcer formation or nerve damage due to positioning.

Heat loss can occur during surgery. The patient is sent to the operating room in a hospital gown, which may be pulled up or removed depending on the body location of the surgery. The body is draped for privacy so that only the surgical area is exposed. The temperature within the operating room is kept rather cool because the air exchange rate is higher within the operating room than in other rooms (to decrease bacterial counts), and the staff are wearing double layers of clothes. Warmers can be set up for the patients during certain procedures when heat loss is expected—a large, open operative site or a long duration of surgery.

At the end of the surgical procedure, the wound is closed. The closure is to hold the wound edges together and to prevent contamination. Closure may be achieved with sutures (either absorbable or nonabsorbable), staples, glue, or skin closure tape. Nonabsorbable sutures and staples will have to be removed in the post-operative period.

Drains may be inserted near the operative site if significant wound drainage is anticipated. Some drains are attached to suction, some have self-suction, and some will drain due to gravity. The wound site is covered with a sterile dressing before the patient is transferred out of the operating room.

ANESTHESIA

Anesthesia can be administered via general or regional routes (for major procedures) or conscious sedation (for minor procedures). General anesthesia renders the patient unconscious and incapable of breathing on his or her own; pain reception is also blocked. These patients must be intubated and mechanically ventilated for the duration of the anesthesia. Regional anesthesia can be achieved through nerve blocks, or epidural or spinal anesthesia. Nerve blocks occur when an anesthetic agent is injected into an area immediately surrounding a particular nerve or nerve bundle. The nerve tissue becomes anesthetized, effectively causing the tissue that it supplies to become pain-free. With epidural anesthesia, an anesthetic agent is injected into the epidural space surrounding the spinal column, usually in the lower lumbar area. The nerves become anesthetized as they leave the spinal column, causing the area of the body supplied by these nerves to become pain-free. This anesthesia is most commonly associated with childbirth but is used for many surgical procedures. Spinal anesthesia is not commonly used; the anesthetic agent is injected into the cerebrospinal fluid. Patient positioning is very important, as gravity will cause the anesthetic agent to travel. The patient must remain flat after the procedure to prevent leakage of cerebrospinal fluid from the puncture site.

4 *The Postoperative Period*

After the surgery, the patient enters the postoperative period. The immediate post-operative period requires close monitoring as the patient emerges from anesthesia.

The patient will then be transferred to either a same-day surgery area for discharge home that day or an inpatient surgical unit for care. After discharge from the hospital, the patient may need home care. Return to full activities may take several weeks.

POSTANESTHESIA CARE

The patient is transferred from the operating room to the postanesthesia care unit (PACU) for close monitoring in the immediate postoperative period. Initial assessment is focused on ABC: airway, breathing, and circulation. Monitor the patient's airway, gas exchange, pulse oximetry, oxygen delivery, accessory muscle use, and breath sounds. The patient can develop stridor due to edema or bronchospasm. The cardiovascular status is checked next. Vital signs are checked every 15 minutes until stabilized; pulse, blood pressure, and cardiac rhythm are monitored.

The surgical wound is checked for signs of drainage or bleeding. The dressing is checked. The drains are checked for output and patency. Tubes that need to be connected to suction (such as nasogastric tubes) are connected. Intravenous fluids are monitored.

Neurologic assessment is performed to check level of consciousness. Following general anesthesia, the patient follows a predictable progression in the return to consciousness. Initially there is muscular irritability, and then restlessness followed by pain recognition and the ability to reason and control behavior. Pupil responses are monitored, looking for bilaterally equal responses to light. Motor responses are monitored, looking initially for purposeful response to painful stimuli and later for response to command. Pain management is begun during this time. As the anesthetic agent wears off, it is important to assess the patient's level of pain. This may be assessed through subjective information in patients who are conscious, or through more objective signs in patients who are still in semiconscious states. Monitor for changes in vital signs (elevated pulse and BP), changes in movement, and moaning. Expected pain levels can be estimated from the type of surgery and give a starting point for those patients as they begin to come out of the anesthesia.

Gastrointestinal status is monitored for presence of nausea or vomiting. This may be a reaction or side effect to anesthesia. Check for abdominal distention and presence of bowel sounds. Monitor drainage from nasogastric tube; note amount and color of drainage.

Monitor laboratory results as indicated. Electrolyte levels, hemoglobin or hematocrit levels, BUN and creatinine, arterial blood gases (ABGs), or other studies may be necessary in the immediate postoperative period. The diagnostic studies necessary will depend on the patient's history, the estimated blood loss during surgery, and the type of procedure performed.

After the initial recovery time, the stable patient who is transferred from the PACU to the same-day surgical area continues to be monitored. Vital signs are taken, although not as frequently. Respiratory and cardiovascular functions are monitored. Cardiac rhythm is no longer monitored. The dressing is checked for any drainage. Bowel sounds are checked. Clear fluids are given if the patient is not experiencing nausea. Patients are monitored for urinary output prior to being discharged to home.

Patients who are admitted to the hospital are transferred from the PACU to a surgical unit. Vital signs, respiration, and cardiovascular status are checked. The dressing is monitored for drainage; drainage tubes are monitored for output. Intravenous lines are monitored for signs of infiltration and proper flow rates. Bowel sounds are monitored.

Patients who are unstable or who have had extensive procedures are transferred to intensive care for close monitoring. Nurses who are used to caring for complex, unstable patients care for these patients. Their vital signs are closely monitored. Some patients will still be on mechanical ventilation.

POSTOPERATIVE COMPLICATIONS

The focus of care that is common for all of these postoperative patients is identification of complications. Common complications involve the cardiac, respiratory, and gastrointestinal areas, and infections.

Just the Facts

 ## *Cardiovascular Complications*

WHAT WENT WRONG?

Patients may develop cardiovascular complications due to the physiological stress of surgery, side effects of the anesthesia or other medications, or comorbidities. Myocardial infarction (MI), cardiac arrhythmias, or hypotension are likely during or in the immediate postoperative period. When getting the patient out of bed for the first time after surgery, it is good practice to have the patient sit on the side of the bed for a minute or two before standing up to ascertain if the patient feels dizzy due to a drop in blood pressure associated with position change. Deep vein thrombosis (DVT) is a later vascular complication associated with inflammation and decreased mobility after surgery.

HALLMARK SIGNS AND SYMPTOMS

- Chest pain which may radiate to back, neck, jaw, or arm due to ischemia in MI
- Shortness of breath due to altered cardiac output and tissue perfusion
- Dizziness or lightheadedness due to diminished cardiac output and cerebral tissue perfusion or cardiac arrhythmia
- Palpitations due to cardiac arrhythmia
- Cardiac arrhythmias due to myocardial irritability—possibly due to ischemia, medication side effect, or electrolyte imbalance
- Low blood pressure due to diminished cardiac output
- Unilateral calf pain and lower extremity swelling due to DVT

INTERPRETING TEST RESULTS

- Elevated troponin levels in MI.
- EKG shows ST elevation or T-wave inversion with lack of oxygen delivery to myocardial tissue.
- Cardiac monitor or EKG shows arrhythmia.
- BP below normal level.
- Doppler ultrasound of extremity shows clot within blood vessel.

TREATMENT

- Monitor cardiac rhythm.
- Administer antiarrhythmic medications to stabilize cardiac rhythm.
- Administer intravenous fluids to expand circulating blood volume to raise blood pressure.
- Administer blood-thinning medications to decrease likelihood of clot enlarging or additional clots forming:
    - heparin

- low–molecular weight heparin
- warfarin

NURSING DIAGNOSES

- Decreased cardiac output
- Ineffective cardiopulmonary tissue perfusion
- Ineffective peripheral tissue perfusion
- Impaired physical mobility

NURSING INTERVENTIONS

- Monitor vital signs for changes.
- Check blood pressure lying down and sitting up for orthostatic change.
- Monitor cardiovascular status for cardiac rhythm, heart sounds, peripheral pulses, capillary refill, and pulse deficit.
- Assess for peripheral edema.
- Ask patient about calf pain or tenderness.
- Monitor intravenous site for signs of infiltration.
- Encourage ambulation and leg exercises to prevent development of DVT.
- Monitor proper use of elastic stockings or sequential compression devices postoperatively.

6 *Respiratory Complications*

Patients with preexisting respiratory disorders, obesity, or thoracic or upper abdominal surgical procedures are at greater risk of developing respiratory complications postoperatively.

WHAT WENT WRONG?

After surgery, patients are not as mobile. This lack of physical activity leads to diminished chest wall and diaphragmatic movement, resulting in a decreased amount of air exchange. Alveolar sacs can collapse, leading to areas of atelectasis.

Pain medications can adversely affect respiratory status by decreasing respiratory drive. Patients at increased risk for respiratory complications may develop pneumonia in the postoperative period due to diminished airflow, increased respiratory secretions, and inflammatory processes. Patients with increased risk for clotting or DVT, or those with hypercoagulable states are at risk for developing a pulmonary embolism.

HALLMARK SIGNS AND SYMPTOMS

- Shortness of breath due to diminished airflow and resultant decreased oxygenation
- Chest pain in the area of atelectasis due to collapse of the alveolar sacs within that area of the lung
- Productive cough due to pneumonia
- Fever due to infection in pneumonia
- Sudden onset chest pain and shortness of breath in pulmonary embolism as clot blocks arterial blood flow within the lung
- Diminished oxygen levels as gas exchange is impaired in atelectasis, pneumonia, or pulmonary embolism

INTERPRETING TEST RESULTS

- Pulse oximetry shows diminished oxygenation.
- Chest x-ray shows area of collapse in atelectasis, infiltrate in pneumonia, wedge infiltrate in pulmonary embolism.
- CT scan shows alveolar collapse in atelectasis, area of infiltrate in pneumonia.
- Spiral CT or helical CT shows clot in pulmonary embolism.
- WBC elevated in bacterial pneumonia.

TREATMENT

- Administer supplemental oxygen.
- Administer antibiotics for pneumonia—initially intravenously, then orally:
  - macrolides
  - fluoroquinolones

- Administer blood-thinning agents to prevent enlarging of clot or development of new clots in pulmonary embolism.
- Mechanical ventilation if necessary.

NURSING DIAGNOSES

- Ineffective breathing pattern
- Ineffective airway clearance
- Impaired gas exchange
- Ineffective cardiopulmonary tissue perfusion

NURSING INTERVENTIONS

- Monitor vital signs for changes.
- Monitor respiratory status: check respiratory rate, rhythm, and depth; check skin color; listen to breath sounds.
- Monitor pulse oximetry level for oxygenation.
- Monitor intravenous site for signs of infiltration.
- Encourage coughing and deep breathing exercises.
- Encourage incentive spirometer use.
- Encourage early ambulation.

7 *Infection*

The skin is the body's first line of defense against infection. During surgery this line of defense is penetrated. Even though the surgical procedure is performed in as aseptic an environment as possible, the possibility of infection still exists.

WHAT WENT WRONG?

Wound infections can develop in the postoperative period. The wound may be contaminated before surgery, such as with penetrating trauma, or may become infected during healing. The surface of the skin has bacteria that are naturally present, referred to as normal flora. These bacteria may enter the wound and cause infection. Nosocomial infections can also occur at the surgical site, caused by bacteria found elsewhere in the hospital. Infection within the surgical wound will slow approximation of the wound edges, delaying wound healing.

HALLMARK SIGNS AND SYMPTOMS

- Increase in pain at surgical wound due to inflammatory process early in infection
- Redness at wound edges that spreads if untreated
- Drainage from wound site due to body's response to bacterial presence (change in color and odor of drainage)
- Fever due to infection
- Elevated white blood cell count

INTERPRETING TEST RESULTS

- Elevated WBC due to body's response to bacterial presence.
- Elevated erythrocyte sedementation rate due to inflammation.
- Culture of wound area will identify organism.
- Sensitivity test will identify appropriate antibiotic treatment.

TREATMENT

- Obtain culture and sensitivity test of wound.
- Administer appropriate antibiotics intravenously.
- Keep wound site clean and dry.

NURSING DIAGNOSES

- Risk for infection
- Impaired skin integrity
- Impaired tissue integrity
- Delayed surgical recovery

NURSING INTERVENTIONS

- Monitor vital signs; look for fever.
- Assess surgical wound for redness, drainage.
- Ask patient about pain at surgical site.
- When obtaining wound culture, remove surface drainage with gauze, then obtain specimen from within wound edge (this will ensure that the organism is actually from the wound and not from the skin).

8   *Gastrointestinal Complications*

Following administration of anesthesia or pain medication, patients may experience nausea, vomiting, constipation, or paralytic ileus.

WHAT WENT WRONG?

Nausea is a common side effect of both anesthesia and pain medications. A patient's reaction to anesthetic agents varies. Some patients have a lot of nausea after anesthesia that may last for several hours. Abdominal surgery may cause direct visceral afferent stimulation, resulting in nausea and vomiting. Medications may act upon the chemoreceptor trigger zone, located within the medulla outside the blood-brain barrier. Once the patient begins vomiting, antiemetic medication may be necessary to break the cycle. Opiod-based medications and decreased activity can both cause slowing of peristaltic activity, leading to constipation. Patients having abdominal procedures are at greater risk for paralytic ileus as a postoperative complication.

HALLMARK SIGNS AND SYMPTOMS

- Nausea as a side effect of medication
- Vomiting due to visceral afferent stimulation or activation of chemoreceptor trigger zone
- Mild, generalized abdominal discomfort and distention with paralytic ileus due to decreased intestinal motility
- Slow bowel sounds with constipation; absent bowel sounds with paralytic ileus due to changes in intestinal motility

INTERPRETING TEST RESULTS

- Electrolyte abnormality due to vomiting.
- Abdominal flat and upright x-ray shows stool in constipation, gas-filled intestinal loops in paralytic ileus.

TREATMENT

- Monitor abdomen for distention; listen for bowel sounds.
- Assess for dehydration as a result of prolonged vomiting.
- Restrict oral intake in paralytic ileus or if nausea and vomiting are present.
- Nasogastric (NG) tube connected to suction to prevent vomiting in paralytic ileus.
- Progress diet as tolerated once bowel sounds return and patient is passing flatus rectally.
- Administer intravenous fluids.
- Administer total parenteral nutrition.
- Administer antiemetics as required.

NURSING DIAGNOSES

- Risk for imbalanced nutrition: less than what body requires
- Risk for imbalanced fluid volume
- Risk for delayed surgical recovery
- Risk for constipation
- Altered bowel elimination

NURSING INTERVENTIONS

- Ask patient about presence of nausea.
- Monitor vital signs for changes.
- Listen to bowel sounds; assess abdomen for distention.
- Monitor intravenous site for signs of infiltration, pain, and redness.

- Monitor intake and output.
- Monitor color and amount of fluid drained from NG tube.
- Ask patient if he or she is passing any flatus rectally or having bowel movement.

Quiz

1. Donna is a healthy, 46-year-old female scheduled for elective surgery next week. You would include in her preoperative preparation:

    (a) a pulmonary function test and chest x-ray.

    (b) a CBC, chemistry panel, and pregnancy test.

    (c) urine culture, thyroid panel, and cortisol level.

    (d) glucose tolerance test, ankle-brachial index, and electrocardiogram (EKG).

2. Lucinda is a 37-year-old with a history of asthma who is scheduled for an appendectomy later today. Because of her asthma, you would include as part of her preoperative teaching her need to perform postoperatively:

    (a) coughing and deep breathing exercises.

    (b) leg exercises.

    (c) wound dressing changes.

    (d) all of the above.

3. Josie is the mother of a healthy 19-year-old having surgery tomorrow. After the surgeon discusses the surgery, risks, and benefits with the patient and her mother, the mother wants to sign the consent form. The most appropriate response to this would be:

    (a) Of course she can sign the consent form; after all the patient is her daughter.

    (b) No, she can't sign the form.

    (c) While you appreciate her concern for her daughter, the patient is a consenting adult and legally has to sign her own consent form.

    (d) Why don't both the patient and her mother sign the form?

4. Which member of the surgical team does not scrub into the operating room?

    (a) The surgeon.

    (b) The circulating nurse.

    (c) The scrub nurse or surgical tech.

    (d) The holding area nurse.

5. Suzette is having a minor procedure performed. Which type of anesthesia is most likely to be used?

    (a) General.

    (b) Epidural.

    (c) Regional.

    (d) Conscious sedation.

6. 65-year-old Dominic is being transferred into the PACU from the OR. Once there, initial assessment will focus on:

    (a) airway, breathing, circulation, and wound site.

    (b) intake, output, and intravenous access.

    (c) abdominal sounds, oxygen setting, and level of consciousness.

    (d) pulse oximeter, pupil responses, and deep tendon reflexes.

7. Denise is recovering from an open cholesystectomy. You know that because of the location of the surgery, she has an increased risk of postoperative:

    (a) myocardial infarction.

    (b) respiratory complications.

    (c) deep vein thrombosis.

    (d) wound infection.

8. Three days after surgery, Mark notices that the wound site is more painful now than it was the day before. When you inspect the surgical site you are looking for redness or inflammation. Other indicators of infection would include:

    (a) elevated RBC and elevated respiratory rate.

    (b) elevated WBC and elevated temperature.

    (c) elevated erythrocyte sedimentation rate and decreased pulse.

    (d) decreased platelets and decreased blood pressure.

9. Paralytic ileus may occur as a postoperative complication. Which of the following patients would cause you the greatest concern about the development of paralytic ileus?

(a) Kim, a 27-year-old postlaparscopic appendectomy.

(b) Joyce, a 39-year-old post–open right hemicolectomy.

(c) Nancy, a 56-year-old postmediastinoscopy.

(d) John, a 47-year-old post–total joint replacement.

10. Steve has developed pneumonia following intrathoracic surgery performed last week. Treatment for postoperative pneumonia would most likely include:

(a) a cephalosporin, such as cefazolin.

(b) a penicillin, such as amoxicillin.

(c) a fluoroquinolone, such as levofloxacin.

(d) a tetracycline, such as doxycycline.

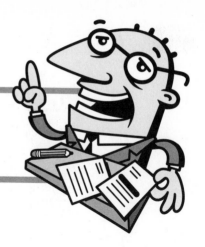

CHAPTER 14

Women's Health

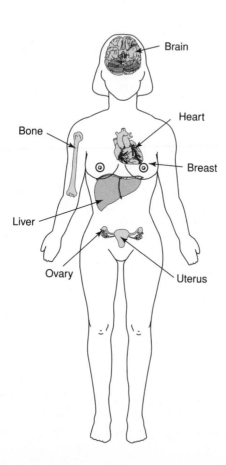

Learning Objectives

1. Breast cancer
2. Cervical cancer
3. Dysmenorrhea
4. Ectopic pregnancy
5. Endometrial cancer
6. Fibroids (leiomyomas)
7. Infertility
8. Menopause
9. Ovarian cancer

10. Ovarian masses, benign
11. Pelvic inflammatory disease (PID)
12. Trophoblastic disease
13. Pregnancy
14. Labor and delivery
15. Postpartum
16. Rh incompatibility
17. Preeclampsia and Eclampsia

Key Terms

Anovulation
Beta hCG serum levels
BRCA1
BRCA2
Cervical intraepithelial
  neoplasia (CIN)
Chemotherapy
Cone biopsy
Corpus luteum
Cryotherapy

Egg follicle
Endometrium
Estrogen
Follicle-stimulating
  hormone (FSH)
Human papillomavirus
  (HPV)
Leiomyomas
Luteinizing hormone
  (LH)

Luteal phase
Mastectomy
Menarche
Menstrual cycle
Menstruation
Oocyte
Papanicolaou (Pap)
  smear
Progesterone

The Female Body

The menstrual cycle is the series of changes a woman's body goes through monthly to prepare for conception and a growing fetus. If fertilization does not occur, the uterus will remove the prepared lining, termed menstrual bleeding. Menstruation begins in the early teens (menarche) and ends around age 50 (menopause). The average age of menarche for African-Americans is 9 to 11 years while for Caucasians it is from 10 to 12 years. The cycle is controlled by hormones from the hypothalamus, pituitary, ovaries, and the uterus. A normal menstrual cycle is 28 days, but only about 25 percent of women actually are on this schedule. The average can run from 21 to 35 days. The menstrual cycle is often divided into three phases, dependent upon the hormones. The beginning of menstruation is the start of the follicular phase which lasts until day 14. As hormone levels are low, the thickened lining of the uterus begins to shed. The cramping that is felt is from small uterine contractions, helping to shed the lining. An egg follicle begins to mature due to growing levels of follicle-stimulating hormone (FSH), which also causes estrogen secretion. The increase in estrogen causes the endometrium to mature and thicken. The last five days of the follicular phase plus the day of ovulation are the most fertile days. Upon ovulation, on day 14, the oocyte, or egg, is released from the follicle due to a surge in luteinizing hormon (LH). The egg is expelled near the opening of one of the fallopian tubes, (oviducts, uterine tubes), located laterally at the top of the uterus. Fertilization usually occurs in one of the tubes. The embryo now travels to the uterus, the primary job of which is to sustain development. A nonpregnant uterus measures about 7 × 5 cm. As it is a muscular organ, it is capable of great stretching. At the distal end of the uterus is the cervix which attaches to the superior portion of the vagina. The luteal phase starts next with LH causing the follicle to secrete progesterone instead of estrogen. Progesterone causes the endometrial lining to begin to thicken in preparation for implantation of a fertilized cell. Progesterone inhibits release of FSH and LH. If fertilization does not occur, the corpus luteum, containing the oocyte, dies, which lowers the level of progesterone. Sloughing of the lining begins about the 28th day of the cycle, resulting in a flow of blood and cellular debris through the vagina. The cycle will begin again. Primary amenorrhea is the absence of menses by age 16. Secondary amenorrhea is the absence of menses for more than 6 months in a woman who previously was menstruating regularly.

Just the Facts

1 *Breast Cancer*

Studies show that by age 80, about 1 in 8 women will have breast cancer. Ten percent of all breast cancers are inherited. Two major genes have been identified—BRCA1 and BRCA2.

WHAT WENT WRONG?

Despite the research and advances in medicine, the cause of breast cancer is unknown. Some studies have implicated a higher-fat diet. Some medications, like estrogen, seem to increase the risk of breast cancer. Exposure to radiation also increases the risk. Childlessness and delayed childbirth also may be factors.

PROGNOSIS

Breast cancer is the second leading cause of cancer death in women and the number one cancer in women. Prognosis depends on the stage at which the cancer is discovered. Those with no involved lymph nodes have the best expectations. With lymph node involvement, survival ranges from 50 to 75 percent for five years.

HALLMARK SIGNS AND SYMPTOMS

- Mass in breast, usually painless
- Nipple inversion, drainage
- Bone pain from metastasis
- Cough from lung metastasis

INTERPRETING TEST RESULTS

- Mammography may show mass.
- Biopsy is confirmative for cancer.
- Ultrasonography to further delineate the mass.
- MRI of breast.
- CT scan to check for metastasis.

TREATMENTS

Treatment for breast cancer is either curative or palliative, depending on the staging of the tumor and involvement of lymph nodes.

- Lumpectomy for small tumors.

- Mastectomy for larger tumors or more than two tumors in the same breast.
- Chemotherapy before surgery to shrink some tumors, or after surgery:
  - cyclophosphamide
  - methotrexate
  - fluorouracil
  - doxorubicin
  - epirubincin
  - vincristine
  - paclitaxel
  - docetaxel
- Hormonal therapy:
  - tamoxifen
  - anastrozole
- Radiation therapy.
- Prophylactic bilateral mastectomy for women with BRCA1 or BRCA2 genes.

NURSING DIAGNOSES

- Body image disturbance.
- Anticipatory grieving.
- Altered sexuality patterns.

NURSING INTERVENTIONS

- Allow patient to voice concerns and questions over treatment plans.
- Monitor incision site, dressing, and drainage.
- Check for signs and symptoms of infection.
- Explain to patient:
  - Disease.
  - Use of affected arm.
  - Use of pain medication, timing, and side effects.
  - Urge follow-up mammography.
  - Discuss low-fat diet.

2 *Cervical Cancer*

The Papanicolaou (Pap) smear has markedly increased early detection of cervical cancer and thus decreased the mortality.

WHAT WENT WRONG?

Abnormal cells, cervical intraepithelial neoplasia (CIN), are the initial indication on a Pap smear, and are more common in women with HIV and those infected with human papillomavirus (HPV), subtypes 16, 18. HPV is more common in women with multiple sexual partners, those having sex at an early age, and those with HIV.

PROGNOSIS

Prognosis is dependent upon the stage at which the cancer is discovered. The five-year survival rate ranges from 60 to 80 percent.

HALLMARK SIGNS AND SYMPTOMS

- Vaginal bleeding due to abnormal cells and ulceration of the cervix
- Postcoital bleeding
- Pelvic pain

INTERPRETING TEST RESULTS

- Pap smear.
- Biopsy to confirm disease and determine staging.
- Cone biopsy which provides a sample of tissue of the lateral margins of the cervix.

TREATMENT

- Cone biopsy may remove enough of the dysplasia.

- Ablation of the lesion with cryotherapy, which freezes the cells.
- Hysterectomy with lymph node biopsy for women with late-stage cancer or those with early-stage cancer who have completed childbearing.
- Radiation.
- Chemotherapy:
  - cisplatin
  - 5-fluorouracil

NURSING DIAGNOSES

- Altered sexuality patterns
- Personal identity disturbance
- Disturbance in self-esteem

NURSING INTERVENTIONS

- HPV vaccine.
- Offer pain and antiemetic medications.
- Abdominal assessment—distention, bowel sounds.
- Check vaginal bleeding.
- Assess urinary retention.
- Intake and output.
- Assess vital signs; check for fever.
- Remove vaginal packing when directed.
- Emotional reassurances.
- Explain to the patient:
  - Need for Pap tests.
  - All procedures.
  - Support through cancer treatments.
  - Use of pain and antiemetic medications.
  - Benefit of early ambulation.
  - Safer sex practices.

3 *Dysmenorrhea*

Menstrual pain occurring after ovulation for which no cause can be discerned is called dysmenorrhea.

WHAT WENT WRONG?

Dysmenorrhea is caused by the changing hormones in the reproductive cycle. Uterine contractions from prostaglandins and blood vessel constriction in the uterine lining cause the discomfort as the enriched lining prepares to be sloughed off.

PROGNOSIS

Dysmenorrhea usually begins one to two years after menarche and becomes more acute with age. Pregnancy often diminishes the severity of dysmenorrhea, as does age. Some women are debilitated for several days per month. A large majority of women experience some degree of discomfort.

HALLMARK SIGNS AND SYMPTOMS

- Cramps from small uterine contractions
  - Nausea from fluctuating hormone levels
  - Headache from declining hormone levels

INTERPRETING TEST RESULTS

- Pelvic exam is normal.
- Hemoglobin and hematocrit may be slightly declined from excessive blood loss.

TREATMENTS

- Over-the-counter preparations.
- Hot water bottles.

- Home remedies.
- Nonsteroidal anti-inflammatory drugs (NSAIDs) have antiprostaglandin activities, which decrease the discomfort:
  - ibuprofen
  - naproxen
  - nabumetone
- Oral contraceptives which inhibit ovulation as well as diminish amount of menstrual flow and dysmenorrhea.

NURSING DIAGNOSES

- Intolerance for activity
- Pain, discomfort

NURSING INTERVENTIONS

- Explain to the patient:
  - The disease.
  - Benefit of exercise.
  - Medication use, timing, and side effects.

4 *Ectopic Pregnancy*

Ectopic pregnancy occurs when the fertilized ovum implants in an area other than the uterus. Most ectopic pregnancies occur in the fallopian tubes; however, other possible sites for ectopic pregnancy include the ovary, cervix, and peritoneum.

WHAT WENT WRONG?

When the fertilized ovum is unable to get to the uterus, it may settle in the fallopian tube. Any blockage, stricture, previous surgery on the tube, infection or inflammation may impede the ovum from its final, proper destination.

PROGNOSIS

Ectopic pregnancy is the greatest cause of maternal death early in the pregnancy if diagnosis cannot be made. Rupture of the involved organ and excessive bleeding into the peritoneum may occur.

HALLMARK SIGNS AND SYMPTOMS

- Severe, lancinating (stabbing) lower pelvic pain from the growing embryo stretching the fallopian tube or other structure
- Backache from pressure on these structures
- Vaginal spotting; bleeding; amenorrhea

INTERPRETING TEST RESULTS

- Beta hCG serum levels will be elevated but not as high as during an intra-uterine pregnancy.
- Ultrasound will show an empty uterus.
- Urine pregnancy test will be positive.

TREATMENTS

Surgery is planned to remove the fertilized egg. Often the egg can be retrieved laparoscopically if the pregnancy is early. Surgery will involve removal of the egg and may involve partial or complete removal of the fallopian tube (called salpingectomy—partial or complete).

NURSING DIAGNOSES

- Body image disturbance
- Anticipatory grieving
- Pain, discomfort

NURSING INTERVENTIONS

- Check vaginal bleeding.
- Check incision site.
- Assess abdomen—bowel sounds, distention.
- Assess voiding patterns.
- Administer pain medication.
- Check vital signs, temperature.
- Explain to the patient:
  - Use of pain medication.
  - Benefit of early ambulation.
  - Increased chance of future ectopic pregnancies.

5 *Endometrial Cancer*

One of the most common gynecological cancers in women, it is most often diagnosed in postmenopausal women.

WHAT WENT WRONG?

Abnormal tissue grows rapidly, affected most often by estrogen. Eventually, this abnormal tissue, hyperplasia, turns into a cancer. Some causes of elevated estrogen levels are exogenous estrogen, polycystic ovarian disease, and estrogen-producing tumors. Risk factors for endometrial cancer include endometrial hyperplasia, tamoxifen, diabetes type II, nulliparity, obesity (estrogen is stored in adipose tissue).

PROGNOSIS

Prognosis is dependent upon the stage and grade of the cancer upon diagnosis. Staging of the tumor (I–IV) can only be done via surgery and grading is based on the histology of the tumor (GI, GII, GIII). In patients with stage IV, the 5-year survival rate is 10 percent.

HALLMARK SIGNS AND SYMPTOMS

- Abnormal bleeding
- Abnormal Pap test (not diagnostic but begs a further work-up)

INTERPRETING TEST RESULTS

- Pap test.
- Endometrial biopsy.
- Endocervical curettage.
- Ca-125.

TREATMENT

- Surgery initially for staging and to remove the tumor—usually hysterectomy, bilateral salpingo-oophorectomy, biopsy of nodes.
- Radiation.
- Hormone therapy:
  - progestins
- Chemotherapy used for cancers that recur outside the pelvis:
  - doxorubicin
  - cisplatin
  - ifosphamide

NURSING DIAGNOSES

- Anticipatory grieving
- Body image disturbance
- Sexual dysfunction

NURSING INTERVENTIONS

- Check vaginal bleeding.

- Check incision site.
- Assess abdomen for bowel sounds, distention.
- Check urinary output.
- Administer pain medication.
- Check vital signs, temperature.
- Emotional reassurance.
- Explain to the patient:
  - Use of pain medication.
  - Benefit of early ambulation.
  - Increased chance of future ectopic pregnancies.

6 *Fibroids (Leiomyomas)*

Leiomyomas are smooth muscle tumors of the uterus. Since they are hormone-receptive, the tumors will change in size with the menses.

WHAT WENT WRONG?

It is unknown what causes the proliferation of these smooth muscle tumors. Fibroids are more common in African-American women.

PROGNOSIS

Since the tumors are hormone-responsive, they will shrink with menopause. However, in patients with large tumors, pain, and excessive bleeding, treatment is necessary.

HALLMARK SIGNS AND SYMPTOMS

- Bleeding, anemia
- Pain, from a large tumor
- Pressure

INTERPRETING TEST RESULTS

- Labwork will show a declining Hgb and Hct.
- Ultrasound, MRI, CT scan, and hysteroscopy will all show a tumor.

TREATMENTS

- Watchful waiting.
- Surgery—myometomy if childbearing is to be preserved, or hysterectomy if childbearing is completed.
- Hormones may help to shrink the tumor.

NURSING DIAGNOSES

- Pain, discomfort
- Fatigue
- Disturbed body image

NURSING INTERVENTIONS

- Monitor CBC to check anemia.
- Check vaginal bleeding.
- Check incision site.
- Administer pain medication.
- Check vital signs, temperature.
- Explain to patient:
  - Use of pain medication.
  - Increased chance of future ectopic pregnancies.
  - Encourage early ambulation.

7 *Infertility*

Infertility is the inability of a reproductive-age couple to conceive after 12 months of unprotected sexual intercourse. More than 50 percent of the time the reproductive tract of the woman is at issue. Primary infertility is when a woman has never had a pregnancy; secondary is when it occurs in a woman who has had one or more pregnancies.

WHAT WENT WRONG?

At fault may be decreased secretion of hormones from the anterior pituitary, failure to ovulate, endometriosis, or past infections causing blockage of the reproductive tract. Structural problems (blocked fallopian tubes, or anovulation), poor sperm motility and/or count, or multifactorial problems can cause infertility. Prior exposure to radiation, medications, exercise frequency, and menstrual cycle and length need to be evaluated.

PROGNOSIS

Infertility affects about 15 percent or more of couples.

HALLMARK SIGNS AND SYMPTOMS

- Inability to achieve conception

INTERPRETING TEST RESULTS

- Semen analysis.
- Menstrual diary.
- Sonogram to view endometrial anatomy.
- Endometrial biopsy to check on hormone status and to determine if the lining is able to support a fertilized ovum, and if leiomyomas are present.
- Labwork: hormone levels—progesterone, LH, FSH, TSH to check on normal uterine, ovarian, pituitary, and thyroid function.
- Hysterosalpingogram to view uterus, fallopian tubes.
- Postcoital test—cervix is checked for patency and whether the mucous is thin enough for sperm to penetrate.

TREATMENTS

- Treatments depend on the cause of the infertility.
- For abnormal sperm findings:
  - Urology referral.
  - Check medications—calcium channel blockers can impair sperm function.
  - Artificial insemination.
- For anovulation:
  - LH/FSH to stimulate ovulation.
  - Bromocriptine for hypothalamic dysfunction.
  - Clomiphene to stimulate ovulation.
- For structural aberrations:
  - Surgery to repair tube.
  - Myomectomy to remove leiomyomas.
  - Surgery to lyse adhesions.
  - In vitro fertilization.

NURSING DIAGNOSES

- Body image disturbance
- Defensive coping
- Risk for parenting

NURSING INTERVENTIONS

- Explain to the patient:
  - Suggest support groups.
  - Encourage questions.
  - Discuss tests.

8 *Menopause*

Menopause is defined as 12 months without a menses. Few follicles are left to mature, levels of hormones decline, ovulation no longer occurs, and the uterine lining no longer needs to thicken in preparation for a fertilized egg.

WHAT WENT WRONG?

Natural progression of life

PROGNOSIS

The average age of menopause in the United States is 51. About 50 percent of American women experience some symptoms of menopause.

HALLMARK SIGNS AND SYMPTOMS

- Lack of menstrual cycle
- Breasts, vagina, and uterus shrink in response to decreased estrogen and progesterone
- Vasomotor flushing due to estrogen levels falling
- Moodiness due to changing hormone levels
- Cardiovascular risks increase due to less estrogen
- Osteoporosis is a risk factor due to less estrogen
- Vaginal mucous dryness from less hormones

INTERPRETING TEST RESULTS

- Increase in FSH during menopause.
- Decrease in LH during menopause.
- Estrogen levels decline.

TREATMENTS

Some women elect to begin hormone replacement therapy (HRT) (in women with a uterus) or estrogen replacement therapy (ERT) (in women without a uterus), to ameliorate the vasomotor flushing and menopausal signs and symptoms, and to decrease the risk of coronary artery disease.

NURSING DIAGNOSES

- Effective management of individual therapeutic regimen

- Decisional conflict
- Personal identity disturbance

NURSING INTERVENTIONS

- Explain to the patient:
  - Bodily changes.
  - Effects of HRT and ERT.

9 *Ovarian Cancer*

Ovarian cancer is the deadliest gynecological cancer because it is usually advanced before it is detected. There is no proven screening test for ovarian cancer. There are no definitive early signs. Some women experience vague abdominal discomfort and bloating.

WHAT WENT WRONG?

A woman who has never had a child or who has had only one or two children, is at higher risk for ovarian cancer. Women with a history of breast cancer, colon cancer, or a family history of these are at a higher risk of ovarian cancer. There is an association between endometriosis and ovarian cancer.

PROGNOSIS

Unfortunately, prognosis for ovarian cancer is poor. Over 75 percent of women are diagnosed at an advanced stage. The prognosis is more grim if the CA-125 level is elevated, and if the disease has spread. The higher the staging, the worse the prognosis. Of stage IV patients, 5 percent survive five years.

HALLMARK SIGNS AND SYMPTOMS

- Bloating from the enlarging tumor
- Pelvic mass

- Dyspnea due to pressure from the diaphragm from an enlarging tumor
- Ascites—abnormal abdominal fluid

INTERPRETING TEST RESULTS

- An elevated CA-125 indicates a tumor may be malignant.
- Transvaginal ultrasound for detection of disease.

TREATMENTS

- Treatment depends on the staging at diagnosis.
- Surgical staging is necessary.
- Complete abdominal hysterectomy, with bilateral salpingo-oophorectomy, omentectomy, and node dissection.
- Complete removal of all visible tumor and metastasis-debulking.
- Chemotherapy:
  - cisplatin
  - carboplatin
  - paclitaxel
- Radiation.

NURSING DIAGNOSES

- Ineffective breathing pattern
- Hopelessness
- Anxiety

NURSING INTERVENTIONS

- Monitor CBC to check anemia.
- Check vaginal bleeding.
- Check incision site.
- Abdominal assessment—check for bowel sounds, distention.

- Check vital signs, temperature.
- Administer pain medication.
- Emotional reassurance.
- Explain to the patient:
  - Benefit of early ambulation.
  - Use of pain medication.
  - Treatments promoted by the oncologist.

10   *Ovarian Masses, Benign*

The most common ovarian cysts are follicular.

WHAT WENT WRONG?

The egg is enclosed in a follicle as it waits to be expelled monthly from the ovary. When the follicle does not open to allow the egg out or the follicle is not reabsorbed, a benign cyst, a fluid-filled sac, may result.

PROGNOSIS

Most cysts resolve in several months. However, a small percentage of patients experience discomfort or pain when the cyst does not resolve.

HALLMARK SIGNS AND SYMPTOMS

- Asymptomatic
- Changes in menstruation
- Unilateral pelvic pain (usually one ovary is involved)
- Sharp pelvic pain, which indicates rupture

INTERPRETING TEST RESULTS

- Pregnancy test.

- Pelvic exam.
- Ultrasound.

TREATMENTS

- Watchful waiting since most cysts resolve.
- Oral contraceptives.
- Surgery to remove the cyst.

NURSING DIAGNOSES

- Pain, discomfort
- Anxiety

NURSING INTERVENTIONS

- Reassure her that a large majority of cysts resolve.
- Explain to the patient:
  - Cause of her pain.
  - The menstrual cycle, pain may be worse during ovulation.
  - Medication use.

11 *Pelvic Inflammatory Disease (PID)*

PID is a variety of inflammation and infection of the upper genital tract, which includes the uterus, fallopian tubes, ovaries and other structures. It includes endometritis, salpingitis, oophoritis, tubo-ovarian abscess, and pelvic peritonitis.

WHAT WENT WRONG?

Bacteria from the cervix and vagina migrate to the upper genital tract. Usual organisms include *Chlamydia trachomatis*, *Neisseria gonorrhoeae*, *Escherichia coli*, and

Bacteroides. Most infections are due to a mix of bacteria. PID occurs most often in sexually active women and is more common in adolescents. PID is more common with multiple sexual partners, a young age, unprotected sex, and a history of sexually transmitted disease.

PROGNOSIS

About one in ten sexually active women will experience PID in her lifetime and 25 percent of those will experience a major complication such as infertility, ectopic pregnancy, abscess, or chronic pain.

HALLMARK SIGNS AND SYMPTOMS

- Abdominal tenderness
- Adnexal tenderness (ovaries and fallopian tubes)
- Cervical motion tenderness (pain on movement of the cervix) due to an infection
- Fever
- Vaginal discharge
- Dyspareunia (pain during intercourse)
- Elevated white blood cell count

INTERPRETING TEST RESULTS

- CBC will show an elevated WBC
- Pregnancy test—beta hCG
- Chlamydia test
- Gonorrhea test
- Venereal Disease Research Laboratory (VDRL) test for syphilis
- Rapid Plasma Reagin (RPR) test for syphilis
- Fluorescent Treponema Antibody (FTA–ABS) test used to confirm syphilis
- Chandelier sign—a great amount of pain is elicited when the cervix is touched (the woman will jump to the chandelier)

TREATMENTS

- Most patients are able to be managed in an outpatient setting with antibiotics:
  - ofloxacin and metronidazole
  - ceftriaxone and doxycycline
  - azithromycin and metronidazole
- Those who are pregnant, who present with an abscess or peritonitis, or with GI symptoms require inpatient treatment.
  - cefotetan and doxycycline
  - clindamycin and gentamycin
  - azithromycin and metronidazole
- Sexual partners must also be treated.

NURSING DIAGNOSES

- Pain, discomfort
- Sexual dysfunction
- Risk of infection

NURSING INTERVENTIONS

- Teach patient about:
  - Spread of the disease.
  - Practicing safe sex.
  - Medication use and side effects.
  - Necessity of treating all partners.

12 *Trophoblastic Disease*

Trophoblastic neoplasias are abnormal cells growing from a shell that forms between the embryo and the endometrium. The four disease entities are called hydatidiform mole (partial or complete), invasive mole, choriocarcinoma, and placental site trophoblastic tumor. A complete mole is formed when an egg that has no DNA is fertilized by a sperm. A partial mole has DNA from both parents and usually fetal parts. An invasive mole is a hydatidiform mole in the endometrium. Choriocarcinomas are tumors composed of trophoblasts with bleeding. Placental site trophoblastic tumors are trophoblasts which intrude the myometrium. All are suggestive of malignancy and require a full metastatic work-up, including CT scan of brain, kidneys, liver, and lung.

WHAT WENT WRONG?

There is thought to be a problem with the genetic material of the zygotes. The chances are increased with an older mother, prior molar pregnancy, and a history of miscarriage.

PROGNOSIS

Prognosis is the best for a woman diagnosed with a hydatidiform mole. Approximately 20 percent of complete mole pregnancies result in further trophoblastic disease. The remaining three diagnoses may point to malignancy. Most non-metastatic malignancies have a good remission rate after treatment.

HALLMARK SIGNS AND SYMPTOMS

- Usual pregnancy signs during the first trimester
- Vaginal passing of a grapelike cluster of vesicles
- Vaginal bleeding
- Abnormally elevted hCG
- Abnormally large uterus
- Absence of fetal heart tones
- Elevated blood pressure

INTERPRETING TEST RESULTS

- Pelvic examination.
- hCG higher than expected serum levels in blood pregnancy test.
- Ultrasound.

TREATMENTS

- Dilation and Curettage (D&C) to remove all trophoblastic cells.
- Frequent testing of hCG levels to ensure no further cells remain.
- Chest x-ray to assess for lung metastasis.
- Liver function tests to assess for liver metastasis.
- Contraception for a full year.
- Chemotherapy till hCG levels return to normal:
  - methotrexate
  - actinomycin-d
- Total abdominal hysterectomy and chemotherapy.

NURSING DIAGNOSES

- Risk of altered parenting
- Anticipatory grieving
- Powerlessness

NURSING INTERVENTIONS

- Educate the patient:
  - Trophoblastic disease.
  - Discuss further testing.
  - Allow for grieving.
  - Provide referrals to counselors, clergy.
  - Discuss need for year-long birth control.

13   *Pregnancy*

Gestational age is measured from the first day of the last menstrual period (LMP). At each prenatal visit, the fundus (the top of the uterus) will be measured as to its location in the abdomen. This information is used to assess the growth of the fetus. Pregnancy is usually divided into trimesters. The first trimester is from 0 to

14 weeks, and starts at implantation. During this time, it is not uncommon to feel more fatigue, nausea, and morning sickness. At two months, the uterus is the size of a grapefruit. At nine weeks, the embryo is called a fetus and is about one inch in length. During the first trimester, most major organs have developed. The second trimester is from 14 to 28 weeks, and is characterized by less breast tenderness, less fatigue, and a diminishing of morning sickness. However, some back pain may begin, as well as stretch marks, heartburn, and hemorrhoids. At 16 weeks, the fundus is halfway between the pubic bone and the umbilicus. At 16 to 18 weeks, fetal movement may be felt. At 27 weeks, the fundus is two inches above the umbilicus. The third trimester is from 28 weeks to birth. Less movement will be felt due to the limited space for the fetus to move about. The mother may feel some respiratory difficulty as the uterus is directly underneath the diaphragm, pushing up the lungs. She may experience some edema, have difficulty sleeping, and an increased urge to urinate due to pressure on the bladder. She may feel Braxton-Hicks contractions, which are mild abdominal cramping.

WHAT WENT WRONG?

Nothing.

PROGNOSIS

Healthy baby after nine months gestation.

HALLMARK SIGNS AND SYMPTOMS

Symptoms and signs are usually due to pregnancy, but none are diagnostic.

- Symptoms:
  - Nausea, vomiting
  - Breast enlargement and tenderness
  - Quickening (feeling fetal movements)
  - Weight gain
  - Absence of menses
- Signs:
  - Abdominal enlargement

- Breast enlargement
- Softening of cervix
- Increased pigmentation and enlargement of areolae
- Chadwick's sign—vagina and cervix show a blue hue from increased vasculature

INTERPRETING TEST RESULTS

- Human chorionic gonadotropin (hCG):
  - plasma hCG—positive 3 to 4 weeks after LMP.
  - urine hCG—positive one week after first missed menses.
  - serum hCG—will also be elevated in ectopic pregnancy, trophoblastic tumors.
- Fetal heart tones—a positive test of pregnancy.
- Ultrasound—confirms pregnancy.

TREATMENTS

- Regular visits with health care provider.
- Prenatal vitamins.
- Routine labwork.
- Ultrasound.

NURSING DIAGNOSES

- Altered nutrition
- Body image disturbance

NURSING INTERVENTIONS

- Discuss bodily changes.
- Stress importance of prenatal vitamins.
- Reinforce diet, exercise.

- Remind of obstetrician appointments.
- Advise patient when to call the obstetrician:
  - Vaginal bleeding, discharge.
  - Several-hour duration of cramping, pain.
  - Fever.
  - Diminished fetal movements.
  - Sustained vomiting.

14 *Labor and Delivery*

Labor is usually shorter in women who have previously had children than in first-time mothers. The average labor is anywhere from 12 to 24 hours. Labor is typically divided into three stages, with the first stage having two phases. The first stage starts with the beginning of labor, which is uterine contractions which result in thinning (effacement) and dilation of the cervix. The first stage of labor ends with full dilation, at 10 cm, and complete effacement. This is the longest part of labor. Contractions are milder, last 60 to 90 seconds, and are 15 to 20 minutes apart in this first phase of labor, termed the latent phase. The active phase occurs when the cervix dilates from 4 to 8 cm, contractions become stronger, last about 30 to 45 seconds, and are closer together. This is often when the membranes rupture, releasing amniotic fluid. A backache is common, as is some vaginal bleeding. When the cervix is fully dilated at 10 cm, the second stage of labor has started. This phase is fetal expulsion. Contractions continue, but feel different. There is pressure on the rectum, and a strong urge to push. The second stage of labor ends with the birth of the baby. Delivery of the placenta, or afterbirth, is the third stage of labor. Contractions will continue, but will be milder, as the uterus contracts, which helps to expel the placenta and slow the bleeding.

WHAT WENT WRONG?

Nothing.

PROGNOSIS

A healthy baby.

HALLMARK SIGNS AND SYMPTOMS

- Bloody show which is the mucous plug, expelled from the vagina
- Rupture of membranes, which releases amniotic fluid (commonly referred to as water breaking)

INTERPRETING TEST RESULTS

- CBC to assess any anemia.
- Blood typing.
- Rh factor.
- Urinalysis to look for protein and glucose.

TREATMENTS

- Some medications may be administered to stimulate uterine contractions:
  - oxytocin
  - prostaglandins
- Pain medications may be administered, but always with the safety of the fetus in mind. The risk versus the benefit must be weighed.
- Analgesia and sedation:
  - stadol
  - butorphanol
  - meperidine
  - fentanyl
  - nalbuphine
- General anesthesia:
  - nitrous Oxide inhalation
- Regional anesthesia:
  - pudendal block
  - paracervical block
  - spinal block

- Epidural analgesia.
- Local infiltration.

NURSING DIAGNOSES

- Anxiety
- Pain, discomfort

NURSING INTERVENTIONS

- Teach the patient:
  - Benefit of continued exercise.
  - Increase fluids, especially in nausea.
  - Observe for signs of dehydration.
  - Eliminate spicy foods to decrease heartburn.
  - Eat small, frequent meals.
  - Increase high-fiber foods to avoid constipation.
  - Prenatal vitamins daily.
  - Support hose for varicose veins.
  - Stool softeners to aid in hemorrhoid pain.
  - Avoid high heels if backache persists.
  - Avoid prolonged sitting.
  - Avoid MMR vaccine in pregnancy.
  - Suggest Lamaze or other labor support groups.

15 *Postpartum*

The time from birth to 6 weeks when involutionary changes occur.

WHAT WENT WRONG?

Nothing.

PROGNOSIS

Return to prepregnant state.

HALLMARK SIGNS AND SYMPTOMS

- Vaginal drainage (lochia) lessens, becomes lighter in color
- Uterus shrinks in size
- Abdomen shrinks
- Breasts enlarge and fill with milk
- Body weight decreases

INTERPRETING TEST RESULTS

- CBC to assess blood loss.

TREATMENTS

- Iron supplementation if indicated.

NURSING DIAGNOSES

- Fatigue
- Disturbance in body image
- Effective breastfeeding

NURSING INTERVENTIONS

- Explain lochia (postpartum vaginal discharge)—color, amount.
- Answer breast-feeding questions.
- Remind patient to call obstetrician if fever develops, or if there is excessive vaginal bleeding, chest pain, or dyspnea.
- Discuss contraception—ovulation may occur before menses resume.

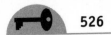

16 *Rh Incompatibility*

WHAT WENT WRONG?

Rh incompatibility is assessed on each mother during pregnancy. An antigen, Rh, may or may not be on the surface of the red blood cell. If a mother is Rh positive, she carried the Rhesus antigen on the RBC. A fetus has antigens from its mother and father. The Rh is problematic when the mother is Rh– and the father is Rh+. When the mother is Rh– and the fetus is Rh+, she may develop antibodies that will cross the placenta and attack the fetal RBCs, which are recognized as foreign.

PROGNOSIS

Prognosis is good as all mothers are tested during prenatal care.

HALLMARK SIGNS AND SYMPTOMS

- Incompatibility with Rh of mother and baby

INTERPRETING TEST RESULTS

- Rh type.

TREATMENT

- RhoGAM is Rh IgG (immunoglobulin) to prevent an immune response by the mother.

NURSING DIAGNOSES

- Safety
- Risk for injury

NURSING INTERVENTIONS

- Retest if unsure of antibody titer.

- Administer RhoGAM.
- Explain Rh status to the mother.

17 *Preeclampsia and Eclampsia*

Preeclampsia is a condition that women may get in the latter half of pregnancy. It is pregnancy-induced hypertension and more often occurs in a first pregnancy. If preeclampsia is left untreated, eclampsia (which is severe) will result.

WHAT WENT WRONG?

The etiology of preeclampsia and eclampsia is unknown. Pre-pregnant hypertension, obesity, and poor nutrition may be contributing factors. First-time mothers have a greater risk of preeclampsia, as do women with a family history of the condition.

PROGNOSIS

Preeclampsia can cause a small baby, premature birth, and learning disabilities. Untreated eclampsia can lead to seizures, coma, and even death of the mother and baby.

HALLMARK SIGNS AND SYMPTOMS

- Preeclampsia (may be asymptomatic):
  - BP > 140/90
  - Proteinuria (presence of excess serum protein in the urine) >300 mg / 24 hours
  - Elevated creatinine
  - Headache
  - Edema
  - Pulmonary edema
  - Hemolysis
  - Rapid weight gain

- Abdominal pain
- Diminished urine output
- Excessive vomiting and nausea
- Eclampsia:
  - As above
  - Seizures

INTERPRETING TEST RESULTS

- Chemistry panel to assess hydration status as well as kidney and liver function.
- CBC to asses anemia and platelet count.
- Urinalysis to look for protein and creatinine in the urine.
- Fetal ultrasound.

TREATMENT

Birth of the baby is the only cure for eclampsia and preeclampsia. Mild preeclampsia with mild hypertension and a small amount of protein in the urine can be managed at home with rest and frequent health care provider checks, depending on the status and gestational age of the baby. All other preeclampsia and eclampsia patients are hospitalized.

- Bedrest.
- Low-salt diet.
- Medications:
  - To control blood pressure:
    - hydralazine
    - labetolol
    - methyldopa
    - nifedipine
  - To control seizures:
    - magnesium sulfate

NURSING DIAGNOSES

- Safety

- Risk for altered parenting
- Altered growth and development

NURSING INTERVENTIONS

- Monitor blood pressure.
- Monitor protein in urine.
- Assist during bedrest.
- Explain to the patient:
  - The disease.
  - Necessity of low-salt diet.
  - All tests.

Crucial Diagnostic Tests

Beta Subunit of Human Chorionic Gonadotropin (β-hCG)

This test, better known as pregnancy testing, is used to detect early pregnancy and to diagnose or to monitor trophoblastic disease and other β–hCG secreting tumors. Using a chemilumnescent or florimetric immunoassay, the test measures the level of β–hCG in a blood sample.

Biopsy

Biopsy is removal of tissue from the body for examination to determine if cellular changes have occurred. It is one of the principal tools used in diagnosing cancer. Core or incisional biopsy involves removal of only a sample of tissue. When an entire lump or suspicious area is removed, the procedure used is an excisional biopsy. Needle aspiration biopsy involves the removal of tissue or fluid with a needle.

After the test—Always monitor the patient for bleeding following a biopsy.

Cancer Antigen 125 (CA 125)

This test measures the amount of the protein, CA 125, in the blood. It is performed to monitor existing endometrial and ovarian cancers. This is not a screening test.

Hysterosalpingogram (HSG)

This is an x-ray test that examines the inside of the uterus and fallopian tubes and the surrounding area. It is used to identify abnormalities, reasons for infertility, tubal pregnancy or infections in the uterus and tubes. A contrast dye is inserted through the vagina into the cervix and x-ray pictures are taken as the dye flows through the uterus and fallopian tubes.

Before the test—Explain to patient NPO for 6–8 hours before the procedure and that it is normal to experience some cramping during and after the test. Obtain informed consent.

After the test—Monitor the patient after the test for any allergic reaction to the dye. Monitor for excessive vaginal bleeding.

Hysteroscopy

This test directly examines the lining of the uterus to determine the cause of abnormal bleeding and infertility. A thin viewing tube called a hysteroscope is moved through the cervix into the uterus via the vagina. A light and a camera are hooked to the hysteroscope so that the lining of the uterus can be viewed on a video screen.

Before the test—Explain to patient that she must be NPO for 6–8 hours before the procedure. Obtain informed consent.

After the test—Monitor for excessive vaginal bleeding.

Mammogram

A radiological study of the breast tissue in which the breasts are positioned and compressed within a special device to allow optimal imaging. At least two images are taken of each breast. This test is used to detect growths within the breast tissue, as part of recommended screening for breast cancer.

Before the test—Explain to patient that she must avoid using lotions, powders and deodorants the day of the tests.

Papanicolaou (Pap) Smear

This test is a screening test for cervical cancer. During the test the doctor takes a sample of cells from the cervix and sends the sample to a laboratory which then checks the sample for changes in the cervical cells.

Rhesus (Rh) Factor

This is a serum test used to check for the presence of a protein, Rh D antigen, on the surface of the red blood cells. It is used to assess for blood compatibility between mother and fetus. This is a nonfasting test.

Semen Analysis

This test evaluates the male aspect of a couple's inability to conceive. The patient must abstain from sex for 2 days and then collect a specimen, which is then microscopically evaluated for volume, sperm motility and count. The specimen must be delivered to the lab within one hour of collection.

Quiz

1. Which of the following is a definitive sign of pregnancy?
    (a) Amenorrhea.
    (b) Positive hCG.
    (c) Morning sickness.
    (d) Fetal heart sounds.

2. The third stage of labor is when:
    (a) contractions reach their peak.
    (b) the head is visible.
    (c) the water breaks.
    (d) the placenta is delivered.

3. Your patient is a 25-year-old female just diagnosed with hydatidiform mole. You would expect:

   (a) a positive hCG.

   (b) weight loss and wasting as with other malignancies.

   (c) Braxton-Hicks contractions.

   (d) a cough.

4. The start of the luteal phase of the menstrual cycle is marked by:

   (a) menstruation.

   (b) pelvic pain.

   (c) ovulation.

   (d) cramping.

5. Which of the following is a finding that is most often associated with endometrial cancer?

   (a) Thickened endometrial lining on ultrasound.

   (b) Irregular periods.

   (c) Young age.

   (d) Dyspareunia.

6. Symptoms of an ectopic pregnancy include:

   (a) hematuria, pelvic pain, and dizziness.

   (b) amenorrhea, pelvic pain, and vaginal spotting.

   (c) constipation, nausea, and fainting.

   (d) fallopian pain, nausea, and breast enlargement.

7. One risk factor that increases a woman's chances of getting breast cancer include:

   (a) family history.

   (b) young age at first birth.

   (c) multiple births.

   (d) underwire bras.

8. Symptoms indicative of cervical cancer include:

   (a) irregular vaginal bleeding.

   (b) bloating.

(c) weight gain and nausea.

(d) dyspareunia.

9. The most important lab value to monitor in a patient with heavy bleeding due to fibroids is:

(a) hemoglobin.

(b) luteinizing hormone.

(c) white blood cell count.

(d) potassium.

10. The main action of luteinizing hormone is:

(a) beginning of menses.

(b) menopause.

(c) ovulation.

(d) pregnancy.

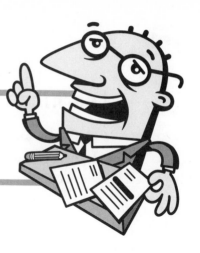

CHAPTER 15

Pain Management

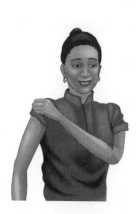

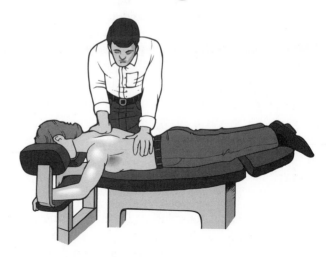

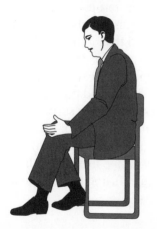

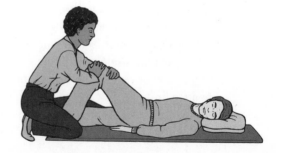

Learning Objectives

1 Acute pain

2 Chronic pain

3 Peripheral neuropathy

4 Phantom limb pain

5 Substance use disorders

6 Drug addiction

Key Terms

Adjuvant modalities
Biofeedback
Electomyography

Endorphins
Enkephalins
Likert scale

Neuroleptics
Serotonin
Serum levels

Pain

Pain is sensed through nerve endings, which are generously spread throughout the internal tissues and the skin. The brain is the only structure without pain receptors. When pain receptors are stimulated, discomfort or pain results, prompting that action be taken to remove the cause of the pain. The pain impulse travels along sensory fibers of the spinal nerves to the spinal cord and then to the brain, which interprets the degree and source of the pain. The brain can then signal nerve fibers to release chemicals to inhibit pain signals. Some of the chemicals—enkephalins, serotonin, and endorphins—are able to suppress pain signals and provide endogenous pain control. Visceral pain is pain from an organ secondary to surgery, cramping, ischemia, stretching, or spasms. Referred pain is the sensation of pain coming from another part of the body than where it actually originates. It is common for heart pain to be felt in the arm, jaw, or back. The pain impulses from the heart travel the same circuit as the receptors in these areas, confusing the interpretation in the brain.

Various individuals can experience different levels of pain with the same injury. Researchers have sought to explain this phenomenon. The gate control theory postulates that there is a "gate" in the spine which controls the impulses from the finger on the hot stove to the brain. The brain controls this gate to allow total or partial signals through. However, the interpretation is based on current emotions, memories, expectations, ideals, and cultural biases. If your mind is busy elsewhere, the pain may be somehow lessened, for example, the Lamaze experience through labor and childbirth. This is one of the more popular pain theories, among others.

Emotional pain can produce many symptoms, as varied in their presentation as the etiology of the pain.

Pain scales are useful tools to assess severity of pain and quality of life. They will help the patient to accurately assess the pain and the impact it is having. Pain scales often are measured on a Likert scale, from 0 (no pain) to 10 (the worst pain ever). The Wong pain scale for children, uses a happy smiling face to a sad, tearful one. Another useful tool is a pain diary, in which the patient records severity, location, activity at the time, precipitating factors, and what, if anything, relieved the pain. It is a helpful tool to asses worsening or alleviating pain and also reactions to pain medications.

Just the Facts

1 *Acute Pain*

Acute pain usually points to an aberration or an illness. It is differentiated from chronic pain by the duration, usually less than 4 to 6 months.

WHAT WENT WRONG

Pain nerves are stimulated by pressure, cuts, heat, cold, stabs, surgery, and so on. Other causes include fractures, burns, and bruises.

PROGNOSIS

Acute pain is usually able to be managed and terminated in less than 4 to 6 months.

HALLMARK SIGNS AND SYMPTOMS

- Intense sharp pain (severe)
- Fleeting, momentary, or ongoing
- Cramping, spasmotic

INTERPRETING TEST RESULTS

- Ultrasound.
- X-rays.
- CT scans.
- MRI.

TREATMENTS

- Surgery.
- Delivery of child.
- Anesthesia.
- Analgesics:
  - acetaminophen
  - aspirin
  - COX-2 inhibitors
  - NSAIDs:
    - celecoxib
    - diclofenac
    - flurbiprofen
    - ibuprofen
    - indomethacin
    - ketorolac
    - nabumetone
    - naproxen
  - Opioids:
    - codeine
    - hydrocodone

- hydromorphone
- levorphanol
- meperidine
- methadone
- morphine
- oxycodone
- Antispasmotics.
- Muscle relaxers.
- Neuropathic pain relievers:
  - tricyclic antidepressants:
    - amitriptyline
    - desipramine
  - nontricyclic antidepressants:
    - bupropion
  - anticonvulsants:
    - carbamazapine
    - clonazepam
    - gabapentin
    - pregabalin
- Anxiolytics.
- Steroids.
- Heat/cold.
- Transcutaneous electrical nerve stimulator (TENS) unit.
- Epidural injection.

NURSING DIAGNOSES

- Acute pain
- Powerlessness

NURSING INTERVENTIONS

- Cold or hot packs.
- Massage.

- Physical therapy.
- Acupuncture.
- Biofeedback.
- Chiropractic.
- Meditation.
- Support groups.
- Prayer.
- Explain to the patient:
  - Diagnoses.
  - Tests and treatments.
  - Use of pain medication, timing, and side effects.
  - Use of alternative therapies.

2 Chronic Pain

Chronic pain is lingering pain after identification of etiology of the initial onset. It may be less intense after 4 to 6 months, or may be the same degree of pain.

WHAT WENT WRONG?

- Arthritis
- Backaches
- Cancer
- Headaches
- Neurogenic pain
- Psychogenic pain

PROGNOSIS

Prognosis for chronic pain is poor. Adjuvant modalities may help ease the long-term effects of chronic pain.

HALLMARK SIGNS AND SYMPTOMS

In addition to the above, other manifestations may include:

- Anger
- Decreased mobility
- Decreased energy
- Depression
- Restlessness or anxiety
- Tense muscles

INTERPRETING TEST RESULTS

- Heart rate, blood pressure, and respiratory rate may be elevated.
- Pain scales.

TREATMENTS

- Anxiolytics.
- Antidepressants.
- Neuroleptics.

NURSING DIAGNOSES

- Chronic pain
- Hopelessness
- Self-esteem, situational low

NURSING INTERVENTIONS

- Recommend counseling or joining a support group.
- Daily exercise.
- Physical therapy.

- Massage.
- Deep breathing and meditation.
- Biofeedback.

3 *Peripheral Neuropathy*

This is the degeneration or disease of the peripheral nerves that affect motor and/or sensory nerves. The peripheral nerves include all but the brain and spinal cord.

WHAT WENT WRONG?

The neuropathies are poorly understood. When peripheral nerves are damaged, the brain becomes confused when processing communication from the damaged nerves. Pain or numbness may be out of proportion to the damage or may be present where skin and tissue are intact. Peripheral neuropathy may affect motor nerves, sensory nerves, or both. It is often a sequelae (secondary result) of poorly controlled diabetes, autoimmune diseases, hypothyroidism, toxic substances, HIV/AIDS, vitamin deficiencies, alcohol abuse, or some infections.

PROGNOSIS

Treating the underlying disease state may help to relieve the pain. Often, treating the pain is the best option.

HALLMARK SIGNS AND SYMPTOMS

Symptoms result from pressure on the nerve or damage to the nerve, either sensory or motor.

- Pain.
- Numbness.
- Tingling.
- Muscle weakness.

- Loss of sensation.
- Burning.

INTERPRETING TEST RESULTS

- History and physical.
- Reflexes.
- Sensation.
- Muscle strength.
- EMG—electomyography.
- Nerve conduction studies.
- Low serum level of vitamin B_{12}, which may be the cause of nerve disturbances.

TREATMENT

Treatment options include management of the underlying disease to ameliorate the neuropathy and treatment of the pain or symptoms caused by the neuropathy.

- Pain relief—see this chapter.
- Antiseizure medication:
  - gabapentin
  - pregabalin
  - carbamazepine—helps neuropathic pain for unknown reasons
- Tricyclic antidepressants:
  - amitriptyline
  - desipramine
  - imipramine—works by blocking the signals sent to the brain
- Lidocaine patch—a topical anesthetic applied directly to the site.

NURSING DIAGNOSES

- Risk for peripheral neurosensory dysfunction
- Alterations of tactile sensory perception

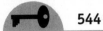
NURSING INTERVENTIONS

- Relaxation.
- Biofeedback.
- Acupuncture.
- Protect feet—loss of sensations will make injuries undetectable.
- Exercise.
- Remove pressure from affected limbs.
- Heat/cold application.

Phantom Limb Pain

Pain, mild to severe, felt in the area where an extremity has been amputated, is called phantom limb pain.

WHAT WENT WRONG?

The nerve endings at the surgical site continue to relay pain signals to the brain. The missing limb could be the result of surgical amputation or trauma.

PROGNOSIS

Some patients experience little or no phantom pain. Other patients' pain diminishes with time. Poor prognosis is associated with ongoing pain for 4 to 6 months.

HALLMARK SIGNS AND SYMPTOMS

- Pain distal or proximal to the amputation
- Itch
- Cramps
- Tingling

TREATMENT

- Physical therapy.
- Analgesics.
- Pain relievers.
- Neuroleptics:
    - gabapentin
    - pregabalin

NURSING DIAGNOSES

- Pain, discomfort
- Powerlessness
- Grieving

NURSING INTERVENTIONS

- Heat.
- Massage.
- Explain to the patient:
    - Nerve conduction.
    - Medications, timing, and side effects.

5 *Substance Use Disorders*

Substance abuse is defined as an irresistable urge for drugs, alcohol, or other substances, including physical, physiological, and psychological longings, and a need for more and greater dosages to satisfy the cravings. Abused substances produce euphoria and intoxication, which include changes in mental status, decreased coordination, and slurred speech. Seizures and loss of consciousness are late signs. Usual abused substances include alcohol, club or illegal drugs, and cigarettes. However, food, caffeine, and sex may be included in some definitions.

WHAT WENT WRONG?

Research shows a varied set of internal and external circumstances leading to drug abuse. There seems to be a genetic factor involved, as well as environmental and social elements. Individuals may slowly begin a habit for pleasure, depression, hunger issues, weight reduction, societal pressures, or to escape from pressure. Teen use often begins early.

PROGNOSIS

Prognosis depends on the drug, its potency, the duration of usage, and genetic factors of the user. Research shows that a history of prolonged abuse changes some brain functions, leading to increased cravings. Substance use disorders may start with one substance and may progress to others; for example, it is not uncommon to begin with marijuana and progress to cocaine or heroin.

HALLMARK SIGNS AND SYMPTOMS

- Removing oneself from sports, work, and friends
- Decrease in grades, interest in school
- Irritability, depression
- Stealing money to support habit
- Hangovers
- Forgetfulness from effects of drug on the brain
- Fever
- Epistaxis from nasal administration, snorting
- Pain at injection sites
- Tremors
- Chest pain
- Abdominal pain
- Discolored, dark urine
- Tobacco:
  - Heart disease
  - Lung cancer

- Emphysema
- Peptic ulcers
- Stroke
- Alcohol:
  - Depression
  - Slurred speech
  - Diminished coordination
  - Decreased inhibitions
  - Irregular heartbeat
  - Anxiety
  - Seizures
  - Liver failure
- Cannabis (marijuana):
  - Diminished memory and coordination
  - Progression to harsher drugs
- Stimulants/amphetamines (cocaine, methedrine, ecstasy, methylphenidate, phenmetrazine, methamphetamines):
  - Change in pupil size
  - Paranoia
  - Heart damage
  - Hyperactivity
  - Tachycardia
  - Hypertension
  - Stroke
  - Psychoses
  - Coma
- Opioids/narcotics (heroin, opium):
  - Change in pupil size
  - Vomiting, diarrhea
  - Confusion
  - Bradypnea
  - HIV/AIDs
- Designer/club drugs:

- Respiratory depression
- Euphoria
- Tremors
- Hallucinations
- Paranoia
- Tachycardia
- Benzodiazepines/barbiturates [Rohypnol, GHB (hydroxybutyrate G)]:
  - Hypotension
  - Sedation
  - Confusion
  - Cramps
- Dissociative anesthetics [PCP (phencyclidine), ketamine]:
  - Impairs memory
  - Aggression
  - Depression
  - Dyspnea
- Hallucinogenics (LSD, mescaline):
  - Hallucinations
  - Tachycardia
  - Delusions
  - Paranoia
- Inhalants (aerosols, solvents, gasoline, lighter fluid, paint thinners, cleaning fluids):
  - Euphoria
  - Confusion
  - Hallucinations
  - Memory loss
  - Vomiting

INTERPRETING TEST RESULTS

For alcoholism, several screening tests are available to assess for dependency. The CAGE screening test is commonly used:

1. Have you ever felt you should **C**ut down on your drinking?
2. Have you ever felt **A**nnoyed by others questioning your drinking?
3. Has your drinking ever made you feel **G**uilty?
4. Do you need a drink first thing in morning for an **E**ye-opener?

In addition, the following tests may be performed.

- Blood alcohol levels.
- Screening tests for drug use:
  - Blood work.
  - Urinalysis.

TREATMENTS

Those treatments for alcohol abuse that include behavior modification seem to be the most effective. Often, a combination of behavior modification, support group, and/or medication may be needed.

- ABCs of emergency support—airway, breathing, circulation.
- Inpatient facilities.
- Outpatient settings.
- Counseling.
- Support groups.
- Abstinence.
- Behavior modification.
- Activated charcoal.
- Toxicity medications:
  - For opiods:
    - naloxone
    - nalmefene
  - For benzodiazepines:
    - flumazenil
  - For alcohol:
    - acamprosate
    - disulfiram

- For acetaminophen:
  - acetylcysteine
- For ethylene glycol:
  - fomepizole

NURSING DIAGNOSES

- Ineffective denial.
- Hopelessness.
- Altered family processes: alcoholism.
- Ineffective individual coping.

NURSING INTERVENTIONS

- Prevent relapse.
- Instruct the patient:
  - Adopt strategies to cope with cravings.
  - Use of medication.
  - Physical symptoms of withdrawal.
  - Benefit of attendance at group sessions.

6 *Drug Addiction*

Drug addiction is the chronic overuse and abuse of legal or illegal substances causing interpersonal, social, and family problems. Addiction occurs when the use of the substance causes an abnormal physical or psychological dependence in which the sudden discontinuance will cause severe trauma. This differs from tolerance in which the desired effectiveness of the drug diminishes over time. Larger quantities of the drug must be used to achieve the same effect. Severe addiction is usually characterized by the inability to carry out work requirements, school responsibilities, or family obligations and duties.

WHAT WENT WRONG?

Some patients who take pain medications other than directed or to achieve a sensation different than pain relief are more at risk for addiction. Addiction is a multifaceted problem caused by peer pressure, genetic factors, social nonconformity, stress, depression, and mental anxiety. Those who have a family member with an addiction or who have themselves had an addiction in the past are at an increased risk. Societal pressures and environmental pressures can influence the probability of becoming addicted. Research has determined that long-term drug use results in changes in brain function, which increases the compulsion to abuse drugs.

PROGNOSIS

People of all ages, young ones in particular, are dying in unprecedented numbers because of their addictions. Most of the deaths are due to addiction to diverted prescription analgesics, alcohol, and benzodiazepines. Since addiction is such a multifaceted problem, treatment prognosis varies greatly. Relapses, unfortunately, are frequent. Studies have shown that females and older patients respond better to treatment programs and have fewer relapses. The greatest incidence of drug addiction occurs in males between the ages of 18 and 25. Active participation in a treatment program increases the chances of success.

HALLMARK SIGNS AND SYMPTOMS

- Tachycardia
- Dilated pupils
- Restlessness
- Weight loss due to poor appetite
- Hypervigilance
- Euphoria
- Death due to overdose

INTERPRETING TEST RESULTS

- Urinalysis for initial diagnoses and to monitor compliance; will determine substance and toxicity.
- Blood tests will identify the drug used up to 12 hours before testing

TREATMENTS

- ABCs of emergency support—airway, breathing, circulation.
- Referral to a specialist in substance abuse.
- Behavioral therapy (counseling, cognitive therapy, and/or psychotherapy).
- Avoidance of situations detrimental to well-being.
- Residential programs.
- Outpatient programs.
- Medications—methadone, naltrexone, and buproprion.
- Antidepressants—paroxetine, fluoxetine, sertraline, amitriptyline, and trazodone.
- Mood stabilizers—olanzapine and risperidone.
- Acupuncture.
- Biofeedback.

NURSING DIAGNOSES

- Altered family process
- Social isolation
- Risk for loneliness

NURSING INTERVENTIONS

- Assess for HIV/AIDS, tuberculosis, and hepatitis.
- Different approaches work for different people.
- Drug abuse is a result of multiple issues and treatment must address all of these issues.
- Explain to the patient:
  - Disease process.
  - Long-term treatment is more effective.
  - Benefit of continued counseling.
  - Treatment, medications, and side effects.

- Detoxification.
- Benefit of avoidance of high-risk behaviors.
- Recovery process is a long-term commitment.
- Strategies for coping.
- Prevention strategies.

Crucial Diagnostic Test

Urine Toxicology Screening

This test detects the presence of drugs in the urine. Urine screening is preferred to blood screening because urine samples contain the substance for several days after its use, whereas blood levels diminish after several hours. Hair and nail samples may also be required for certain tests. The test is done to detect commonly used drugs, such as alcohol, anabolic steroids, amphetamines, barbiturates, benzodiazepines, cannabinoids, cocaine, methamphetamines, opiates, phencyclidine, propoxyphene.

Before the test—Obtain informed consent if the specimen is needed for medical/legal purposes. Urine specimen collection must be monitored to ensure the specimen has not been altered in any way. Be aware of which prescription medications the patient is taking as some may alter the test results.

Quiz

1. You are caring for a patient who borrowed pain medication from a friend at a beauty salon. She seems to be experiencing side effects of the medication. Your most appropriate response would be:

   (a) Stop the medication and call the friend's practitioner.

   (b) Continue the medication if pain relief is adequate.

   (c) Instruct the patient as to the proper use of the medication.

   (d) Take the medication with milk.

2. The most appropriate assessment of the efficacy of administered pain medication would be:

   (a) The nurses visual assessment.

   (b) Changes in blood pressure, pulse, and respiratory rate.

   (c) The nurse's verbal assessment.

   (d) The patient's perception measured on a pain scale.

3. Prior to giving a requested pain medication, you would:

   (a) wait longer; the patient did not appear to be uncomfortable.

   (b) administer after the family left.

   (c) assess the vital signs.

   (d) call the doctor.

4. An elderly patient has a two-year history of back pain from arthritis. You would encourage:

   (a) lifestyle modification and NSAIDs.

   (b) use of narcotics for pain management.

   (c) diagnostic tests.

   (d) vigorous physical therapy.

5. It would not be unusual for a patient with chronic pain to be taking:

   (a) tricyclic antidepressants.

   (b) antibiotics.

   (c) antidiabetic medications.

   (d) hypertensive medications.

6. A two-day postoperative right-below-the-knee amputation patient complains of severe right foot pain. Your appropriate nursing response would be to:

   (a) refer the patient to psychiatry.

   (b) explain to the patient the pain is not real because the foot is not there.

   (c) medicate the patient for pain.

   (d) encourage guided imagery or another diversion technique.

7. Your postdischarge instructions for a 65-year-old male with peripheral neuropathy from diabetes would include:

   (a) Walk barefoot to increase the stimulation.

   (b) Wear socks and shoes.

   (c) Check feet weekly for wounds.

   (d) Soak feet in hot water daily.

8. On the first postoperative day after a fractured femur, the patient is resting quietly, watching TV. Your nursing interventions would include:

   (a) asking the patient what their pain level is on a scale of 1 to 10.

   (b) administering an ordered dose of opioid.

   (c) encouraging ambulation.

   (d) telling the next shift nurse not to give any pain medication.

9. A mother is concerned about her teenaged son who is depressed and irritable. His school teachers have called, concerned about his declining grades. You would ask:

   (a) if you can recommend a psychiatrist.

   (b) if he has a fever.

   (c) about any family history of substance use disorders.

   (d) about any allergies.

10. An elderly patient with chronic arthritis asks you for suggestions for pain relief. You advise

   (a) increasing caffeine.

   (b) marijuana.

   (c) decreasing caffeine.

   (d) guided imagery.

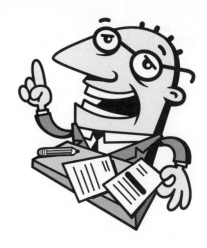

Final Exam

1. A 55-year-old smoker who is normally in good health reports having had a
   bad cough for the past three weeks. He does not have crackles, rhonchi, and
   discolored, blood-tinged sputum. What would you expect his physician to
   rule out?

   (a) Asthma.

   (b) Pneumonia.

   (c) The flu.

   (d) Lung cancer.

2. The patient experiences sudden pain in his right calf while sitting at home.
   He is diagnosed with deep vein thrombosis (DVT). The first intervention
   is to:

   (a) apply ice packs to the affected area every 4 to 6 hours.

   (b) increase dietary intake of foods rich in vitamin K.

   (c) monitor platelet counts daily.

   (d) use intermittent warm soaks of the affected area.

3. While you are talking with the patient she becomes confused and begins slurring her words. What would you expect the physician to do?

(a) Assess if the patient had an ischemic or hemorrhagic CVS.

(b) Administer TPA since this is within three hours of the CVA.

(c) Tell the patient to go home, get rest, and to call the physician in the morning if the symptoms continue.

(d) Admit the patient and place her on bed rest.

4. The patient asks when she should take bisphosphonate medications for treatment of osteoporosis. You tell her:

(a) on a full stomach.

(b) just before getting into bed.

(c) first thing in the morning on an empty stomach with a full glass of water, 30 to 60 minutes before eating, and without lying down.

(d) with an acidic liquid such as orange juice.

5. Mary tells you that she has an undiagnosed case of hypothyroidism. What symptoms would you expect her to present?

(a) Polydipsia and polyphagia.

(b) Fatigue and cold intolerance.

(c) Weight loss and hyperglycemia.

(d) Tachycardia and diarrhea.

6. You are caring for a patient who has had a transurethral resection of the prostate for benign prostatic hypertrophy. There is continuous bladder irrigation set-up. You would notify the physician if you noted:

(a) any signs of hematuria.

(b) a change from clear red output to thicker, bright red output.

(c) a decrease in the amount of blood in the urine.

(d) the development of uremic pruritis.

7. A patient with a history of asthma is scheduled for an appendectomy. Because of her asthma, you would include as part of the preoperative teaching the need to perform postoperatively:

(a) coughing and deep breathing exercises.

(b) leg exercises.

(c) wound dressing changes.

(d) all of these.

8. When assessing the patient, you notice that there is contraction of his facial muscle after tapping the facial nerve anterior to his ear. This is a sign of:

(a) hyponatremia.

(b) hypokalemia.

(c) hypomagnesemia.

    (d) hypocalcemia.

9. A patient is diagnosed with Bell's palsy and has signs of unilateral facial paralysis and is unable to close his right eye. What eye care is required?

    (a) The patient will need to instill artificial teardrops and use an eye patch.

    (b) None, since the symptoms will go away in a few weeks.

    (c) Increase fluid intake to prevent dryness of the eye.

    (d) Wear sunglasses.

10. Upon hearing that he has acute pericarditis, the patient asks how he could have contracted the disease. The best response is:

    (a) The upper respiratory viral infection that you experienced a couple of weeks ago could have led to acute pericarditis.

    (b) It is a genetic condition that you received from your father.

    (c) It is a genetic condition that you received from your mother.

    (d) It is the weakening of the left side of your heart.

11. Bob presents with emphysema. He has difficulty breathing and has a barrel chest. He asks why increasing oxygen therapy doesn't relieve his difficulty breathing. You respond by saying:

    (a) You must lie on your right side for oxygen therapy to work properly.

    (b) Your barrel chest has decreased, causing your lungs to overly expand.

    (c) You must take deeper breaths when receiving oxygen therapy.

    (d) Your difficulty in breathing is due to air trapped in your lungs, reducing the lungs' ability to exchange oxygen and carbon dioxide. Increasing oxygen does not resolve the trapped air.

12. Mary asks how the pulmonary function test ordered by her physician is performed. You respond by saying:

    (a) You breathe into a spirometer to measure your lung capacity.

    (b) You breathe through a mouthpiece into a spirometer until all air in your lungs is expelled; then you take a deep breath through the mouthpiece. This is done three times and a computer calculates the capacity of your lungs.

    (c) A computer is used to measure your volume and vital capacity.

    (d) A tube is inserted into your lungs while you're asleep to expand your lungs to their full capacity.

13. The joints most commonly involved with rheumatoid arthritis include the:
    (a) spine, from the sacrum to the cervical spine.
    (b) symmetrical involvement of major joints.
    (c) small joints of hands and feet.
    (d) slightly movable joints of the axial skeleton.

14. Tom presents with sudden difficulty breathing, tachypnea, tachycardia, and localized chest pain. The physician suspects a pulmonary embolism and would order what test?
    (a) EKG.
    (b) Helical CT scan.
    (c) ECC.
    (d) Vital capacity.

15. A father asks you how to prevent another asthmatic attack in his son. You respond by:
    (a) saying asthmatic attacks cannot be prevented.
    (b) asking his son's physician to change his medication.
    (c) instructing him to move his family immediately to a dry climate.
    (d) helping him identify triggers that cause asthmatic attacks and showing him how to avoid them.

16. The primary mode of treatment for ankylosing spondylitis is:
    (a) relaxed posture for comfort.
    (b) physical therapy.
    (c) strict bedrest.
    (d) respiratory therapy.

17. Signs of clotting and bleeding concurrently indicate:
    (a) hemophilia.
    (b) multiple myeloma.
    (c) disseminated intravascular coagulation.
    (d) polycythema vera.

18. A nurse criticizes the attending physician and suggests that a different physician should care for the patient. What is your best response?
    (a) Call the nurse away from the patient and remind him that the patient can still hear even if unconscious.
    (b) Report the nurse to the attending physician.

(c) Ask the nurse why he has such feelings.

(d) Simply nod your head in agreement.

19. For your patient with a CD4 count < 200, the most important nursing assessment would include:

(a) bowel movements.

(b) urinary output.

(c) fever.

(d) blood pressure.

20. Patients returning from the operating room should be monitored for atelectasis. Why is this important?

(a) Immobility, anesthesia, and lack of deep breathing places the patient at risk for collapsed lung.

(b) All postoperative patients are at risk for infection.

(c) Postoperative patients might have received too much oxygen during surgery.

(d) Postoperative patients don't receive enough oxygen during surgery.

21. Tom is diagnosed with congestive heart failure and asks why fluid accumulates in his lungs. You respond by saying:

(a) Because of the excessive volume of IV fluid that is being administered.

(b) The right side of your heart is weakened and is losing the capability to pump blood to your lungs.

(c) You stand too long at work.

(d) The left side of your heart is weakened and is losing the capability to pump blood to your lungs.

22. Joan is apprehensive about undergoing bronchosopy. You respond by saying:

(a) The thought of this procedure seems to be disturbing you. You will be sleeping during this procedure. I'll ask your physician to visit you again and answer any questions that you might have regarding the procedure.

(b) Your physician has performed this procedure frequently.

(c) I had it performed three years ago and I was fine.

(d) You won't feel a thing. You'll be fine.

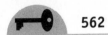

23. The best treatment for mononucleosis is:

    (a) antibiotics.

    (b) physical therapy.

    (c) nonsteroidal anti-inflammatories (NSAIDs).

    (d) rest and fluids.

24. It is important to teach a patient who is receiving immunosuppressive therapy for a bone marrow transplant to:

    (a) avoid other people with signs of infection.

    (b) report signs of infection, such as sore throat or fever.

    (c) take the medications as directed.

    (d) all of the above.

25. Bob, who has Huntington's disease, tells you that he sees the same symptoms of the disease in his 13-year-old son. You respond by saying:

    (a) Your son probably has the early symptoms of the disease.

    (b) Symptoms usually appear between the ages of 30 and 50; however, you may want to ask your physician about genetic testing that can detect if your son has the gene that is associated with Huntington's disease.

    (c) Symptoms usually appear before the age of 30; you may want to ask your physician about genetic testing.

    (d) Huntington's disease is genetically transmitted.

26. What is the priority intervention for a patient admitted to your unit diagnosed with advanced ALS?

    (a) Develop a method of communication.

    (b) Provide six small meals high in protein and assist with feeding.

    (c) Don't involve the patient in decisions about his health care because he does not have the mental status to respond.

    (d) Provide six normal meals high in protein and assist with feeding.

27. Your patient is often fatigued as a result of having anemia. She asks you why she is fatigued. You respond by saying:

    (a) Destruction (hemolysis) of the red blood cells.

    (b) Paleness (pallor) of the skin.

    (c) Lack of nutritional intake of essential nutrients, such as iron or B_{12}.

    (d) Decreased oxygen-carrying capability of the blood.

28. Your patient's physician told him that he has hemophilia. You are asked to teach the signs and symptoms of this disease. You respond by saying:

    (a) Clot formation, especially in the veins of the lower extremities.

    (b) Low blood counts and fatigue due to lack of adequate red blood cell production.

    (c) High blood counts and clot formation under the nails.

    (d) Excessive bleeding after minor trauma.

29. What cell ingests invading or foreign cells?

    (a) Macrophage.

    (b) T-cell.

    (c) B-cell.

    (d) Erythrocyte.

30. The patient asks you what the clip on his finger is for. The best response is:

    (a) This is a cardiac monitor that alerts us to any arrhythmia that you might experience during the night.

    (b) This measures your temperature.

    (c) This is pulse oximetry and is used to give us an idea of how much oxygen is in your blood.

    (d) This tells us the number of red blood cells you have. These cells provide oxygen throughout your body.

31. Your patient is experiencing exacerbations of systemic lupus erythematosus. What would you expect the physician to prescribe?

    (a) Antiemetics.

    (b) Corticosteroids.

    (c) Antineoplastics.

    (d) Antibiotics.

32. Joan is a data-entry specialist who types most of the day. She has an increased risk for:

    (a) osteomyelitis.

    (b) osteoporosis.

    (c) fracture of the overused area.

    (d) carpal tunnel syndrome.

33. Anne asks how a chest x-ray would help the physician examine her heart. You respond by saying:

    (a) A chest x-ray is used to rule out that a fractured rib caused your pain.

    (b) The chest x-ray is an error. I'll cancel the order.

    (c) A chest x-ray is used to detect the size and position of the heart.

    (d) All patients who are admitted must have a chest x-ray.

34. Which of the following would have the highest priority in septic shock?

    (a) Monitoring temperature.

    (b) Monitoring pupillary reaction.

    (c) Monitoring ABC (airway, breathing, circulation).

    (d) Monitoring ANA and RF levels.

35. Mary presents difficulty breathing, fatigue, orthopnea, and palpitation, and is diagnosed as having aortic insufficiency. After undergoing aortic valve repair, what medication would you expect her physician to prescribe?

    (a) Ativan.

    (b) Haldol.

    (c) Heparin.

    (d) Thorazine.

36. A confirmatory lab test for HIV includes:

    (a) western blot.

    (b) low WBC.

    (c) comprehensive metabolic panel.

    (d) enzyme-linked immunosorbent assay (ELISA).

37. A patient with sickle cell anemia will be given supplemental oxygen and which of the following?

    (a) IV fluids to adequately hydrate.

    (b) Narcotic pain management when pain is severe.

    (c) Transfusion of red blood cells to correct anemia.

    (d) All of the above.

38. Anne returned from carpal tunnel surgery. Her hand and arm must remain elevated above the heart after the surgery. She asks you why. You respond by saying:

    (a) to reduce lymphatic drainage.

    (b) to restrict hand movements.

(c) to decrease possibility of nosocomial infection.

(d) to reduce postoperative swelling.

39. Chronic Hepatitis C may be treated with:
    (a) sulfasalazine.
    (b) interferon and ribavirin.
    (c) metronidazole or ciprofloxacin.
    (d) acetaminophen.

40. Priority treatment of a fracture is:
    (a) surgical reduction of the fracture.
    (b) immobilization of the area.
    (c) insertion of an internal fixation device.
    (d) reduction of the fracture.

41. Roger presents with blurred and double vision, muscle weakness, and intolerance of temperature changes. In order to rule out multiple sclerosis, the physician will likely order:
    (a) CBC showing a very low WBC count.
    (b) Endocrine function study showing a low growth hormone and high T3 and T4.
    (c) CT scan showing plaque formation.
    (d) Fasting glucose test showing a result over 300 mg/dl.

42. Patients with rheumatoid arthritis typically have pain:
    (a) with activity.
    (b) only upon awakening.
    (c) late in the evening.
    (d) all day without remission.

43. Mary, who is scheduled for a thoracentesis, asks why there is so much fluid in the pleural space. You respond by saying:
    (a) Your body is unable to remove fluid, resulting in a build-up of fluid in the pleural space around your lungs.
    (b) An error occurred and you were administered too much IV medication.
    (c) This is the result of oxygen therapy.
    (d) This is a normal side effect of bumetanide, which is medication ordered by your physician.

44. Bob is diagnosed with idiopathic thrombocytopenic purpura (ITP). You realize that he has an increased risk of bleeding and you must monitor:

    (a) WBC and bleeding time.

    (b) PT and PTT.

    (c) platelet count and RBC.

    (d) iron and ferritin levels.

45. Tom reports a history of carpal tunnel syndrome. What else would you expect to find in his history?

    (a) Crepitus (grating feeling on palpation over joint during range of motion) due to loss of articular cartilage and bony overgrowth in joint.

    (b) Excessive forward curvature of the thoracic spine (kyphosis) due to pathologic vertebral fractures and collapsing of the anterior portion of the vertebral bodies in the thoracic area.

    (c) Pain and numbness or tingling sensation in the hand over the palmar surface of the thumb, index, and middle fingers, and lateral aspect of the ring finger, that is worse at night.

    (d) Acute onset of excruciating pain in joint due to accumulation of uric acid within the joint.

46. Joan is diagnosed with a gastric ulcer. What symptoms would she exhibit?

    (a) Epigastric pain worse before meals, pain on awakening, and melena.

    (b) Decreased bowel sounds, rigid abdomen, rebound tenderness, and fever.

    (c) Boring epigastric pain radiating to back and left shoulder, bluish-gray discoloration of periumbilical area, and ascites.

    (d) Epigastric pain that is worse after eating and weight loss.

47. You have been caring for a patient with osteomyelitis. In preparing the patient for discharge, you include teaching about:

    (a) the importance of multiple-week treatment with antibiotics.

    (b) the side effects and interactions of the medications.

    (c) symptoms that necessitate a call to the physician, nurse practitioner, or physician assistant.

    (d) all of the above.

48. Following a bone marrow transplant the patient has an increased risk for:

    (a) bleeding.

    (b) infection.

(c) clot formation.

(d) nausea and vomiting.

49. Joan asks you why she is being administered so many arterial blood gas tests. You respond by saying:

(a) This test determines if your liver and kidneys are functioning properly.

(b) This test determines if you have sufficient WBC to fight infection.

(c) This test determines if you are hyperglycemic, which is a side effect of your medication.

(d) This test determines how well your tissues are oxygenated.

50. Tom is diagnosed with an aortic aneurysm. He asks why this didn't show up on his annual physical examination. You respond by saying:

(a) It did show and your physician did not want to alarm you.

(b) You probably don't remember that your physician told you about your condition

(c) Aortic aneurysms are asymptomatic.

(d) Aortic aneurysms are always symptomatic.

51. Anne asks how she developed iron deficiency anemia. You respond by saying:

(a) insomnia.

(b) an increase in iron intake.

(c) heavy menses or an inadequate intake of iron.

(d) low salt intake.

52. Tom has Guillain-Barré syndrome and asks what causes his burning, prickling feeling. You respond by saying:

(a) You are lying too long on the affected side.

(b) This is in response to your medication.

(c) The myelin cover of the nerve endings is absent.

(d) This is secondary to dysphagia.

53. An inflammatory bowel disorder in which the patient develops abdominal pain, bloody diarrhea, tenesmus (feeling of incomplete defecation), and weight loss is:

(a) Crohn's disease.

(b) diverticulitis.

(c) ulcerative colitis.

(d) appendicitis.

54. Tom arrives in the ER and is unable to move his legs as a result of an automobile accident that occurred 30 minutes ago. You respond by saying:

    (a) Swelling due to the initial trauma prevents you from moving your legs.

    (b) There are good rehabilitation centers that will help restore sensation to your legs.

    (c) Swelling due to the initial trauma may make the injury seem move severe than it actually is. A more accurate assessment will be made once the swelling goes down.

    (d) You should have been wearing your seatbelt.

55. When assessing a patient for anaphylaxis, you would be alert for:

    (a) chest pain and indigestion.

    (b) hives and dyspnea.

    (c) hypertension and blurred vision.

    (d) headache and photophobia.

56. A patient with a history of pulmonary embolism asks how to lower the risk of experiencing another pulmonary embolism. You respond by saying:

    (a) Take vitamin K with heparin.

    (b) Avoid confined spaces.

    (c) Avoid sitting and standing for too long and don't cross your legs.

    (d) Jog five miles each day.

57. Bob reports chest pains when performing strenuous work. The pain goes away when he sits. What is he likely to be experiencing?

    (a) Indigestion.

    (b) Stable angina.

    (c) Unstable angina.

    (d) Prinzmetal's angina.

58. Mary is diagnosed with a brain tumor and is unable to speak. Where is the tumor probably located?

    (a) Occipital Lobe.

    (b) Cerebellum.

    (c) Frontal Lobe.

    (d) Parietal Lobe.

59. Mary is diagnosed with gastroesophageal reflux disease. You need to teach Mary to:

    (a) avoid coffee, tea, and other caffeine-containing beverages.

    (b) take histamine 2 blockers, such as ranitidine, as directed.

(c) avoid acidic foods such as citrus or tomato.

(d) all of the above.

60. The first priority to care for the patient with a new fracture includes assessing:

(a) respiratory rate and effort, as well as pulse.

(b) the fracture site for bleeding.

(c) for signs of infection at the wound site of an open fracture.

(d) for circulation and sensation distal to the fracture site.

61. John presents with bronchitis. He thinks that he might have chronic bronchitis and asks you to explain the difference between them. You respond by saying:

(a) Acute bronchitis lasts for three consecutive months and is reversible.

(b) Acute bronchitis lasts seven to ten days.

(c) Chronic bronchitis lasts three consecutive months in two consecutive years. This results in a blockage of the airways which cannot be reversed. Acute bronchitis is caused by a viral or bacterial infection and lasts about ten days. Blockage of the airways is reversible in acute bronchitis.

(d) I'll ask your physician to explain the differences during his rounds.

62. Sam is diagnosed with having a myocardial infarction after experiencing chest pain and pain radiating to his arms, jaw, and back. He asks what a myocardial infarction is. You respond by saying:

(a) You had a heart attack.

(b) Your aortic valve was malformed at birth, causing a disruption in blood flow.

(c) All patients who are as overweight as you will have a heart attack

(d) One or more arteries that supply blood to your heart are blocked, thereby preventing blood from flowing to your cardiac muscles.

63. Tim presents with an acute episode of gout. You expect the physician to prescribe:

(a) nonsteroidal anti-inflammatory medications and colchicine.

(b) allopurinol and aspirin.

(c) antibiotics and acetaminophen.

(d) bisphosphonates and calcium.

64. Gregory has gastrointestinal bleeding and is experiencing hematochezia. You recognize this as:

    (a) vomiting of bright red or maroon blood.

    (b) passage of black, tarry stool.

    (c) passage of red or maroon-colored stool.

    (d) coffee ground emesis.

65. Sue is diagnosed with congestive heart failure. What medication would you expect to administer to strengthen myocardial contractility?

    (a) Nitroprusside.

    (b) Digoxin.

    (c) Nitroglycerine ointment.

    (d) Furosemide.

66. Tom reports abdominal pain that started over the periumbilical area and moved to the right lower quadrant area. Tom probably has:

    (a) Crohn's disease.

    (b) cholecystitis.

    (c) appendicitis.

    (d) diverticulitis.

67. Joan is diagnosed with a ruptured aneurysm. She wonders why this wasn't picked up in her annual physical. You respond by saying:

    (a) The physician must have misread the x-ray.

    (b) The aneurysm must have developed since the physical.

    (c) Aneurysms are often asymptomatic.

    (d) Don't be too concerned because this happens all the time.

68. Build-up of bile salts may cause the systemic symptom of:

    (a) hypotension.

    (b) pruritis (itching).

    (c) ecchymosis (bruising).

    (d) urticaria (hives).

69. Mary, who is diagnosed with osteomyelitis, may not heal properly unless she has:

    (a) debridement and drainage of the area.

    (b) immobilization of the area.

    (c) ice packs alternating with moist heat, applied externally.

    (d) internal fixation device inserted.

70. Treatment of the patient with appendicitis includes:
    (a) transfusion to replace blood loss.
    (b) bowel prep for cleansing.
    (c) surgical removal of appendix.
    (d) medications to lower pH within stomach.

71. Patients with pernicious anemia are treated with:
    (a) oral iron.
    (b) oral folic acid.
    (c) parenteral vitamin B_{12}.
    (d) oral prednisone.

72. Patients with a paralytic ileus typically have:
    (a) intravenous fluid replacement and a nasogastric tube connected to suction.
    (b) surgical correction of the problem.
    (c) endoscopic injection of botulinum toxin or esophageal dilation.
    (d) endoscopy to allow biopsy followed with broad-spectrum antibiotics.

73. Joan has osteoporosis. She has an increased risk for:
    (a) infection in the bone.
    (b) peripheral blood clot formation.
    (c) fracture formation.
    (d) painful joint inflammation.

74. On assessment of the abdomen in a patient with peritonitis, you would expect to find:
    (a) a soft abdomen with bowel sounds every 2 to 3 seconds.
    (b) rebound tenderness and guarding (protecting).
    (c) hyperactive, high-pitched bowel sounds and a firm abdomen.
    (d) ascites and increased vascular pattern on the skin.

75. Steve, who is diagnosed with pneumonia following recent intrathoracic surgery, will likely be prescribed:
    (a) cephalosporin, such as cefazolin.
    (b) penicillin, such as amocicillin.
    (c) fluoroquinolone, such as levofloxacin.
    (d) tetracycline, such as doxycycline.

76. Following treatment with fluoxetine, a selective serotonin reuptake inhibitor for depression, Mary hardly sleeps, is hyperactive, easily distracted, and appears elated. You would expect her physician to:

   (a) continue the selective serotonin reuptake inhibitor.

   (b) start a mood stabilizer.

   (c) switch to a tricyclic antidepressant.

   (d) add a monoamine oxidase inhibitor.

77. To clean a wound, it is best to use:

   (a) hydrogen peroxide to bubble away the debris.

   (b) tap water.

   (c) saline.

   (d) It is best not to disturb a healing wound.

78. Instructions for a patient at risk for testicular cancer include:

   (a) restrict potassium, phosphate, sodium, protein in diet.

   (b) self-catheterization of ileal reservoir.

   (c) testicular self exam.

   (d) change in color of urine is to be expected.

79. Paralytic ileus may occur as a postoperative complication. Which of the following patients would cause you the greatest concern about the development of paralytic ileus?

   (a) Kim, a 27-year-old post-laparscopic appendectomy

   (b) Joyce, a 39-year-old post-open right hemicolectomy

   (c) Nancy, a 56-year-old post-mediastinoscopy

   (d) John, a 47-year-old post-total joint replacement

80. Felicia's family is concerned because Felicia states that she is hearing voices. This is a sign of:

   (a) bipolar disorder.

   (b) schizophrenia.

   (c) panic disorder.

   (d) bulimia nervosa.

81. Your postoperative patient develops a cellulitis in her leg. Your nursing treatments would include:

   (a) keeping both her legs elevated as much as possible.

   (b) encouraging ambulation as much as possible to help with the blood flow.

(c) application of ice four times a day for one hour each to reduce inflammation.

   (d) application of moisturizing lotion three times daily to keep the skin moist.

82. A patient with a second-degree burn has a greater risk for:

   (a) constipation.

   (b) infection.

   (c) hypotension.

   (d) hyperglycemia.

83. Alex is a 78-year-old married man with sudden onset of confusion and disorientation; he is exhibiting combative behavior. He has no previous psychiatric history. A psychiatric consultation has been called. You suspect Alex has:

   (a) delirium.

   (b) psychosis.

   (c) depression.

   (d) panic disorder.

84. Sue is having a minor procedure performed. Which type of anesthesia is most likely to be used?

   (a) General.

   (b) Epidural.

   (c) Regional.

   (d) Conscious sedation.

85. Sue has a mild dermatitis rash and asks for advice. You respond by saying:

   (a) Wash the area with an antiseptic soap frequently to keep the area clean.

   (b) Use an antifungal ointment.

   (c) Use talcum powder to soothe the inflamed skin.

   (d) Use a mild steroidal cream.

86. Karen is suspected of having a hormone imbalance. What would you expect to monitor?

   (a) Electrolyte levels.

   (b) Thyroid studies, FSH, and LH.

   (c) Caloric intake.

   (d) All of the above.

87. Which member of the surgical team does not scrub in the operating room?

    (a) The surgeon.

    (b) The circulating nurse.

    (c) The scrub nurse or surgical tech.

    (d) The holding area nurse.

88. Mary has been dieting and exercising daily. Her weight is well below the recommended minimum for her height. Assessment for Mary would include looking for:

    (a) ecchymosis and extraocular movements.

    (b) temporal wasting and irregular heart rhythm.

    (c) peripheral edema and rales.

    (d) periorbital edema and chorea.

89. Steps to prevent a pressure ulcer may include:

    (a) not disturbing the patient.

    (b) changing the position of a bed-bound patient every 4 hours.

    (c) vigorously rubbing the skin with alcohol.

    (d) avoiding pressure on the heels of a bed-bound patient.

90. When assessing a skin lesion, you look for A—asymmetry, B—irregular borders, C—variegated colors, D—diameter, and E—

    (a) edema.

    (b) erythema.

    (c) elevation.

    (d) ever-changing.

91. Mandy is a 17-year-old female. On physical examination you note partial erosion of her tooth enamel and callus formation on the posterior aspect of the knuckles of her hand. This is indicative of:

    (a) a connective tissue disorder; she should be referred to dermatology.

    (b) self-induced vomiting; she likely has bulimia nervosa.

    (c) self-mutilation; this correlates with anxiety.

    (d) a genetic disorder; her siblings should also be tested.

92. Three days after surgery, Mark notices that the wound site is more painful now than it was the day before. When you inspect the surgical site you are looking for redness or inflammation. Other indicators of infection would include:

    (a) elevated RBC and elevated respiratory rate.

    (b) elevated WBC and elevated temperature.

(c) elevated erythrocyte sedimentation rate and decreased pulse.

(d) decreased platelets and decreased blood pressure.

93. You are caring for a patient with an infected wound. You would expect:

(a) to prepare for sutures to close the wound.

(b) to use steri-strips to hold the edges together.

(c) to leave the wound open.

(d) to cover the wound with a loose, fluffy dressing.

94. Donna is a healthy, 46-year-old female scheduled for elective surgery next week. You would include in her preoperative preparation:

(a) a pulmonary function test and chest x-ray.

(b) a CBC, chemistry panel, and pregnancy test.

(c) urine culture, thyroid panel, and cortisol level.

(d) glucose tolerance test, ankle-brachial index, and electrocardiogram (EKG).

95. When staging a pressure ulcer, you correctly recognize a stage II ulcer as:

(a) redness, with no break in the skin.

(b) shallow ulcer with red base.

(c) dermis involvement with eschar.

(d) bone visible with no drainage.

96. Josie is the mother of a healthy 19-year-old having surgery tomorrow. After the surgeon discusses the surgery, risks, and benefits with the patient and her mother, the mother wants to sign the consent form. The most appropriate response to this would be:

(a) Of course she can sign the consent form; after all, the patient is her daughter.

(b) While you appreciate the concern for her daughter, the patient is a consenting adult and legally has to sign her own consent form.

(c) No consent form must be signed.

(d) Why don't both the patient and her mother sign the form?

97. Appropriate treatment for a patient with cellulitis includes:

(a) petrolatum and vitamin A&D ointment.

(b) antibiotics, such as cephalexin, and over-the-counter analgesics.

(c) weight-bearing exercises and diuretics, such as furosemide.

(d) wet to dry dressings and steroids.

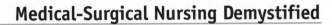

98. Sixty-five-year-old Dominic is being transferred into the PACU from the OR. Once there, initial assessment will focus on:

   (a) airway, breathing, circulation, and wound site.

   (b) intake, output, and intravenous access.

   (c) abdominal sounds, oxygen level, and level of consciousness.

   (d) pulse oximetry, pupil responses, and deep tendon reflexes.

99. Patient teaching for risk reduction of skin cancer should include:

   (a) Having suspicious moles checked by a dermatologist.

   (b) Daily sun exposure every one-half hour.

   (c) Daily sun exposure of 1 hour to build tolerance.

   (d) Applying moisturizer.

100. Denise is recovering from an open cholesystectomy. You know that because of the location of the surgery, she has an increased chance of postoperative:

   (a) myocardial infarction.

   (b) respiratory complications.

   (c) deep vein thrombosis.

   (d) wound infection.

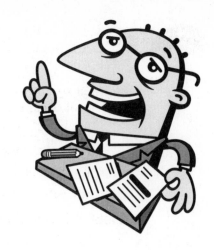

Answers to Quiz and Exam Questions

Chapter 1

| 1. b | 2. a | 3. d | 4. b | 5. b |
| 6. a | 7. a | 8. d | 9. a | 10. b |

Chapter 2

| 1. b | 2. a | 3. b | 4. c | 5. c |
| 6. c | 7. a | 8. c | 9. a | 10. b |

Chapter 3

| 1. c | 2. a | 3. b | 4. a | 5. b |
| 6. c | 7. c | 8. d | 9. c | 10. d |

Chapter 4

1. b	2. d	3. a	4. a	5. b
6. b	7. c	8. d	9. d	10. c

Chapter 5

1. b	2. d	3. a	4. a	5. c
6. b	7. a	8. b	9. c	10. a

Chapter 6

1. c	2. b	3. a	4. d	5. a
6. d	7. b	8. a	9. d	10. a

Chapter 7

1. c	2. b	3. d	4. a	5. b
6. c	7. d	8. b	9. a	10. a

Chapter 8

1. a	2. a	3. d	4. a	5. b
6. c	7. a	8. a	9. d	10. d

Chapter 9

1. b	2. a	3. c	4. c	5. a
6. c	7. d	8. d	9. a	10. b

Chapter 10

1. d	2. a	3. b	4. b	5. b
6. c	7. d	8. d	9. a	10. c

Chapter 11

1. b	2. a	3. c	4. b	5. c
6. a	7. d	8. b	9. d	10. c

Chapter 12

1. a	2. d	3. b	4. d	5. c
6. c	7. b	8. b	9. b	10. d

Chapter 13

1. b	2. a	3. c	4. d	5. d
6. a	7. b	8. b	9. b	10. c

Chapter 14

1. d	2. d	3. a	4. c	5. b
6. b	7. a	8. a	9. a	10. c

Chapter 15

1. a	2. d	3. c	4. a	5. a
6. c	7. b	8. a	9. c	10. d

Final Exam

1. d	2. d	3. a	4. c	5. b
6. b	7. a	8. d	9. a	10. a
11. d	12. b	13. c	14. b	15. d
16. b	17. c	18. b	19. c	20. a
21. d	22. a	23. d	24. d	25. b
26. a	27. d	28. d	29. a	30. c
31. b	32. d	33. c	34. c	35. c
36. a	37. d	38. d	39. b	40. b
41. c	42. a	43. a	44. c	45. c
46. d	47. d	48. b	49. d	50. c
51. c	52. c	53. a	54. c	55. b
56. c	57. b	58. c	59. d	60. a
61. c	62. d	63. a	64. c	65. b
66. c	67. c	68. b	69. a	70. c
71. c	72. a	73. c	74. b	75. c
76. b	77. c	78. d	79. b	80. b
81. a	82. b	83. a	84. d	85. d
86. d	87. d	88. b	89. d	90. d
91. b	92. b	93. c	94. b	95. b
96. b	97. b	98. a	99. a	100. b

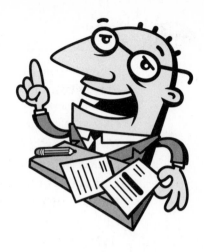

Glossary

CHAPTER 1

ABG: A test that measures the arterial blood gas.

ANA complement: Antinuclear antibody test that measures the amount of auto-immune antibodies.

antecubital fossa: Triangular cavity of the elbow joint.

AST/ALT: Enzymes released by liver tissue when the liver is damaged. Their levels are used as a measure of liver function.

BNP: A test that measures the presence and severity of heart failure.

Bradycardia: A heart rate lower than 60 beats per minute.

cardiac troponin levels: A troponin test checks for elevated levels of these proteins which are released when there is damage to the heart or skeletal muscle.

Cardiomyopathy: A disease of the heart muscle.

Complete Blood Count (CBC): A test used to determine the general health of the patient.

CK isoenzymes: Enzymes released if there is damage to the heart muscle.

CK-MB: An enzyme released by damaged cardiac tissue 2 to 6 hours following an infarction.

Creatine Kinase (CK): Enzyme released if there is damage to the heart muscle.

Creatinine: A waste product from protein metabolism and muscle that is removed by the kidneys in urine. Creatinine is tested to determine kidney function.

CXR: Chest x-ray.

DVT: Deep vein thrombosis.

endocarditis antibiotic prophylaxis: Antibiotic given to prevent a bacterial infection.

Erythrocyte Sedimentation Rate (ESR): See sed rate.

Fowler's position: A position where the client is semi-sitting with knees flexed.

Guaiac: A test to locate hidden (occult) blood in stool.

HTN: Hypertension.

Hypoxia: Decreased oxygen to tissues.

IM: Intramuscular.

Internationalized Normalized Ratio (INR): A medical blood test used to determine the coagulation capability of a patient's blood.

Ischemia: Reduced blood flow due to an obstructed vessel.

Lactate Dehydrogenase (LDH): Enzymes released when there is tissue damage in the heart, liver, kidney, skeletal muscle, or lungs.

LDH isoenzymes: A test to check the level of lactate dehydrogenase in the blood.

Myoglobin: A protein in the heart and skeletal muscles. A rising level of myoglobin is an early indication of a myocardial infarction.

NPO: Nothing by mouth.

Partial Throboplastin Time (PTT): A medical blood test used to measure the coagulation capability of a patient's blood.

Percutaneous Coronary Intervention (PCI): Commonly referred to as angioplasty where the diameter of a narrow blood vessel is increased.

Prothrombin Time (PT): A medical blood test used to determine the coagulant capability of the patient's blood.

PT/PTT/INR: Tests that help detect and diagnose bleeding disorders. Also used to determine the effectiveness of anticoagulants.

RA: Rheumatoid arthritis.

radiopaque dye: Makes structures visible on x-rays.

sed rate: The rate at which red blood cells settle in a test tube. A high rate indicates inflammation.

Troponins: Proteins in cardiac and skeletal muscles.

CHAPTER 2

Alpha 1-antitrypsin deficiency: A lack of a liver protein that leads to emphysema and liver disease.

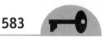

Beta 2-agonist: A bronchodilator that relaxes muscles around the airway thereby opening the airway during an asthma attack or in COPD.

Cardiac glycoside: Medication that improves cardiac output and reduces distention of the heart.

Caseous granulomas: Destructive tissue that enters the bronchus causing tuberculous bronchopneumonia.

Chronic Obstructive Pulmonary Disease (COPD): A lung disease where excess mucus in the airways interferes with gas exchange in the lungs resulting in frequent coughing.

Computerized Tomography (CT) scan: A three-dimensional image of the body structure created from a series of cross sectional images of the patient.

D-dimer: A blood test to diagnose conditions that cause hypercoagulability, a tendency to produce inappropriate blood clots.

Eosinophils: White blood cells that respond to allergic diseases, parasitic infections, and other disorders.

Exudate: Fluid from the circulatory system that enters into areas of inflammation.

FEV$_1$: A measurement of the volume of air exhaled in the first second.

Ghon's complex: Infection caused by Mycobacterium tuberculosis that usually results in primary tuberculosis.

Granulomaous: Inflamed granulation tissue associated with ulcerated infections.

Helical CT scan: Computerized tomography scan produced by a scanner with a continuously rotating gantry. This innovation enabled a very quick scan time.

Histamine: A substance that is released from mast cells that causes itching, sneezing, and nasal congestion related to an allergic reaction.

Incentive spirometer: A device that improves the functioning of lungs by exercising breathing muscles. It is used to prevent development of pneumonia following surgery.

Indurated area: A raised thick or hardening area.

Induration: The process of becoming extremely firm or hard.

Leukotrienes: A substance, released by mast cells during an allergic reaction, which constricts the bronchial passages in an asthma attack.

Mast cells: These are cells that make and release histamine during an allergic reaction.

Mediastinum: The middle section of the chest cavity.

Pulmonary Function Test (PFT): A test that measures how well the lungs take in and exhale air and how efficiently they transfer oxygen into the blood.

Postural drainage: The patient is positioned with the head lower than the chest allowing gravity to clear secretions from the lungs.

Prostaglandins: A hormone-like substance that dilates and constricts blood vessels as well as contracts and relaxes smooth muscles during an immune response.

Serous fluid: Pale yellow and transparent body fluid.

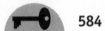

CHAPTER 3

Bamboo spine: Spinal fusion gives a bamboo-like appearance on an x-ray.

Buccal mucosa: Inner lining of the cheeks and lips.

CMV: Herpes virus found in healthy individuals without causing symptoms.

Coagulopathies: A defect in the body's blood-clotting mechanism.

IgM antibody: The first immunoglobulin antibody made in response to an infection.

Lymphadenopathy: Disease of the lymph nodes.

NSAID: A medication that is an anti-inflammatory and pain-killer such as ibuprofen.

ROM: Range of motion.

Sicca complex: Dryness of mucous membranes in the absence of connective tissue disease.

Synovial: A cavity filled with synovial fluid.

CHAPTER 4

Ataxia: Loss of muscle coordination.

Bilirubin: A substance, part of bile, that is formed when red blood cells are broken down.

DDAVP: Medication that mimics the action of an antidiuretic hormone.

Demyelination: The loss or breakdown of myelin, which is the protective coating on nerve cells.

Erythropoiesis: Formation of red blood cells.

Mean Corpuscular Hemoglobin (MCH): The amount of oxygen-carrying hemoglobin inside red blood cells.

Mean Corpuscular Volume (MCV): The average size of red blood cells.

Myeloid: Relating to bone marrow.

Parenteral: Any type of injectable medication.

Parietal cells: Stomach cells that produce hydrochloric acid.

Petechiae: Small red, purple, or brown spots on the skin or mucosa.

Proprioception: Subconscious awareness of position, posture, movement, and changes in equilibrium.

Red Cell Distribution Width (RDW): A calculation of various sizes of red blood cells.

Reagent: Substance used to produce a chemical reaction.

Reticulocytes: Immature red blood cells without a nucleus that are normally found in the circulation.

Romberg test: A neurological test to detect poor balance.

Shilling test: Determines vitamin B_{12} deficiency.

CHAPTER 5

ADL: Activities of daily living.

Afferent: Nerve signals which travel from the peripheral nervous system to the central nervous system.

Aphasia: Unable to speak, write and/or understand due to brain damage.

Arachnoid mater: The middle portion of the meninges that encloses the brain and spinal cord.

Bi-Level Positive Airway Pressure (BiPAP): Device used to provide oxygen to a person who has sleep apnea.

Coninuous Positive Airway Pressure (CPAP): Device used to provide oxygen to a person who has sleep apnea.

Diabetes insipidus: A condition characterized by excessive thirst and increased urination.

Efferent: Nerve signals which travel from the central nervous system to the peripheral nervous system.

Lumen: The hollow area of a tube.

NG: Nasal gastric.

Nystagmus: Rapid involuntary eye movement.

Petechial: Small purple spot caused by a hemorrhage.

Pia mater: The inner portion of the meninges that encloses the brain and spinal cord.

Postcal stage: The final stage of an epileptic seizure in which the patient gradually recovers. Also known as ictal.

Stenosis: Abnormal narrowing of a passage.

Vagal: Related to the vagus nerve.

CHAPTER 6

C-Reactive Protein (CRP): Increases during the inflammatory process and is part of an early defense system against infections.

Haversian canals: Tubes around the channels in the region of a bone called compact bone.

Uricosuric agent: Medication that increases the excretion of uric acid.

CHAPTER 7

A & D Ointment: All purpose skin protection ointment.

ALT: Serum glutamic-pyruvic transaminase is an enzyme that is elevated in liver disease.

AST: Serum glutamic-oxaloacetic transaminase is an enzyme that is elevated in liver disease.

Cast: A cylindrically-shaped aggregation of some particulate in the urine. There are several different types, such as hyaline casts, red blood casts, etc.

Colostomy: An opening into the colon usually from outside the body.

Encephalopathy: A degenerative brain disease.

Fecalith: Hard mass of fecal matter.

Fistulas: Abnormal connection between vessels or organs that normally do not connect.

Glomerulonephritis: Inflammation of the kidney.

HAV: Hepatitis A.

HBeAg: A test that measures hepatitis B antigen.

HBsAg: A test that measures hepatitis B surface antigen.

HBV: Hepatitis B.

HCV: Hepatitis C.

HDV: Hepatitis D.

hepatocellular: Liver cells.

IgM: A class of immunoglobulin involved in fighting blood infections.

IgG: A class of immunoglobulin that is the most common serum antibody. It is passed from mother to fetus.

Manometry: Measures pressure of the rectum and anus muscles.

polyarteritis nodosa: Inflammation of the arteries caused by an autoimmune disease.

Polycast: Presence of many casts in the urine.

RIBA-2: Recombinant immunoblot assay.

septicemia: Blood poisoning.

CHAPTER 8

Dysmetabolic syndrome: Abnormalities in serum insulin/glucose levels.

Ectopic: Tissue growing in an unusual location.

CHAPTER 9

Cryptorchism: Absence of one or both testes from the scrotum.

Hematuria: Blood in urine.

Hydronephrosis: Enlarged kidney resulting from urine accumulation in the upper urinary tract caused by a blockage of the urinary tract.

Median sulcus: Shallow midline groove.

Stoma: A surgical opening in the abdominal wall.

CHAPTER 10

Atopic: Predisposition to allergies.

Radioallergosobent test (RAST): A test used to measure allergic reactions in the blood.

CHAPTER 11

Ketones: By-product of fat metabolism.

mEq/L: Milliequivalents per liter.

mOsm/L: Osmolarity per liter.

paresthesia: Numbness, prickly sensation or tingling of the skin.

Rhabdomyolysis: Degeneration of skeletal muscle.

SLE: Systemic lupus erythematosus.

CHAPTER 12

Caries: Tooth decay.

Echhymosis: Bruise.

Hypoxia: Oxygen reduction.

NMDA: Receptors in the brain.

CHAPTER 13

Asepsis: Without infection.

Atelectasis: Collapse of part or all of the lung.

Chemo receptors Trigger zone: This is the part of the brain responsible for nausea.

Cholecystectomy: Surgical removal of the gallbladder.

Laparoscopic: A surgical procedure performed through small incisions in the abdominal wall using a camera transmitting images to a video monitor.

Paralytic ileus: Movement loss in the small intestine.

Stridor: High-pitched respiratory sound usually occurring in inspiration.

CHAPTER 14

Adnexal: An appendage of an organ.

Beta HCG: A fragment of the human chorionic gonadotropin (hCG) complex used to determine pregnancy.

Brain hormone (BH): Hormone that causes stimulation of growth.

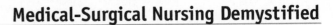

CA 125: A cancer marker for ovarian cancer.

Dyspareunia: Painful intercourse.

Dysplasia: Noncancerous abnormal cells.

I&O: Intake and output of fluids.

Laparoscopically: A surgical procedure, using a camera transmitting images to a video monitor, performed through small incisions in the abdominal wall.

Myomectomy: A surgical procedure to remove fibroids from the uterus.

MMR: Measles, mumps, and rubella vaccine.

Nulliparity: Never pregnant.

Peritonitis: Inflammation of the peritoneum.

RhoGAM: Rh immunoglobulin prevents an Rh-negative mother's antibodies from attacking the fetus's Rh-positive cells.

Rapid Plasma Reagin Test (RPR): A new test to diagnose Syphillis.

Salpingitis: Inflammation of the fallopian tubes.

Venereal Disease Reference Laboratory (VDRL): Older test to diagnose Syphillis.

CHAPTER 15

Adjutant modalities: Additional methods of treatments given in addition to the primary treatment

Epistaxis: Nosebleed.

INDEX

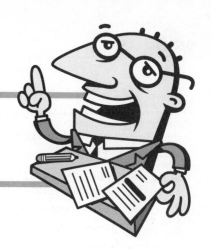

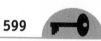

www. GOINSULIN.com